Cognitive Deficits in Brain Disorders

Edited by

John E Harrison BSc PhD CPsychol
Chief Executive and Principal Consultant
Cambridge Psychometric Consultants
Ely UK

Adrian M Owen PhD
Senior Scientist
Medical Research Council Cognition and Brain Sciences Unit
Cambridge UK

Martin Dunitz

© 2002 Martin Dunitz Ltd, a member of the Taylor & Francis group

First published in the United Kingdom in 2002
by Martin Dunitz Ltd, The Livery House, 7-9 Pratt Street, London NW1 0AE

Tel.:   +44 (0)20 7482 2202
Fax.:   +44 (0)20 7267 0159
E-mail: info.dunitz@tandf.co.uk
Website: http://www.dunitz.co.uk

Although every effort has been made to ensure that all owners of copyright material have been acknowledged in this publication, we would be glad to acknowledge in subsequent reprints or editions any omissions brought to our attention.

Although every effort has been made to ensure that drug doses and other information are presented accurately in this publication, the ultimate responsibility rests with the prescribing physician. Neither the publishers nor the authors can be held responsible for errors or for any consequences arising from the use of information contained herein. For detailed prescribing information or instructions on the use of any product or procedure discussed herein, please consult the prescribing information or instructional material issued by the manufacturer.

A CIP record for this book is available from the British Library.

ISBN 1-85317-921-3

Distributed in the USA by
Fulfilment Center
Taylor & Francis
7625 Empire Drive
Florence, KY 41042, USA
Toll Free Tel: 1-800-634-7064
Email: cserve@routledge_ny.com

Distributed in Canada by
Taylor & Francis
74 Rolark Drive
Scarborough
Ontario M1R 4G2, Canada
Toll Free Tel: 1-877-226-2237
Email: tal_fran@istar.ca

Distributed in the rest of the world by
ITPS Limited
Cheriton House
North Way, Andover
Hampshire SP10 5BE, UK
Tel: +44 (0)1264 332424
Email: reception@itps.co.uk

Composition by Wearset, Boldon, Tyne and Wear

Printed and bound in Great Britain by Biddles Ltd, Guildford and King's Lynn

Contents

Contributors' profiles

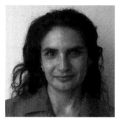

Sharon Abrahams

Dr Abrahams is a Lecturer in Neuropsychology in the Department of Psychology, Institute of Psychiatry, King's College London and the Division of Psychological Medicine, Guy's King's and St Thomas' School of Medicine, London, UK. Dr Abrahams' current research includes the investigation of cognitive and cerebral dysfunction in motor neurone disease using structural and functional imaging techniques and the investigation of spatial memory deficits in patients with localized damage to the hippocampus.

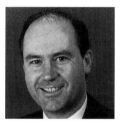

Patrick F Bolton

Dr Patrick Bolton is a University Senior Lecturer in Child and Adolescent Psychiatry in the Developmental Psychiatry Section, University of Cambridge. His research interests include the genetics and brain basis of autism and social communication disorders. In addition to his basic research, he is keen on putting research findings into clinical practice and has helped develop a national service for children with complex developmental disorders.

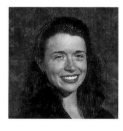

Nancy D Chiaravalloti

Nancy D Chiaravalloti, PhD, is a research fellow in the Neuropsychology and Neuroscience Laboratory at Kessler Rehabilitation Research and Education Corporation (West Orange, NJ, USA) and Instructor of Physical Medicine and Rehabilitation at the University of Medicine and Dentistry of New Jersey – New Jersey Medical School (Newark, NJ, USA). Dr Chiaravalloti's main areas of research include cognitive functioning and cognitive rehabilitation following anterior communicating artery aneurysm, stroke, and multiple sclerosis, including the application of virtual reality and neuroimaging to cognition.

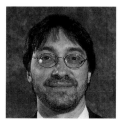

John DeLuca

John DeLuca is Professor of Physical Medicine and Rehabilitation, and Neurosciences at the University of Medicine and Dentistry of New Jersey – New Jersey Medical School (Newark, NJ, USA). He is also Director of Neuroscience Research at the Kessler Rehabilitation Research and Education Corporation

(West Orange, NJ, USA). Dr DeLuca's main areas of research include the examination of cognitive functioning following anterior communicating artery aneurysm, traumatic brain injury, and multiple sclerosis. His recent investigations have also utilized technology including virtual reality and neuroimaging in the evaluation of cognition and rehabilitation.

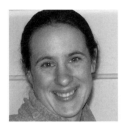

Rebecca Elliott

Rebecca Elliott is Lecturer in Neuropsychology and Functional Brain Imaging at the Neuroscience and Psychiatry Unit, University of Manchester. Her current research focuses on using functional neuroimaging to investigate the neural basis of motivational processes in both normal subjects and psychiatric patient populations.

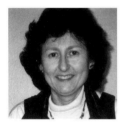

Laura H Goldstein

Laura Goldstein is a reader in neuropsychology in the Department of Psychology, Institute of Psychiatry, King's College London and an honorary consultant clinical psychologist at the Maudsley Hospital, London, UK. Dr Goldstein's current research includes the cognitive and psychological consequences of motor neurone disease and other neurological conditions, the psychosocial aspects of epilepsy and the application of cognitive behavioural techniques to the treatment of epileptic seizures. She is also Programme Leader of the Postgraduate Diploma in Clinical Neuropsychology at the Institute of Psychiatry.

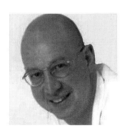

John E Harrison

Dr Harrison is Principal Consultant at Cambridge Psychometric Consultants, and Honorary Research Psychologist at Radcliffe Infirmary, Oxford, UK. Dr Harrison has more than 10 years experience of neuropsychological assessment, gained primarily during post-doctoral research fellowships at Cambridge University and the Charing Cross and Westminster Medical School. He has for the past few years worked within the pharmaceutical industry and in 2000 established Cambridge Psychometric Consultants (website: www.ceepcee.com) through which he provides advice on the use of cognitive testing in the drug development process. Dr Harrison holds Chartered Psychologist status with the British Psychological Society and has authored/co-authored more than 30 scientific articles, as well as recently authoring *Synaesthesia: The Strangest Thing* (Oxford University Press).

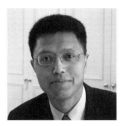

Masud Husain

Masud Husain is a Wellcome Trust Senior Fellow in Clinical Science and Honorary Consultant Neurologist at Charing Cross Hospital, Imperial College, London, UK. His research focuses on the mechanisms underlying visual neglect following stroke.

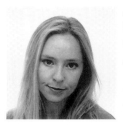

Joanna L Iddon

Dr Iddon, former Head of Neuropsychology at CeNeS Pharmaceuticals (1997–2001), is Research Associate and Neuropsychologist at Addenbrooke's Hospital in Cambridge and at the Chelsea and Westminster Hospital in London, UK. Dr Iddon consults to the pharmaceutical industry and is currently developing a number of her own clinical projects, applying the research concepts of neuropsychology to the real world. Dr Iddon's main fields of interest are the cognitive assessment and profiling of hydrocephalus, age-related cognitive decline, mild cognitive impairment, Alzheimer's disease, schizophrenia, Parkinson's disease and drug addiction.

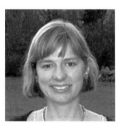

Ingrid S Johnsrude

Ingrid Johnsrude received her PhD in Psychology from McGill University, where she studied with Professor Brenda Milner. She is currently a research fellow at the MRC Cognition and Brain Sciences Unit in Cambridge, UK. Dr Johnsrude's current work explores the functional organization of auditory cortex and its importance for speech comprehension.

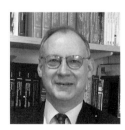

Christopher Kennard

Professor Kennard is Head of the Division of Neuroscience and Psychological Medicine at Imperial College School of Medicine, and Clinical Director for the West London Neurosciences Centre, Hammersmith Hospital Trust based at Charing Cross Hospital, London, UK. He has developed a Clinical Neuro-ophthalmology Unit with special research interest in the neurological control of eye movements and disorders of higher visual function. Professor Kennard is also Editor of the *Journal of Neurology, Neurosurgery and Psychiatry*. He is Chairman of the Royal College of Physicians Joint Committee on Neurology and a Non-Executive Director on the West London Mental Health Trust Board.

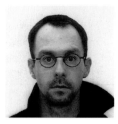

Andrew D Lawrence

Andrew Lawrence, PhD, is a postdoctoral scientist at the MRC Cognition and Brain Sciences Unit, Cambridge, UK. Dr Lawrence's research focuses on the role of the basal ganglia and midbrain dopamine systems in the regulation of affect and action.

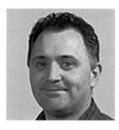

Paul Maruff

Paul Maruff is Associate Professor in the School of Psychological Science at LaTrobe University and is also Head of the Neuropsychology Laboratory at the Mental Health Research Institute of Victoria, Australia. His research uses ocular motor, attentional and neuropsychological methodologies to understand and define cognitive deficits in neuropsychiatric disorders such as obsessive compulsive disorder, schizophrenia and attention deficit disorder.

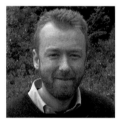

Adrian M Owen

Adrian M Owen is a Senior Scientist at the Medical Research Council Cognition and Brain Sciences Unit and Assistant Director for Activation Studies at the Wolfson Brain Imaging Centre, University of Cambridge, UK. Dr Owen's research combines neuropsychological methods with structural and functional brain imaging (PET and fMRI), to investigate the executive functions of the frontal lobe and the cognitive sequelae of Parkinson's disease and related neurodegenerative disorders.

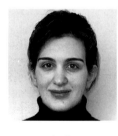

Alidz LM Pambakian

Dr Pambakian is a Clinical Lecturer in the Division of Neuroscience and Psychological Medicine at the Imperial College School of Medicine, and a Specialist Registrar at the West London Neurosciences Centre, Hammersmith Hospital Trust, based at Charing Cross Hospital, London, UK. Her particular interest is clinical neuro-ophthalmology and her recent research has centred on the investigation of patients with visual field defects and their rehabilitation.

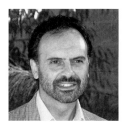

Christos Pantelis

Dr Pantelis is Associate Professor and Head of the Cognitive Neuropsychiatry Research and Academic Unit in the Department of Psychiatry, The University of Melbourne, Australia. He is also co-ordinator of the Applied Schizophrenia Division at the Mental Health Research Institute of Victoria and Clinical Director of the Adult Mental Health Rehabilitation Unit, Sunshine Hospital, dealing with treatment resistant psychoses. His research has focussed on the neuropsychology and neurobiology of schizophrenia, obsessive-compulsive disorder and attention deficit hyperactivity disorder. Dr Pantelis is co-editor of *Schizophrenia: A Neuropsychological Perspective*. His recent work examines the neurobiology of the transition phase to psychosis.

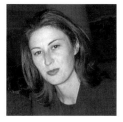

Rosemary Purcell

Rosemary Purcell is a psychologist based at the Victorian Institute of Forensic Mental Health and the Department of Psychological Medicine, Monash University, Victoria, Australia. Her primary research interests include the neuropsychology of obsessive-compulsive disorder, the clinical management of anxiety disorders and, more recently, the nature and impact of stalking. She is co-author of *Stalkers and their Victims*, and winner of the American Psychiatric Association's 2001 Manfred S Guttmacher Award.

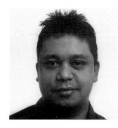

Shibley Rahman

Shibley Rahman is an MB/PhD student at the University of Cambridge, UK. His principal research interests are the cognitive deficits found within the frontotemporal dementias and the dementia of Alzheimer type, and how these are amenable to therapeutic interventions.

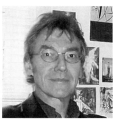

James Russell

Dr James Russell is Reader in Cognitive Development in the Department of Experimental Psychology, University of Cambridge, UK. Most of his research has concerned cognition in normally-developing children, but more recently he has been working on executive dysfunction in children with autism in the hope that this will shed light on the contribution of agency to the development of self-awareness. He has also written extensively on philosophical issues in psychology.

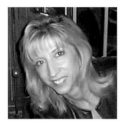

Barbara J Sahakian

Barbara J Sahakian, BA, PhD, DipClinPsych, is Reader in Clinical Neuropsychology at the University of Cambridge, UK, and is based in the Department of Psychiatry at the School of Clinical Medicine. Her research interests include neuropsychology, neuropsychiatry, neuroimaging and cognitive psychopharmacology. She was one of the first researchers to suggest that patients with dementia of the Alzheimer type exhibit deficits in certain forms of attention and that this attentional dysfunction could be ameliorated using pharmacotherapy, such as cholinesterase inhibitors. Dr Sahakian has over 150 publications in scientific journals, including *Nature, Science, The Lancet, British Medical Journal, Brain* and *Psychological Medicine.*

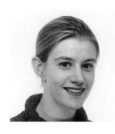

Isabel Stow

Isabel Stow studied Experimental Psychology at Robinson College, Cambridge, UK. She then worked as a Research Psychologist at CeNeS Ltd, Cambridge, where she conducted research primarily using the Cambridge Automated Neuropsychological Test Administration Battery (CANTAB). This included research looking at cognitive dysfunction in Parkinson's disease and early Alzheimer's disease. She is now studying for her Clinical Psychology Doctorate at the University of East Anglia.

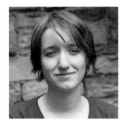

Rachel Swainson

Rachel Swainson, PhD, investigated the potential for neuropsychological assessment in aiding early detection and differential diagnosis of Alzheimer's disease whilst at the University of Cambridge Department of Psychiatry. Dr Swainson is currently at the University of Nottingham, UK, researching neural mechanisms of behavioural selection and control.

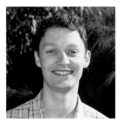

Stephen J Wood

Stephen Wood gained his PhD in 1998 from the University of London, UK, where he studied the relationship between neuropsychological function and medial temporal lobe damage in children with temporal lobe epilepsy. Since then he has been involved in continued studies of epilepsy, phenylketonuria and schizophrenia, with a strong interest in the paediatric and developmental fields.

Contributors' contact details

Sharon Abrahams PhD DClinPsy
Lecturer in Neuropsychology
Department of Psychology
Institute of Psychiatry
London UK

Patrick F Bolton BSc MA PhD MB BS
FRCPsych
University Senior Lecturer in Child
Psychiatry
University of Cambridge
Cambridge UK

Nancy D Chiaravalloti PhD
Department of Physical Medicine and
Rehabilitation
University of Medicine and Dentistry of
New Jersey
Newark NJ
Research Fellow
Kessler Medical Rehabilitation
Research and Education Corporation
West Orange NJ
USA

John DeLuca PhD
Department of Physical Medicine and
Rehabilitation, and Neurosciences
University of Medicine and Dentistry of
New Jersey
Newark NJ
Director of Neuroscience Research
Kessler Medical Rehabilitation
Research and Education Corporation
West Orange NJ
USA

Rebecca Elliott PhD
Neuroscience and Psychiatry Unit
University of Manchester
Manchester UK

Laura H Goldstein PhD MPhil
CPsychol
Department of Psychology
Institute of Psychiatry
London UK

John E Harrison BSc PhD CPsychol
Chief Executive and Principal
Consultant
Cambridge Psychometric Consultants
Ely UK

Masud Husain DPhil MRCP
Wellcome Trust Senior Fellow in
Clinical Science
Imperial College School of Medicine
Division of Neuroscience and
Psychological Medicine
Charing Cross Hospital
London UK

Joanna L Iddon PhD CPsychol
Department of Academic
Neurosurgery
Addenbrooke's Hospital
Cambridge UK

Ingrid S Johnsrude PhD
Research Fellow
MRC Cognition & Brain Sciences Unit
Cambridge UK

Christopher Kennard
Professor of Clinical Neurology
Imperial College Medical School
London UK

Andrew D Lawrence PhD
MRC Cognition & Brain Sciences Unit
Cambridge UK

Paul Maruff PhD
School of Psychological Science
LaTrobe University
Melbourne
Australia

Adrian M Owen PhD
Senior Scientist
Medical Research Council Cognition
and Brain Sciences Unit
Cambridge UK

Alidz LM Pambakian MRCP
Lecturer in Neurology
Imperial College Medical School
London UK

**Christos Pantelis MD MRPsych
FRANZCP**
Cognitive Neuropsychiatry Research
& Academic Unit
Department of Psychiatry
Melbourne University & Sunshine
Hospital
Melbourne Victoria
Mental Health Research Institute of
Victoria
Parkville Victoria
Australia

Rosemary Purcell
Department of Psychological Medicine
Monash University
Parkville Victoria
Australia

Shibley Rahman
Department of Psychiatry
University of Cambridge
Cambridge UK

James Russell MA PhD
Reader in Cognitive Development
Department of Experimental
Psychology
University of Cambridge
Cambridge UK

Barbara J Sahakian
Department of Psychiatry
University of Cambridge
Cambridge UK

Isabel Stow
Research Psychologist
Lifespan Healthcare Cambridge NHS
Trust
University of East Anglia
Cambridge UK

Rachel Swainson
Department of Psychiatry
University of Cambridge
Cambridge UK

Stephen J Wood MD PhD
Cognitive Neuropsychiatry Research
& Academic Unit
Department of Psychiatry
Melbourne University & Sunshine
Hospital
Melbourne Victoria
Mental Health Research Institute of
Victoria
Parkville Victoria
Australia

Preface

Two years ago, we sat in the University Arms in Cambridge, discussing the enterprise of neuroscience, when the topic of cognitive dysfunction in neurological disease came up. We had both worked in various academic and clinical establishments and had been fortunate in working alongside a number of excellent clinicians, many of whom were enthusiastic about, but relatively inexperienced in, the world of neuropsychology. We had both often been asked if we could recommend a text that would summarise the cognitive consequences of different neurological and psychiatric diseases. Our response to all of these earnest requests had been 'no', in spite of a belief that somewhere out there such a book must, or should, exist. Rather than continue to ponder the absence of such a volume, we decided then and there to try and fill this obvious gap and this book is the result of that discussion. While the idea sprang from requests from clinicians, we firmly believe there is much within these pages that will appeal to and inform psychologists and others working within the broad field of neuroscience.

We have been very fortunate in attracting a cast of eminent contributors, many of whom have direct experience of both testing and managing the care of patients with the disorders discussed within this publication. Consequently, as well as providing a review of what is known about the cognitive deficits associated with these disorders, useful insights are often provided about the patient's experience of the disorder and its clinical relevance.

Other than vague directions about length, structure and topic, we were concerned to give each contributor a free hand in the writing of their chapter. The result is that, as well as differences in style, the chapters vary greatly in emphasis. However, a recurrent theme and novel aspect of this book is that each contributor has attempted to relate cognitive function to the underlying brain pathology. This enterprise has been something of a psychologist's graveyard for more than 100 years, so much so that many psychologists still concern themselves exclusively with cognitive function and pay little or no heed to the organ in which these functions are housed. While all of our contributors have sought to relate cognitive function to neural structure, many go a little further and speculate about the specific role of particular brain areas. The assumption, of course, is that deficits in cognitive performance following brain disease or injury have the potential to inform us about normal cognitive function. To provide some balance, we have chosen to discuss the potential hazards of this approach in Chapter 1, together with some of the other challenges involved in the assessment of cognitive function in patients with CNS disease or injury.

In Chapter 1 we have also taken the opportunity to introduce a number of approaches and statistical techniques which, while common in therapeutic development, are seldom used in mainstream neuroscience. The opening chapter is thus inevitably eclectic in nature and something of a 'melange'. We hope for some indulgence from you with respect to this, and can only comment that no matter how violently you may disagree with some of its more controversial assertions, rest assured that previous versions were considerably more extreme!

John E Harrison
Adrian M Owen
Cambridge
UK

1
Research issues in the neuropsychological investigation of brain disease

John E Harrison and Adrian M Owen

Linking psychology with physiology

A popular view of the study of human psychology is to posit a link between 'brain', 'behavior' and 'cognition'. In this model, explanations of human psychology can be couched in behavioral terms, i.e. the outward manifestation of a person's psychology. Equally, descriptions can be couched in terms of the underlying cognition that provides the substrates for the observed behavior. Finally, theories can also be posited in terms of the neural substrates of behavior. Of the tripos of 'behavior', 'cognition' and 'biology', only the first may be directly measured. This tripos can best be understood by way of a real example, as would occur with an individual's performance on a psychological test. In this scenario, performance on a popular neuropsychological assessment measure, such as a spatial working memory task, can be described: (1), behaviorally (i.e what the subject was observed to do); (2) cognitively (the cognitive skills needed to perform the task); or (3) biologically (a description of the brain areas required to perform the task). Most scientists would agree that the domains of behavior and cognition are properly the domain of the psychologist, though they would be less sure that 'brains' are their natural territory. Nevertheless, the prefix 'neuro' serves to remind us that for most students of human behavior (though not, perhaps, members of the lay public) all psychological events have physiological correlates. The attachment of the prefix 'neuro' to 'psychology' also suggests that at least some psychologists lay claim not just to the 'mind' but also to its physical seat, the brain. Both authors of this chapter have engaged in this linkage between structure and function, as we have taken the view that a complete explanation of behavior requires reference to the organ that houses cognition. However, the jump from the 'psychological' to the physiological requires that a number of important methodological and theoretical hurdles be addressed, and we begin by considering a number of these issues in detail.

Neuropsychologists enjoy a slightly ghoulish existence, often waiting for misfortune and accident to provide them with appropriate material for study. This study material takes many forms but is most often restricted to cases where there is clear evidence of brain trauma or disease. Neuropsychologists interested in linking brain, cognition and behavior ideally seek small, circumscribed lesions that selectively degrade one, and only one, area of cognition. However, such instances are extremely rare, a circumstance which has two consequences: first, much of the neuropsychological literature is based on single case studies; and second, where possible, groups of patients with similar patterns of brain damage are grouped together so that the study might benefit from the use of traditional inferential statistics (statistical methods for determining individual abnormal performance or significantly changed performance also exist and are dealt with in detail later in this chapter).

A fundamental difficulty with basing science on 'serendipitous' brain damage is that, in contrast to other branches of science, control of the independent variable is wrestled from the grip of the investigator. This difficulty is sometimes addressed by grouping patients according to, for example, (1) which 'lobe' has been damaged, (2) whether the damage is unilateral or bilateral, (3) whether 'anterior' or 'posterior' cortex has been damaged, and (4) whether the damage is in the left or right hemisphere. However, it is important to recognize that there is no necessary reason why individuals grouped in this fashion might be expected to exhibit similar patterns of psychological damage. This point is well illustrated by the work of Ojemann et al.[1] In a number of neurosurgical recording studies, Ojemann and colleagues have provided compelling evidence that the functional anatomy of the human brain is extremely heterogeneous. For example, they observed that at least one temporal lobe and one frontal lobe site were required for language. Other subjects had either exclusively frontal or temporal lobe sites, and yet others had sites in the frontal and parietal, but none in the temporal, lobes. The authors stated that: 'the data from these 117 patients reveal that there is a large variation in the localization of essential language areas between individuals'.

There are a number of other difficulties associated with the assumption that cognitive deficits are related in a direct way to measurable brain damage and, further, that this relationship can inform us about 'normal' cognitive functioning. Marshall[2] lists three problems with making inferences from impaired to normal functioning:

- the possibility of widespread brain reorganization subsequent to damage
- the uncovering of normal, but normally unused, mechanisms after the destruction of brain areas that usually inhibit their operation
- the (sometimes 'conscious') adoption of (normally unnecessary) strategies by the patient to circumvent the use of an impaired subsystem.

Comorbid neuropsychiatric disorder and false-positive diagnosis are two further impediments for research neuropsychologists to contend with. In the following section we describe some of these difficulties in more detail and make a number of recommendations for investigators seeking to evaluate cognitive dysfunction in neurological and psychiatric patient populations.

Misdiagnosis

By necessity, many neurological and psychiatric disorders are categorized not by etiology, as is common in other areas of medicine, but by the signs and symptoms of the disease. Unfortunately, even for apparently well-specified disorders such as Parkinson's disease (PD), a false-positive in vivo diagnosis rate of approximately 25% prevails.[3,4] This causes difficulties at all levels of research, including studies of the cognitive sequelae of PD. However, it is particularly problematic for studies investigating the neural correlates of cognitive deficits caused by the disease. Idiopathic PD is caused by an unknown process that causes marked degeneration of the substantia nigra. For the neuropsychologist interested in discovering the role of the substantia nigra in normal subjects, the study of PD, with its neatly circumscribed pathology, holds considerable promise for achieving that end. Unfortunately, other diseases that involve pathological damage to neural areas in addition to the substantia nigra are often misdiagnosed as idiopathic PD. Thus, in a study of 20 'Parkinson's disease' patients, approximately 5 will not have the disorder of interest and pathological damage extending beyond the substantia nigra.

Co-morbid neurological disease

Neurological disease tends to afflict older people. Sometimes, neurological diseases co-occur, so an older patient with one neurological disorder may also have an increased risk for another disorder, simply by virtue of their age. Thus a study of an individual or group with one disorder may be confounded by the co-occurrence of a second disorder. If the second disorder has consequences for cognitive function, then an investigation of the first disorder will be confounded. This may be manageable in a group study, but in a study of a single subject such a circumstance would be fatal to the investigation.

One remedy for the twin problems of misdiagnosis and comorbid disease is to stringently screen subjects before entering them into the study. Clearly, screening can only be conducted for characteristics that are known, or suspected, to impair cognition, and so such a list is unlikely to be exhaustive. In the following section we consider some of the issues.

An obvious first precaution is to arrange for all subjects entered into the study to receive some form of brain imaging. Magnetic resonance imaging (MRI) is preferable though expensive, and so computer tomography (CT) may constitute an affordable solution. Patients with evidence of brain changes beyond the pathology of interest could then be excluded. This of course assumes that the observed lesions have had a deleterious effect on cognition, an assumption that may not hold. Nevertheless, exclusions of this kind seem to us to be a sensible method of excluding 'rogue' forms of pathology.

Screening out patients receiving psychoactive medication also seems to us a sensible precaution, even when the medication regimen is composed entirely of agents designed to manage the disease of interest. Clearly, there will be occasions when this is undesirable, or unethical, but when the opportunity arises it would be helpful to withdraw all psychoactive medication prior to assessing the patient. A convention in clinical trials is to withhold medication for a period equal to five times the compound's half-life, a criterion that may also be appropriate for investigations of cognitive function.

Inferring neurophysiological damage on the basis of psychological test performance

A characteristic of the contemporary neuropsychological literature is a tendency to speculate on the locus of possible neural damage based on test performance. This often seems to be a useful function, as speculations of this kind made by psychologists can provide useful leads for neurophysiologists and anatomists to follow up. However, some difficulties are associated with asserting the location of neural damage based upon psychological test performance. This danger is best illustrated with reference to functions traditionally viewed as sensitive to damage to the frontal lobes.

Much of the original 'frontal lobe' cognitive literature is based upon the performance of patients who have experienced traumatic damage to, or surgical removal of, anterior portions of their brains. For example, Milner[5] suggested that normal performance on the Wisconsin Card Sorting Test (WCST) required the integrity of dorsolateral prefrontal cortical (DLPFC) areas. Subsequent research has shown that damage to DLPFC does not necessarily lead to poor performance on the WCST and that damage to other neural locations can also lead to poor performance. Consequently, the WCST has quite poor levels of sensitivity and specificity as a test of DLPFC function. In spite of this, substantial numbers of both neurological and psychiatric disorders have been declared to feature frontal dysfunction solely on the basis of poor WCST performance. This is clearly not warranted, especially in the absence of direct evidence of lesion or neurotransmitter dysfunction in these regions. Note that even finding evidence of this kind in the presence of cognitive dysfunction does not prove that the two are related, merely that they might be.

The advent of functional neuroimaging has sometimes provided corroborating evidence for the involvement of frontal lobe involvement for a number of psychological tests such as the WCST. However, these studies also show significant, and often greater, activation of other brain areas. Typically, for example, studies of the functional anatomy of WCST performance will also typically show posterior parietal lobe, thalamus, basal ganglia, primary visual area and cerebellar activation. Thus based on this evidence the WCST could also be described as a putative test of cerebellar function. It would be interesting to know if this is in fact the case.

The death of refutation?

An additional issue worth addressing with regard to the localizationist perspective is some consideration of the degree of veracity that attaches to theories of specific neural locations. For example, a number of theorists have posited a role for the right prefrontal lobe in memory, specifically the retrieval rather than encoding processes. Other roles for this structure include design fluency, as well as involvement in visuospatial working memory, planning, attentional set-shifting, and numerous other aspects of 'executive' function. However, while right prefrontal lobe structures can be activated fairly reliably in traditional paradigms, it remains the case that patients with right prefrontal lobe damage, through either trauma or surgery, remain competent at cognitive tasks allegedly reliant upon the integrity of this brain region. Clearly, there might well be a number of reasons for this; as previously discussed, some relocation of function might account for this preservation. Equally, the activation of prefrontal lobe structure tasks might reflect the activation of a whole network of neural structures, a network that may exhibit 'graceful degradation'—that is to say, substantial damage to the network can be endured without significant reductions in levels of function. Whatever the case, our point is simply this—finding just one patient with right prefrontal brain damage who can satisfactorily perform on tests held to be reliant upon these structures should constitute decisive refutation of theories founded upon this association. However, in neuropsychology, such a demonstration almost never rings the death knell of a structure–function association. Instead, theories appear to die of 'neglect', in that they fall from vogue or favor, or from 'obesity', in that they simply become too large and encompassing to have any useful predictive value. It is our opinion that, as a general rule of thumb, as one advances from posterior to anterior neural structures, individual variation in function as related to structure becomes more marked. By the time one reaches the frontal lobes, what becomes interesting is not the homogeneity of structure–function relationships, but the heterogeneity.

We now turn to the consideration of a number of methodological problems associated with the assessment of cognitive deficits in neuropsychological populations.

Working within the discipline of neuropsychology brings a number of challenges. First, most psychologists will have been taught scientific methods and, consequently, the techniques associated with examining and reporting data, such as descriptive and inferential statistics. However, faced with a paucity of experimental material, many neuropsychologists are forced to study and report on individual patients. Frequently, patients will be assessed on more than one occasion, often after a surgical or pharmacological intervention has been made. In these circumstances, a decision has to be made as to whether any change in score at retest is due to measurement error or to a 'real' effect of the therapeutic intervention. We know of a number of methods by which such a decision can be made, and a section of this chapter is devoted to a discussion of the merits of these techniques.

When groups of patients can be tested, the theory under investigation is usually that patients will be impaired on the selected outcome measure. We, and others, have long suspected that failures to find a difference are for the most part not submitted for publication. A consequence of this is that the published literature almost certainly presents a false view, in the sense that it is composed predominantly of those studies which have found a significant effect. One of the difficulties with showing patients to be normal is that one is seeking to prove the null hypothesis. In spite of the philosophical difficulties that this presents, a method has been proposed for establishing equivalence, an account of which is also provided later in this chapter.

Determining abnormality—statistical methods for single subjects

The two questions most often arising from neuropsychological studies of individuals are:

- Is performance on the 'task of interest' sufficiently poor to be abnormal?
- Has there been a significant change between assessment A and assessment B?

Determining abnormality

In our view, the first of these two questions is easily dealt with. We are aware of two methods for determining whether the test score of any individual is abnormal. Additionally, the criteria for deciding abnormality are statistical in nature. The two methods we suggest are as follows.

Standard or 'Z' scores

If one knows the value of the estimated population mean and standard deviation (SD) for a normally distributed test of interest, any individual score can be described in terms of where in the distribution it falls. Scores falling more than 2 SDs below the estimated population mean constitute levels of performance found in only the bottom 2.3% of the population. A 'Z' score more than 3 SDs below the mean indicates that this score is found in only 0.15% of normal subjects. The only important caveat to be attached to the use of 'Z' scores is the importance of the reference population. For example, it might well be that, for commercially available tests, neurologically and psychiatrically impaired subjects may have been screened out. Clearly, here the reference population is a normal healthy population as opposed to one that is representative of all individuals. It is our experience that the normal healthy and normal distribution are sometimes mistaken for one another.

Percentile scores

Individual performance can also be expressed as a percentile score. This method can be used successfully when the population data are not normally distributed, as percentiles can be calculated using a ranking methodology. However, it is also the case that in normally distributed data sets certain percentile scores can be expected to fall at certain standard score values, as illustrated in Figure 1.1.

Scores approximately 2 SDs below the mean equate to the 2nd percentile, suggesting that they can be taken to be statistically abnormal.

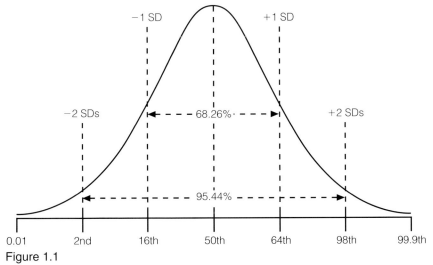

Figure 1.1

The normal or 'Gaussian' distribution with standard deviation (SD)/percentile equivalent scores.

This criterion is designed to be analogous to inferential testing of a two-tailed hypothesis at a significance level of 0.05. Psychology, in contrast to most other areas of science, seems to have a predilection for one-tailed hypothesis testing (see Altman[6] for a critique of this approach). Consequently, investigators are often willing to accept percentile scores equal to, or less than, the 5th percentile as evidence of abnormality.

Significant change

The question of what constitutes 'real' change between test and retesting is, by comparison with deciding on abnormality, a rather more complex issue. It is also heavily reliant upon the psychometric characteristics of the test of interest, especially its 'reliability'. In the following section we will discuss this issue and explain why it is conceptually important for deciding whether retest score changes are due to real effects or to measurement error.

Test reliability

Technically, reliability measurement is an attempt to estimate the measurement error attached to the use of a test or instrument. When applied to psychological tests, reliability most often relates to either the internal consistency (do items in the test measure the 'same thing') or to temporal consistency. The latter form is referred to as 'test-retest reliability' and is most often reported as the degree of correlation between first test and retest performance. The first challenge is to calculate reliability coefficients for the outcome measures of interest and then to determine whether retest performance improves, deteriorates, or remains the same. One consequence of using a correlation coefficient as a reliability measure is that a uniform change in performance across a group will tend to yield a high correlation coefficient, even though subjects may not all have improved or declined by the same rate. With psychometric measures, there appears to be a high a priori expectation that performance will necessarily improve with repeated administrations of the test. Improvements in performance as a result of repeated exposure may be due to the adoption of a strategy or a practice. In these circumstances, changes in performance can be viewed as being due to a real effect, rather than simply due to measurement error. However, when assessing the performance of an individual at retest, we need to know whether any change associated with retest performance is due to a real effect (e.g. due to physical degeneration (a worsening of performance) or due to practice or recovery (an improvement)). A number of methods have been proposed to assist in making this decision.

Techniques for deciding real change versus measurement error

When evaluating individual performance we are seeking to determine whether an individual's change in score is due to a real effect or to measurement error. Several methods exist for determining this difference, some of which are discussed below. In addition to a brief description, we have included in Appendix A two worked examples including our favored technique, which is described first.

Standard error of prediction[7,8]

This technique relies upon using the standard error of prediction to calculate a confidence interval (CI) for first test performance. If the retest performance score falls within the upper and lower bounds of this CI, then retest change can be judged to be due to measurement error. Scores beyond the CI bounds are likely to be due to the influence of a real effect. This decision is subject to the usual twin statistical hazards of making type 1 and type 2 errors. When deciding whether retest change is due to measurement error or a real effect, the decision is biased towards rejecting the hypothesis that the change is due to measurement error. Consequently, we would suggest that only scores falling within 66% CIs be interpreted as likely to be due to measurement error. A step-by-step procedure for determining whether an individual's retest change is due to error or effect is described below.

- **Step 1.** The vast majority of statistical techniques assume that observations are independent. Measures obtained from the same subject, even on vastly different occasions, are clearly not independent. For this reason, techniques have been devised to allow for the calculation of 'true scores' for which an allowance has been made for measurement error and the score actually obtained for a subject. Brophy[8] prescribes the following formula for calculating the true score:

$$T = M + r(X - M)$$

where X is the obtained score, M is the mean of the scores on the test, and r is the reliability coefficient of the test.

- **Step 2.** Calculate the standard error of the 'true' score obtained from step 1, using the appropriate standard error of prediction to plot the appropriate confidence interval. The standard error of prediction for each outcome measure can be calculated using Knight's[7] suggested formula:

Standard error of prediction $= SD \sqrt{(1 - r_{ii}^2)}$

where SD is the standard deviation and r_{ii} is the reliability coefficient.

- **Step 3.** Determine whether the retest scores fall within or beyond the CI calculated in step 2—scores falling within the CI can be judged to be due to change consistent with measurement error. Scores beyond the CI limits are likely to be due to a real effect.

Edwards–Nunnally[9]

This method is very similar to that described above, requiring the regression of an observed score towards the estimated population mean. Further similarity can be found in the construction of a CI around the first test result and then establishing whether the retest 'true' score falls within or beyond this CI. However, Edwards and Nunnally specify the standard error of measurement (SEM) as the appropriate error term, in contrast to the use of the standard error of precision, a specification that has been criticized as inappropriate.[10]

Jacobson–Truax[11]

This technique expresses performance as a ratio derived by dividing the difference between test and retest scores and then dividing by the standard error of the observed difference. Ratios greater than 1.96 should be taken as evidence of a real change.

Hsu–Linn–Lord[12]

This method is essentially indistinguishable from the Brophy–Knight method described above.

Nunnally–Kotsch[13]

This technique is marked out from the others by virtue of its reliance upon a second measure of reliability, a coefficient reflecting the degree of internal consistency of the adopted test. This reliability is a statistic obtained by either calculating a coefficient based on a 'split-half' reliability analysis or by calculating Cronbach's α statistic.[14]

Hierarchical linear modeling—a method for the future?

Speer and Greenbaum,[15] in a review of the available techniques for determining whether real change has occurred, provide a useful critique of the available methods. They suggest that of the numerous techniques available, the Jacobson–Truax method is easily computed and is the best validated. Nevertheless, while computational simplicity is appealing, the Jacobson–Truax method has been criticized for not regressing observed scores towards the population mean to obtain 'true' scores. Speer and Greenbaum cite Rogosa's[16] view that regression is not an inevitable requirement. However, it is our view that when using imperfectly reliable tests it is important to make a correction to the observed score.

Of the other techniques reviewed, both the Edwards–Nunnally and Nunnally–Kotsch methods have been criticized[7,8,12] for using an inappropriate standard error term, a criticism that we view as valid.

Determining normality—a method for showing equivalence

A number of the chapters contained in this book will show that considerable controversy exists regarding the nature, extent and replicability of studies examining cognition. One very good example of this is the reporting of reaction time data in patients with PD, a literature so substantial that it has spawned several review articles. Two tasks, simple reaction time (SRT) and choice reaction time (CRT), have been extensively used with PD patients. Studies to date have reported either a PD deficit selective to SRT, a deficit selective to CRT, a global deficit of both tasks, and no difference between patients and matched controls on either task. Reviews of the area have been hampered by authors' broad use of the term reaction time task to describe their methods. Further confusion is introduced by the marked variation in the inclusion and exclusion criteria adopted by different investigators. The latter issue is dealt with extensively in Chapter 10. A further difficulty is the so-called 'file drawer problem', a reference to journal editors' reluctance to accept null findings, a policy that has encouraged authors to leave manuscripts containing such findings in the 'bottom drawer'. This situation has given rise to suggestions that the reported literature in some areas of research have become prone to publication bias. This issue has been deemed to be of such importance that some researchers have recommended methods for determining whether evidence of such bias can be mustered.[17]

One major problem in showing the performance of neuropsychiatric patient groups to be equivalent to those of matched control subjects is that one comes up against the philosophical problem of seeking to prove the null hypothesis. In circumstances where the mean performance of the patient group is observed to be superior to that of matched controls, this is taken to be reasonable evidence of equivalence. However, when patient performance is observed to be inferior to that of matched controls, there remains the suspicion that the failure to find statistical evidence of patient impairment is due to the study having been under-powered. An alternative interpretation is that the assumed superiority of either group is simply due to measurement error as opposed to a 'real' effect. Thus a small advantage in patient's reaction time score is often viewed as being due to measurement error, whereas the same advantage in controls is often seen as putative evidence of patient impairment.

Showing equivalence is an issue that has also challenged those working in the pharmaceutical industry. Some new chemical entities may be indicated for use in a disorder where efficacious drugs are already prescribed. However, the new compound may be cheaper, or have a better side-effect profile. The issue is thus not whether the new compound constitutes superior therapy, but whether it is as good. This situation is analogous to showing that the performance of a patient group is equivalent to that of a control group. The essence of the methodology adopted in pharmaceutical equivalence trials is to pre-specify a range of difference scores for which equivalence could be claimed (see Jones et al[18] for an excellent treatment of this topic). A critical further aspect of the method is that the 95% CI for any observed group difference is required to fall within the specified range of equivalent differences. A hypothetical illustration of this method is shown in Figure 1.2, which illustrates an attempt to demonstrate equivalence between a patient group and a matched, normal healthy control group on a simple reaction time task. Lines 1, 2, 3 and 4 depict the mean difference and associated 95% CI for four different possible outcomes.

Example (1) shows a small advantage in favor of the control group. However, this difference is not a statistically significant effect, as the CI includes the zero point (a 95% CI that does not include a zero difference is de facto statistically significant at the 5% level, one-tailed). Equivalence has not been demonstrated, as the upper boundary of the observed CI exceeds the declared range of equivalence.

Example (2) illustrates a small advantage for the patient group, though, as with (1), the associated CI includes the zero point and exceeds the range of equivalence, thus it is neither a statistically significant nor an equivalent effect.

Example (3) shows an advantage for the control group. Associated with this difference is a 95% CI that does not include a zero difference,

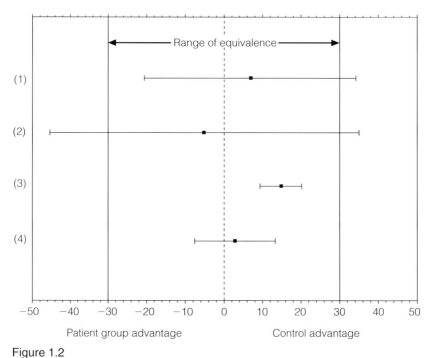

Figure 1.2

Possible observed outcomes in a between-group study of simple reaction time, shown as difference in means with associated 95% confidence interval.

implying a statistically significant effect. Furthermore, because the observed CI falls within the range of equivalence, this observation would be declared as showing equivalence.

Example (4) is included to show an outcome that would also be interpreted as showing equivalence, as the boundaries of the 95% CI fall within the equivalence range. No significant difference between the two groups is implied, as the observed CI includes the zero point.

This methodology, while useful, does impose some challenging disciplines upon the investigator. Perhaps the most difficult discipline to accept is the scenario suggested in (3), where the researcher is required to treat a statistically significant difference as evidence of equivalence. In the following section we deal with these issues and seek to show that consideration of power necessarily entails consideration of a psychologically relevant difference.

'Power' and psychologically relevant differences

Equivalence studies require precise calculations to be made about the number of subjects required to ensure that the standard error of the difference yields a sufficiently small value to permit the 95% CI to fall within the equivalence range. This inevitably requires the investigator to perform a power calculation in order for the precision of any point estimate to be sufficiently good. Power calculations should always be conducted prior to starting a study to ensure that the experiment is sufficiently well powered to detect a real effect, if such an effect exists. Reducing type 2 errors is likely to have the effect of making reviews of patient performance easier to conduct. However, in addition to the unfortunate legacy of under-powering is the danger attached to experiments that detect statistically significant differences for effects of a modest magnitude.

The example of the equivalence study outlined above carried the requirement that the investigator specified what mean difference would be required for an effect to be declared of sufficient interest. This is analogous to the notion of the 'clinically significant difference', i.e. whether the improvement in a patient's status is sufficiently large enough to engender a worthwhile change in their levels of function. This dual requirement for both a statistically and a clinically significant change is commonplace in clinical trials, as, clearly, mere statistical significance may have no practical benefit for sufferers of whatever disorder the new drug is designed to treat. Specifying a clinically relevant difference often presents a difficult challenge but has the advantage of providing a target efficacy level and a means of showing equivalence. It also requires investigators to determine and defend what magnitude a change in function has to have in order to be of sufficient importance.

The goal of most studies of cognitive function in patient groups is to demonstrate that a decline in function has reached such a level that it provides a statistically significant difference between the performance of the patients and control groups. However, it not always evident that statistically significant differences have major cognitive importance. An example of this might be a study of digit span in a neurologically or psychiatrically impaired group. The effective scoring range on such a task is fairly limited and, consequently, so too is any variance attaching to mean performance. Partially as a result of these characteristics of the task, some studies of digit span have reported statistically significant differences between control and patient groups of as little as 0.5. While this difference passes the widely accepted test of significance at the 0.05 level, it is difficult for us to accept that a mean difference so small that it is less than a one-point difference has any psychological relevance. However, and importantly, it might do. We recognize the difficulty of determining what constitutes a large enough difference. We would suggest that such an issue is worth consideration, if only because the methodology for showing equivalence between patients and controls requires it.

References

1. Ojemann G, Ojemann J, Lettich E. Cortical language localization in left, dominant hemisphere: an electrical stimulation mapping experiment in 117 patients. *J Neurosurg* (1989) **71:** 316–26.

2. Marshall JC. The description and interpretation of aphasic language disorder. *Neuropsychologia* (1986) **24(1):** 5–23.

3. Hughes AJ, Daniel SE, Kilford L, Lees AJ. Accuracy of clinical diagnosis of idiopathic Parkinson's disease, a clinico-pathological study of 100 cases. *J Neurol Neurosurg Psychiatry* (1992) **55:** 181–4.

4. Rajput AH, Offord K, Beard CM, Kurland LT. Epidemiological survey of dementia in parkinsonism and control population. *Adv Neurol* (1984) **40:** 229–34.

5. Milner B. Effects of different brain lesions on card sorting: the role of the frontal lobes. *Arch Neurol* (1963) **9:** 90–100.

6. Altman D. *Practical Statistics for Medical Research* (London: Chapman & Hall, 1991).

7. Knight R. On interpreting the several standard errors of the WAIS-R: some further tables. *J Consult Clin Psychol* (1983) **51:** 671–3.

8. Brophy AL. Confidence intervals for true scores and retest scores on cinical tests. *J Clin Psychol* (1986) **42(6):** 989–91.

9. Speer DC. Can treatment research inform decision makers? Non-experimental method issues and examples among older adults. *J Consult Exp Psychol* (1994) **62:** 560–8.

10. Hsu LM. Regression towards the mean associated with measurement error and the identification of improvement and deterioration in psychotherapy. *J Consult Clin Psychol* (1995) **63:** 141–4.

11. Jacobson NS, Truax P. Clinical significance: a statistical approach to defining meaningful

change in psychotherapy research. *J Consult Clin Psychol* (1991) **59:** 12–19.

12. Hsu LM. Reliable changes in psychotherapy: taking into account regression towards the mean. *Behav Assess* (1989) **11:** 459–67.

13. Nunnally JC, Kotsch WE. Studies of individual subjects: logic and methods of analysis. *Br J Clin Psychol* (1983) **22:** 83–93.

14. Cronbach LJ. Coefficient alpha and the internal structure of tests. *Psychometrika* (1951) **16(3):** 297–334.

15. Speer DC, Greenbaum PE. Five methods for computing significant individual client change and improvement rates: support for an individual growth curve approach. *J Consult Clin Psychol* (1995) **63(6):** 1044–8.

16. Rogosa DR. Myths about longitudinal research. In Schaie KW, Campbell RT, Meredith WM et al (eds) *Methodological Issues in Aging Research* 171–209. (New York: Springer, 1988).

17. Rosenthal R. The file drawer problem and tolerance for null results. *Psychol Bull* (1979) **86:** 638–41.

18. Jones B, Jarvis P, Lewis JA, Ebbutt AF. Trials to assess equivalence: the importance of rigorous methods. *BMJ* (1996) **313:** 36–9.

Appendix A

Example 1

A head-injured patient who made 40 paired associate learning (PAL) errors preoperatively is observed to make 32 errors postoperatively, apparently showing signs of improvement. The researcher's requirement is to determine whether this improvement is due to a real effect or simply due to measurement error. A predicted true score is obtained by using the mean test score (PAL total errors = 14.8) and the reliability score for the test ($r = 0.68$). Substituting these scores into the equation given in step 1 yields:

$$14.8 + 0.68(40 - 14.8) = 31.936.$$

The researcher then calculates a 66% CI for the true score using the standard error of prediction (SEP) for PAL errors (SEP = 13.91), yielding a CI of 18.03–45.85. The retest score of 32 falls within this interval, suggesting that the apparent improvement is consistent with variation due to measurement error.

Example 2

A patient with PD makes 51 between errors on the spatial working memory task prior to receiving a novel dopamine agonist. After administration of the compound, his between error score reduces to 20. The researcher wishes to determine whether this change is likely to be due to the effect of the drug. A predicted true score is calculated using the mean and reliability scores for the test (22.3 and 0.7 respectively). Substituting these scores into the step 1 equation yields:

$$22.3 + 0.7(51 - 22.3) = 42.39.$$

A 66% CI is then calculated around the true score using an SEP of 12.54 yielding a CI of 29.85–54.93. The retest score falls beyond the lower bound of this CI suggesting that the improvement is due to the effect of the compound.

2

The neuropsychological consequences of ruptured aneurysms of the anterior communicating artery

John DeLuca and Nancy D Chiaravalloti

With advances in technology and medicine, survival from surgery for cerebral aneurysms has increased significantly over the past three decades. With increased survival come questions about quality of life. Over the last 20 years, questions regarding the quality of life of these individuals have been at the forefront of research with patients surviving aneurysms of the anterior communicating artery (ACoA). Through retrospective reviews[1] as well as prospective studies of cognitive/behavioral status and abilities post-surgery,[2,3] neuroscientists have been able to identify frequently observed cognitive sequelae of ACoA aneurysms. It is now well known that aneurysms at the ACoA frequently lead to neurobehavioral impairments.[4,5] Outcome studies have demonstrated that cognitive and behavioral impairments may range from no impairment to subtle cognitive and emotional problems to profound amnesia, confabulation, or abulic states.[6-8]

In addition to the recognition of the wide range of cognitive problems following ACoA aneurysm, recent progress in ACoA research has begun to refine the identification of the neuropathological underpinnings of the major behavioral problems associated with these aneurysms.[7,9] Research on the course of recovery and effectiveness of rehabilitation in regaining function, however, has lagged behind.

The purpose of this chapter is to provide an overview of the neurobehavioral and neuroanatomical features associated with ACoA aneurysm rupture. We begin with basic background information about ACoA aneurysms, followed by a description of what has been referred to as the 'ACoA syndrome'. A brief discussion of resulting specific neuropsychological and neurobehavioral symptoms of ACoA aneurysms follows. Finally, a brief review of cognitive rehabilitation and outcome studies is presented.

ACoA: background information

An intracranial aneurysm is an abnormal enlargement of a blood vessel resulting from a flaw in the blood vessel wall. Cerebral aneurysm is fairly common, with a prevalence of 2.3–5% in adults.[10,11] The prevalence of aneurysms is also higher in females, individuals with a family history of subarachnoid hemorrhage (SAH), suspected pituitary adenomas, autosomal dominant polycystic kidney disease, and artherosclerosis.[11]

The ACoA lies at the anterior portion of the circle of Willis, interconnecting the two anterior cerebral arteries just rostral to the optic chiasm. Approximately 85–95% of all aneurysms develop at the anterior portion of the cerebral arterial supply, primarily at the circle of Willis.[12] ACoA aneurysm rupture may markedly alter the hemodynamic circulation of the anterior portion of the circle of Willis, often resulting in cerebral infarction.[10] The ACoA is one of the most common sites of cerebral aneurysm in humans and is the most frequent site of cerebral infarct following aneurysm rupture.[10] Infarcts are often observed along the distribution of the anterior cerebral arteries, and the small perforating arterial branches directly off of the ACoA itself.[3,13] The vascular territory of these ACoA branches involves the paraterminal gyrus (including the septal nuclei), the genu of the corpus callosum, anterior cingulum, optic chiasm, columns of the fornix, substantia inominata, anterior hypothalamus, mesial anterior commissure, and nucleus basalis of Meynert.[14]

ACoA aneurysm rupture typically requires neurosurgical repair of the vessel. Neurobehavioral consequences of this surgery have been associated with several factors. However, definitive relationships have not yet been firmly established. Such factors include: timing of surgery,[15,16] side of surgical approach,[17] surgical technique (e.g. trapping versus clipping of aneurysm),[3] and peri-surgical complications such as hydrocephalus, vasospasm, duration of temporary clipping, blood loss during surgery, duration of surgery, intracranial pressure, edema, and SAH.[15,18–20]

The 'ACoA syndrome' and other cognitive sequelae

Numerous studies on aneurysms of the ACoA have revealed wide variability in cognitive and behavioral consequences, ranging from no difficulties, to subtle cognitive deficits, to profound global cognitive impairment, as seen in Table 2.1. The most profound deficits observed following ACoA aneurysm include a severe memory deficit, confabulation, and personality change. These three features have been widely referred to as the 'ACoA syndrome' (see DeLuca and Diamond[5] for a review) and have been the focus of much neurobehavioral research, as described below.

Table 2.1   Frequently observed cognitive sequelae of aneurysms of the anterior communicating artery (ACoA)

ACoA syndrome	Severe memory deficit
	Confabulation
	Personality change
Other Neuropsychological Deficits	Decreased cognitive flexibility
	Decreased verbal fluency
	Poor problem solving
	Mild impairment in intelligence (decrease in PIQ)
	Executive dyscontrol
	Decreased verbal fluency
	Poor new learning
	Difficulty organizing a stimulus
Other Neurobehavioral Dysfunction	Alien hand syndrome
	Akinesia
	Abulia

Amnesia

Although there were isolated reports of neurological dysfunction following ACoA aneurysm in the literature during the 1950s, systematic research examining cognitive deficits only began during the 1960s in the USA. This early work was focused primarily on documenting the existence and nature of the 'ACoA syndrome'.

Lindqvist and Norlen[21] reported that Korsakoff syndrome was observed in 17 of 33 ACoA cases they examined. Similarly, Talland et al[22] discussed the similarities between ACoA amnesics and Korsakoff's amnesia, and hypothesized that the ACoA amnesia resulted from lesions of the same diencephalic structures as demonstrated in Korsakoff patients.

Very little progress was made during the 1970s in understanding the cognitive aspects of ACoA aneurysm. By the mid-1970s, Luria 'seemed to favor an explanation [of the observed amnesia] in terms of either arterial spasm or, in patients with permanently severe amnesia, hemorrhage spreading to the region of the floor of the third ventricle'.[3] Interestingly, characteristically ahead of his time, it was Luria who first suggested that the nature of the amnestic disorder following ACoA aneurysm was qualitatively different from that seen in the typical mesial–temporal amnesic.[23] By the mid-1970s it was discovered that the ACoA had significant perforating branches.[24] These small arterial branches were found to perfuse, among other structures, the basal forebrain.[24]

Gade[3] showed that when a 'trapping' surgical technique (clipping the aneurysm at each junction with the anterior cerebral artery, effectively cutting off circulation) was used for ACoA aneurysm repair, 9 of the 11 patients examined demonstrated an amnestic syndrome. In contrast, only

6 of 37 patients who underwent a 'ligation' procedure (clipping the aneurysm at its neck) showed an amnestic syndrome. As a result, Gade[3] was the first to suggest that the amnestic syndrome observed following ACoA aneurysm was due to reduced blood supply through the perforating branches of the ACoA, which supply the region of the basal forebrain.

Armed with CT scanning, the 1980s produced several case reports documenting not only the amnesia, confabulation and personality changes, but also the purported neuroanatomical substrates of these behavioral features. Volpe and Hirst[25] reported two cases of severe anterograde amnesia who did not confabulate and had normal CT scans. These authors speculated that ischemic changes resulting from cerebral vasospasm constitute the likely mechanism for the amnestic syndrome, involving either orbitofrontal or mesial–temporal structures.

Alexander and Freedman[13] presented a series of 11 ACoA cases, all of whom were amnesic, were confabulatory, and exhibited personality changes. They argued, as did Gade,[3] that the ACoA syndrome may be caused by infarction along the distribution of the ACoA perforating arteries, and that the observed amnesia may be caused by damage to the septal–hippocampal system. Importantly, Alexander and Freedman reported that gross infarction of the frontal lobes was not a requirement for the ACoA syndrome to be manifested. Vilkki[26] examined five ACoA cases and also concluded that frontal lobe damage was not necessary for amnesia to be expressed.

Damasio et al[27] specifically implicated the basal forebrain as the area responsible for the amnesia. Further support for this contention was provided by the post-mortem case presented by Phillips et al.[28] These authors reported an ACoA amnesic with a lesion largely confined to the basal forebrain bilaterally (septal gray, nucleus accumbens, and diagonal band of Broca) but sparing the nucleus basalis of Meynert. There was also involvement of the inferior limb of the internal capsule and globus pallidus. Other case reports of severe memory impairments were also reported during the 1980s.[29,30] While there was some evidence that ACoA amnesics showed a differential pattern of impairment from diencephalic and/or mesial–temporal amnesics,[31] this was not always supported.[32]

In contrast to the case report literature, several group-comparison studies were reported during the 1980s, many of which did not support the concept of a focal lesion to explain impaired memory performance following ACoA aneurysm. While several group studies found that aneurysms at the ACoA were particularly susceptible to cognitive impairments,[4,30] others have concluded that memory difficulties following ACoA aneurysm resulted from diffuse cerebral involvement rather than a discrete lesion.[33–35] Such studies compared a group of ACoA aneurysm patients with patients who had aneurysms elsewhere in the brain, for example posterior communicating artery (PCoA), middle cerebral artery (MCA), internal cerebral artery (ICA). However, these studies differed methodologically from the case reports mentioned above, which may explain the discrepant conclusions. That is, the case studies presented the most severe ACoA patients during the acute phase, while the group studies tended to include in their sample all ACoA subjects, both those with and without cognitive problems, often mixing relatively acute and chronic subjects.

In summary, by the end of the 1980s, group studies suggested that diffuse cerebral involvement could explain the cognitive impairments following ACoA aneurysm. In marked contrast, the case report literature clearly supported a 'focal lesion' hypothesis to explain the 'Korsakoff-like' amnesia observed following ACoA aneurysm rupture. Damage to the basal forebrain was seen as a primary cause for the amnesia. However, an important question remained: why are ACoA patients amnesic despite the absence of damage to the areas traditionally known to cause amnesia, namely medial–temporal and diencephalic structures, on CT scans? The role of these important brain regions remained unclear.

In the 1990s, the number of reports examining ACoA aneurysm patients continued to increase. Several studies were conducted identifying subgroups of individuals with impaired memory within the ACoA population. Stenhouse et al[36] reported three ACoA subgroups in a sample averaging 54 months post-surgery: (1) 'pervasive global impairment'; (2) 'focal frontal damage'; and (3) 'recovered'. Tarel et al[37] also reported three groups, those with: (1) amnesia, (2) memory impaired on neuropsychological tests; and (3) no memory disorders. Bottger et al[6] reported seven specific patterns of cognitive impairment in patients who were discharged from a rehabilitation hospital. Thus, by the 1990s, the notion of behavioral heterogeneity following ACoA aneurysm was beginning to be incorporated into research.

Irle et al[38] subdivided 30 ACoA subjects into five groups according to lesion sites based on CT scans: (1) striatum, (2) basal forebrain, (3) striate plus basal forebrain, (4) basal forebrain plus frontal, and (5) striate, basal forebrain, plus frontal. These groups were compared with two control groups: an ACoA group without demonstrable lesions on CT scan, and normal controls. The basal forebrain and striate groups were not impaired relative to controls in immediate memory performance. However, the memory deficit in the basal forebrain plus frontal group was moderate, whereas the deficits in the striate plus basal forebrain, and striate, basal forebrain, plus frontal groups were severe. These authors concluded that combined striate and basal forebrain lesions 'appear necessary and sufficient to produce amnesia' following ACoA aneurysm rupture. This idea that lesions of the basal forebrain plus damage to adjacent structures produced greater cognitive and behavioral difficulties was also reported by Eslinger and Grattan.[39]

Several additional group studies also suggested 'localized' cerebral dysfunction to explain both anterograde[2] and retrograde[7] amnesia.

However, other group studies came to different conclusions. Tidswell et al[9] examined consecutive admissions to a neurosurgical unit, comparing 20 ACoA patients with 17 patients with non-anterior aneurysms. No significant group differences were found on measures of memory, executive or other cognitive functions. Similar findings were reported by Richardson[20] and Hutter and Gilsbach,[1] who also compared ACoA with another aneurysmal SAH group from the acute setting. These latter authors suggested that cognitive deficits in ACoA patients were due to secondary consequences of the SAH (e.g. vasospasm, brain swelling, bleeding, ischemia), downplaying the role of the basal forebrain in memory. These group studies are in marked contrast to the report of Bottger et al,[6] which showed debilitating cognitive problems following ACoA aneurysm. However, one important contrast is the sample examined. While Bottger et al examined only subjects who were admitted to a rehabilitation unit because of clear neurobehavioral problems, the other authors examined virtually all patients referred to the acute hospital for surgery. Difficulties in contrasting such heterogeneous samples when attempting to identify cognitive problems associated with ACoA aneurysm have been discussed previously by DeLuca and Diamond.[5]

Bottger et al[6] examined 30 ACoA patients admitted to rehabilitation at a mean of 5 months and again at 14 months post-surgery. These authors found that memory disturbance was closely associated with lesions of the medial septum and the nucleus of the diagonal band of Broca. This is consistent with the postmortem findings of Phillips et al.[28] Bottger et al[6] also found that frontal lesions were associated with attentional, executive and psychopathological dysfunction. These authors could not confirm the findings of Irle et al,[38] which suggested that only lesions of the basal forebrain, in conjunction with striatal lesions, resulted in severe amnesia. While Bottger et al[6] found no relationship between the striatum and memory performance, it was not clear from their paper that striatal lesions were specifically examined. However, the case reported by Abe et al[40] also does not support the contention of Irle et al[38] that lesions outside the basal forebrain are required for significant amnesia. This patient showed significant anterograde amnesia up to 30 months post-surgery. MRI of the brain at 30 months showed a discrete lesion of the basal forebrain, including the diagonal band of Broca, septal nucleus, lamina terminalis, and anterior hypothalamus. Involvement of the nucleus basalis of Meynert was minimal (similar to the findings of Phillips et al[28]) and there was no damage to the diencephalon or medial–temporal lobes. Single photon emission computed tomography (SPECT) showed hypoperfusion in the midline frontobasal region bilaterally, corresponding to the basal forebrain region on magnetic resonance imaging. Importantly, SPECT also revealed markedly reduced blood perfusion in the hippocampus bilaterally, relative to the cerebellum. This is of major significance, because it provides direct evidence supporting the hypothesis that ACoA amnesia may result from disruption of critical bidirectional connections between the basal forebrain and the hippocampus. Abe et al conjectured that the diagonal band of Broca played a major role in ACoA amnesia.

Confabulation

Confabulation can be defined as statements or actions that involve unintentional but obvious distortions of memory.[41] A phenomenon first observed by Korsakoff in individuals with a long history of alcohol abuse, confabulation is one of the core features of the ACoA syndrome. Reference to a Korsakoff-like amnesia in ACoA patients was initially made due to the presence of both amnesia and confabulation.[22] Because of the similarities with Korsakoff's syndrome patients, the neuropathological mechanism of confabulation was initially attributed to lesions of the mammilary bodies and dorsal–medial nucleus of the thalamus.[22] However, subsequent studies showed that this idea was too simplistic.

Early studies implicated frontal lobe damage in the neuropathology of confabulation.[42,43] Luria[44,45] specifically highlighted lesions in the medial zones of the frontal lobes as the source of confabulation, citing the extensive connections with the limbic system as the major factor. Vilkki[26] showed that only ACoA amnesics *with* frontal lesions were confabulators.

Several studies provided support for distinct neuropathological causes of amnesia and confabulation.[26,27,43] However, the idea that frontal lesions in isolation were not sufficient to cause confabulation in ACoA patients led to a 'dual-lesion' hypothesis. This hypothesis suggested that lesions in both the frontal lobes and the basal forebrain were necessary for confabulation to be manifested. Support for this hypothesis was provided by DeLuca,[46] who indeed found that confabulation was observed only in those ACoA subjects with both frontal lobe and presumed basal forebrain lesions. There is some evidence from the tumor literature suggesting that lesions restricted to the basal forebrain do not produce spontaneous confabulation.[47] Additional supporting evidence is found in the amnesia literature, where amnesics without frontal lobe involvement do not confabulate.[48]

Fischer et al[49] divided nine acute ACoA patients into two groups, 'spontaneous' confabulators and 'provoked' confabulators. The authors concluded that the type and severity of confabulation noted are largely dependent upon both impairments in memory and the extent of executive system compromise. They concluded that 'spontaneous' confabulation required disruption of both the basal forebrain and frontal systems, supporting the dual-lesion hypothesis. More restricted lesions to either the basal forebrain or orbital frontal structures can result in 'provoked' or transient confabulatory responses.

Schnider et al[50] classified amnesic patients (including ACoA) into 'spontaneous' and 'provoked' confabulators. They reported that confabulators did not show an increased tendency to fill in gaps in memory, a notion sometimes associated with confabulation.[42] Provoked confabulation was associated with decreased verbal learning and verbal fluency. Schnider et al[50] concluded that provoked and spontaneous confabulation are separate disorders, with distinct neuroanatomical mechanisms. This conclusion is in contrast to that of DeLuca and Cicerone,[30] who examined confabulation in ACoA sequentially both when subjects were disoriented and when they became oriented to person, place and time. DeLuca and Cicerone[30] found that improvement in orientation was often associated with a change from spontaneous to provoked confabulation in the same subject. This suggests that severity of confabulation can be viewed on a continuum from more severe (i.e. spontaneous) to less severe (i.e. provoked), rather than being different in kind with separate mechanisms.

Several investigators suggest that spontaneous confabulation is a result of a difficulty in recognizing the temporal order of events during the retrieval of stored information.[50] Moscovitch and Melo[41] postulate that it is strategic retrieval (i.e. active, systematic memory search) that is impaired in confabulation, due to damage to ventromedial frontal structures, as opposed to associative retrieval (passive, automatic search through memory). They suggest that defective temporal order processing is not the cause of confabulation, but a symptom of a more fundamental problem in the strategic retrieval and defective monitoring of output.[41] This hypothesis is supported by Johnson et al,[51] who compared the performance of a confabulating ACoA patient with that of three patients with frontal lobe lesions who did not confabulate. The confabulating ACoA patient was also impaired on tasks measuring memory for temporal duration and speaker identification, suggesting that source memory impairments alone are not sufficient to result in confabulation. However, the ACoA confabulator showed severely impaired autobiographical memory relative to frontal controls.

In summary, the literature on ACoA aneurysm is somewhat consistent in implicating frontal structures as necessary, but not sufficient, sites of neuropathology in confabulation. However, cases of non-amnesic ACoA patients with frontal lobe lesions who do not confabulate suggest that frontal lobe and basal forebrain involvement are both required for spontaneous confabulation to be manifested. Additionally, the literature on ACoA confabulation no longer supports the premise that confabulation represents a tendency to 'fill in the gaps' in memory. Rather, confabulation is hypothesized to result from a deficit in strategic retrieval and monitoring at output, which may explain associated findings such as deficits in temporal order and speaker identification, as well as difficulty in searching for autobiographical memory information.

Personality

Personality changes following ACoA aneurysm have been documented in the literature since the 1950s. Early references to 'improved personality' or becoming 'remarkably good-natured' after ACoA rupture were not uncommon. Personality changes vary dramatically among patients, with some, for instance, showing decreased initiation, apathy, lack of concern, flattened affect, and less of a tendency to worry, while others may display increased irritability, fatuousness, socially inappropriate behavior, and unpredictable aggression.[13] Other changes include an increase in emotional lability, talkativeness, selfishness, euphoria, childlike behavior, laziness, and indifference.[34] Importantly, several investigators have noted that personality change can occur in the absence of confabulation or amnesia.

Studies investigating personality changes following ACoA aneurysm have been relatively sparse for a number of reasons, perhaps most notably the limited tools available for assessing change in personality from premorbid status. The few studies that have been completed have methodological limitations and allow few inferences to be drawn.

As with amnesia and confabulation, early studies attributed personality changes to diencephalic regions, due to similarities with Korsakoff's syndrome.[22] Luria[44,45] attributed personality changes with pathology in the mediobasal region of the frontal lobes, noting the relationship between these frontal structures and the limbic system in the alteration of personality. The important role of orbital frontal regions, particularly areas perfused by the anterior cerebral arteries, in altered personality following ACoA aneurysm has been well documented over the years.[27,52]

Alexander and Freedman[13] and Phillips at al[28] both discussed the potential role of the medial forebrain bundle (MFB) in contributing to aspects of personality change. Because the MFB is thought to modulate cerebral arousal due to the ascending influence of the reticular activating system, disruption of the MFB (which runs through the septal area and lateral hypothalamus) was hypothesized to contribute to decreased arousal, and be manifested as apathy. However, Irle et al[38] suggested that the 'motivational changes' (e.g. decreased energy, apathy) may be associated with basal forebrain/hypothalamic lesions, while the 'cognitive personality changes' (e.g. impaired judgment, self-criticism) may be associated with ventromedial frontal lesions. They noted that ACoA patients with striatal lesions showed higher elevations on the Minnesota Multiphasic Personality Inventory (MMPI) than ACoA patients without such lesions.

Several investigators have noted that personality alterations were frequently chronic and resistant to change, often resulting in long-term management problems, and serving as a significant obstacle to successful social reintegration.[34,53] In fact, chronic, persistent personality changes have been shown to lead to poorer outcome in terms of employment status, return to the home[13] and intellectual performance.[54]

In summary, there is general agreement suggesting that personality changes following ACoA aneurysm are a result of frontal lobe dysfunction, particularly in the mediobasal zones along the distribution of the anterior cerebral artery. The potential role of the ascending fibers of the MFB as well as lesions which include the striate region are in need of replication and extension.

Specific neuropsychological sequelae

Specific neuropsychological deficits often observed in ACoA patients are described in this section. It should be noted that not all ACoA patients will present with difficulties in all domains discussed below. See DeLuca and Diamond[5] for a more detailed description of neuropsychological sequelae.

Intellectual functions

The majority of studies suggest that intelligence is largely preserved following aneurysms of the AcoA,[2,6,36] although some patients can show mild impairment.[38] While performance IQ is often decreased compared to relatively intact verbal IQ,[30,55] this is not always observed.[13,38] Some studies have also found that ACoA patients show a decrease in overall intelligence as compared with a premorbid estimate of intelligence[29,36] based on the National Adult Reading Test (NART). Therefore, despite the fact that IQ remains within normal range, some preliminary data suggest that there may be a reduction from premorbid intellectual abilities.

Attention and concentration

In general, the literature suggests that attentional skills remain relatively intact or mildly diminished in ACoA patients. Multiple studies have noted that most ACoA patients score within the normal range on measures such as the Digit Span and Mental Control subtests of the Wechsler Memory Scale (WMS).[5] However, more difficulty has been observed in some ACoA patients on tests of complex concentration such as the Stroop and Trail Making Test.

In contrast, ACoA patients show a significant susceptibility to interference, which Luria[56] reported as a key feature of ACoA amnesia. The pattern of impaired performance has also been suggested to differ from that seen in diencephalic and mesial–temporal amnesics.[57] Several studies document increased susceptibility and/or release from proactive interference[25,31] and impaired performance on the Brown–Peterson distractor task.[29]

Memory

The neuropathology of memory has been presented above. Memory performance ranges from amnesic, to mild impairment, to normal performance. In general, immediate recall is far less impaired than delayed recall, particularly among amnesic ACoA patients. Additionally, there is some suggestion that ACoA patients show particular difficulty in discriminating temporal context during recall. Very few studies have been conducted on retrograde memory, yielding mixed results. While some studies suggest that the degree of retrograde memory impairment is significantly less than that observed in diencephalic or mesial–temporal amnesics, one study found no group differences.[58] Still others find no retrograde impairment whatsoever, even among amnesics. D'Esposito et al[7] showed that retrograde memory impairments resulted from severe executive dysfunction secondary to bifrontal lesions. The few studies examining implicit memory reported intact performance in ACoA patients.

Executive functions

Deficits in executive control functions, believed to be mediated by the frontal lobes, constitute a major difficulty among ACoA patients. Stenhouse et al[36] reported two groups of impaired ACoA subjects: a group with 'global' cognitive impairment, and a group demonstrating more specific deficits in executive functions (Wisconsin Card Sorting Test Performance, WCST). Several authors have reported executive impairment (e.g. reduced cognitive flexibility, poor concept formation, poor planning) in a subset of ACoA patients, particularly among amnesics.[2,6,59,60] Studies comparing WCST performance of ACoA subjects with amnesia from other etiologies have shown more impairment in ACoA subjects as compared with herpes encephalitis,[61] Korsakoff's patients, or patients with mesial–temporal lobe resection.[32]

Several authors have shown that severity of confabulation is related to deficits in executive functioning.[36,46,62] Fischer et al[49] reported that among amnesic ACoA patients, 'spontaneous' confabulation was observed only among those who had frontal/executive impairments as well as basal forebrain lesions. ACoA amnesics with damage restricted to the basal forebrain showed 'provoked' confabulation.

Executive dysfunction plays a significant role in the memory abilities of ACoA patients. For instance, D'Esposito et al[7] showed that retrograde amnesia was only observed among amnesic ACoA subjects who also had severe executive dysfunction, associated with bifrontal lobe lesions on MRI. Diamond et al[63] showed that anterograde memory was significantly influenced by executive dysfunction, through their use of an organizational strategy to facilitate encoding on the Rey Complex Figure Test. These authors found that organizational strategy facilitated both immediate and delayed recall in the amnesic group to the level observed in non-amnesic ACoA subjects. However, not all amnesic subjects benefited from the organizational strategy. The ability to utilize an organizational intervention to improve memory appeared to be related to the degree of executive impairment as measured by the WCST.

Performance on tests of verbal fluency, also believed to be sensitive to frontal lobe pathology, is variable among all ACoA patients, even amnesics. Some ACoA patients show significantly impaired performance, while others do not.[6,13,28,32,33] ACoA subjects also appear to display impaired performance[31,61] on the Cognitive Estimates Test (CET),[64] another executive test believed to be sensitive to frontal lobe pathology.

Visuospatial/perceptual and constructional abilities

Perceptual skills are generally reported to be intact following ACoA aneurysm. However, some studies have reported some visuo-constructional disorganization and impaired visuoperceptual abilities[33,59,60] following ACoA aneurysm.

Language

Language functions (i.e. expressive, receptive, naming, repetition, reading, writing) have been shown to be preserved in the amnesic ACoA case study literature (see DeLuca and Diamond[5] for a review). Some studies have reported deficient spontaneous speech, impaired speech initiation[13,26] or, rarely, akinetic mutism.[21] Paraphasic or neologistic speech errors have not been reported. The only area of language which more consistently reveals defective performance is verbal fluency (see above). However, this deficit is primarily attributable to initiation deficits (i.e. executive), as opposed to language system dysfunction.

Other neurobehavioral dysfunction

A less frequent symptom following ACoA aneurysm is 'alien hand syndrome' (AHS). AHS is marked by apparently purposeful but uncontrollable movements of one hand (usually the left), which often interferes with the actions of the other hand. Although rare, several reports of AHS following ACoA aneurysm have been reported.[65,66] Exact neurological involvement in AHS is as yet undetermined, but various mechanisms have been postulated, including a combination of a partial callosectomy and mesial frontal lesions,[65] or involvement of the anterior corpus callosum.[67]

Also rare following rupture of the ACoA is akinesia, or absence of movement, presumed to be due to damage to the dopamine system or its projections.[34,68] Sudden paraplegia or paresis has been documented following ACoA aneurysm but is also extremely rare,[69,70] while ideomotor dysfunction has generally not been reported.[33]

Recovery and rehabilitation

Studies have shown that up to 84% of ACoA survivors are able to return to work.[35,71] Despite such apparently encouraging results, it should be noted that significant neuropsychological, psychological and psychosocial consequences are often observed in SAH patients, even in the absence of obvious neurological deficits,[59] with some evidence for particular difficulties in ACoA patients.[4,60]

Table 2.2   Surgical factors potentially affecting outcome following aneurysm of the anterior communicating artery (ACoA)

Timing of neurosurgery	Haley et al, 1992;[15] Hori and Suzuki, 1979[71]
Surgical technique	Hutter and Gilsbach, 1996;[17] Gade, 1982;[3] Artiola i Fortuny and Prieto-Valiente, 1981[18]
Duration of surgery	Hutter and Gilsbach, 1996[17]
Duration of temporary clipping	Hutter and Gilsbach,1996[17]
Induced focal perfusion	Fasanaro et al, 1989[72]

A wide range of recovery has been documented following ACoA aneurysm, both in the time post-surgery for observing improved cognitive functioning[9,34] and in the pattern and degree of recovery.[36] Recovery following ACoA aneurysm has been shown to be related to a variety of surgical (Table 2.2) and post-surgical (Table 2.3) factors. Individual outcome, functional status and employment status can be affected by a variety of factors, including premorbid functional status, premorbid employment status,[73] and the premorbid work environment to which the individual is returning.[74,75] For example, Storey[74,75] noted that ACoA individuals returning to work in large corporations are better able to make the transition back to the workplace than those returning to a self-employed status. Vilkki et al[76] also examined return to work as an outcome measure, reporting that multiple factors influence one's ability to return to work,

Table 2.3   Factors potentially complicating physical and cognitive outcome following aneurysm of the anterior communicating artery (ACoA)

Ischemia	Hutter and Gilsbach, 1992[1]
Infarction	Alexander and Freedman, 1984;[13] Damasio et al, 1985;[27] Gade, 1982[3]
Increased intracranial pressure	Takaku et al, 1979[16]
Edema	Hutter and Gilsbach, 1992[1]
Hydrocephalous	Artiola i Fortuny and Prieto-Valiente, 1981[18]
Vasospasm	Kassell et al, 1990;[19] Haley et al, 1992;[15] Artiola i Fortuny and Prieto-Valiente, 1981;[18] Vilkki, 1985;[26] Stenhouse et al, 1991[36]
Subarachnoid hemorrhage (SAH) following aneurysm rupture	Takaku et al, 1979[16]

including cognitive abilities (memory, cognitive flexibility), personality factors, and emotional issues.

Additional neurobehavioral factors that have been shown to affect recovery include postoperative cognitive abilities,[6] postoperative personality changes[13,34] and postoperative emotional issues.[76] For example, Bottger et al[6] administered comprehensive neuropsychological evaluations to 30 patients, 2–13 months after ACoA surgery. Utilizing multiple regression analysis, these authors noted memory and attentional processes at discharge (2–13 weeks post-injury) to be good predictors of functional outcome, as measured by the Glasgow Outcome Scale (GOS). However, executive dysfunction, psychopathology and neuropathology were not related to outcome.

Studies examining the time frame for neurobehavioral recovery range in their estimations from 1–2 months post-aneurysm[9] to 6 months post-aneurysm.[34] For example, Okawa et al[34] noted that, in most of their cases, postoperative confabulation began to disappear 1–3 months following surgery, disappearing completely within 6 months. However, confabulation can persist well beyond this time frame in some ACoA patients.[62] The regaining of cognitive functions also shows this variability. For example, in 10 patients sustaining ACoA aneurysm, D'Esposito et al[7] noted significant recovery in specific cognitive functions, such as executive functions and retrograde amnesia, during the first 3 months following the lesion. Fukunaga et al[77] also noted significant cognitive recovery within 3 months of surgery, with minimal change in anterograde memory. Richardson,[20] however, found that most cognitive gains occurred within the first 6 weeks post-surgically, with little change noted between the 6-week and 6-month postoperative assessments.

In addition to the length of time required for recovery, the degree and pattern of cognitive recovery have also been shown to differ among individuals. For example, Stenhouse et al[36] examined the long-term cognitive deficits of 27 patients who had sustained rupture and repair of ACoA aneurysm through neuropsychological examination 12–84 months post-surgery. Of the patients in their sample, 41% reportedly returned to their premorbid level of functioning, showing no evidence of cognitive impairment. However, other individuals in the sample showed persisting intellectual and memory impairment as compared with a control group. Alexander and Freedman[13] reported that most patients continued to improve for months following ACoA aneurysm, during which time confabulation, denial and confusion cleared. However, these authors also noted that patients who demonstrated significant personality changes, such as apathy, disinhibition, and unpredictable aggression, had a poorer prognosis for outcome, as discussed previously. Personality change significantly influencing outcome has been reported by other investigators as well.[53] Richardson[20] specifically noted that cognitive recovery moves from broad cognitive impairments to few specific cognitive deficits over time.

Very few studies have been performed evaluating cognitive rehabilitation efforts with ACoA patients, especially those with severe impairments. Vilkki[26] reported that one ACoA patient was able to return to part-time work after 'rehabilitation.' Wilson[78] reported three ACoA amnesics who showed 'fairly substantial improvement' after receiving cognitive rehabilitation 5–10 years earlier. Awareness training has also been shown to significantly reduce confabulation[79] and improve awareness of impaired memory.[80]

DeLuca and Locker[55] reported the case of an ACoA amnesic who received intensive cognitive rehabilitation for more than 1 year. This patient was able to return to his premorbid career as a college professor and return to a lifestyle similar to his premorbid one. Examining neuropsychological test data before and after rehabilitation, these authors attributed the significant functional and employment gains noted to significant improvements in executive functioning.

Given the paucity of studies examining the effectiveness of cognitive rehabilitation in ACoA patients, this area is clearly ripe for further investigation. As of yet, little research has focused on the influence of rehabilitation on long-term outcome of ACoA aneurysm surgery. However, despite this paucity of research, studies overall indicate improvements in mortality, morbidity and postoperative functional status following such pathology over the past decade. With continued research in neuroscience and rehabilitation medicine, it is likely that improvements in therapy and intervention will result in significantly more positive outcomes for the majority of these individuals.

Conclusions and future directions

This chapter has outlined the key behavioral and neuropathological features of what has been termed the 'ACoA syndrome'. It is clear, however, that our knowledge has progressed to the point where reference to such a syndrome has little clinical utility and is no longer applicable. There is a wide range of neurobehavioral consequences following ACoA aneurysm rupture, ranging from few to many, mild to moderate, and transient to long-lasting. The physical consequences are rare following ACoA aneurysm, leaving the behavioral signs as the key clinically relevant features. Therefore, an accurate behavioral descriptor of the consequences of ACoA aneurysm, individualized for each patient, is clearly preferred and clinically appropriate.

The consequences of the neurobehavioral changes following ACoA aneurysm can be potentially devastating, significantly altering the lives of the patient, family and friends. While several authors have reported optimistic post-surgical prognoses (e.g. return to work in up to 84% of patients), it should be recognized that significant neuropsychological,

psychological and psychosocial consequences are observed even in those ACoA patients with 'good recovery' or 'no neurological' symptoms. Nevertheless, many patients do indeed return to happy, productive and meaningful lives following successful surgery. We believe that an understanding of the neurobehavioral features following ACoA aneurysm by healthcare professionals can significantly improve the functional outcome in ACoA patients.

Clearly, much research is needed to continue to improve our understanding of the neurobehavioral features following ACoA aneurysm rupture. Little work has been done on rehabilitation methods to improve cognitive and behavioral impairments and optimize employment opportunities. Studies on the effectiveness of cognitive rehabilitation techniques are particularly relevant. For instance, what may prove effective with ACoA amnesics may have little benefit in patients with other cognitive problems (e.g. executive dysfunction) or more mild symptoms. In addition, relative to cognitive problems, much less research has been conducted on the personality changes which have proven to be particularly devastating for long-term prognosis. Because the problem is primarily in *changes* in personality, existing instruments designed to measure personality constructs are of little clinical utility. Improved methods to assess personality change are needed, as well as improved rehabilitation strategies to aid not only the patient, but also family, friends, employers, employees and all other significant people in the patient's life. Lastly, improved technology such as functional neuroimaging can significantly improve our understanding of the neuropathological mechanisms responsible for the behavioral symptoms following ACoA aneurysms.

Working with ACoA patients can also be particularly fruitful in more theoretically oriented cognitive neuroscience research. For instance, contrasting basal forebrain amnesics with mesial–temporal and diencephalic amnesics holds the promise of significantly improving our understanding of the neural mechanisms involved in declarative and non-declarative memory systems in the brain.

While research over the last 40 years has been very productive in our understanding of brain-behavioral mechanisms following ACoA aneurysm, the next 10 years hold the promise of being even more exciting and fruitful.

References

1. Hutter BO, Gilsbach JM. Cognitive deficits after rupture and early repair of anterior communicating artery aneurysms. *Acta Neurochir (Wien)* (1992) **116(1):** 6–13.

2. DeLuca J. Cognitive dysfunction after aneurysm of the anterior communicating artery. *J Clin Exp Neuropsychol* (1992) **14(6):** 924–34.

3. Gade A. Amnesia after operations on aneurysms of the anterior communicating artery. *Surg Neurol* (1982) **18(1):** 46–9.

4. Bornstein RA, Weir BK, Petruk KC, Disney LB. Neuropsychological function in patients after subarachnoid hemorrhage. *Neurosurgery* (1987) **21(5):** 651–4.

5. DeLuca J, Diamond BJ. Aneurysm of the anterior communicating artery: a review of neuroanatomical and neuropsychological sequelae. *J Clin Exp Neuropsychol* (1995) **17(1):** 100–21.

6. Bottger S, Prosiegel M, Steiger HJ, Yassouridis A. Neurobehavioural disturbances, rehabilitation outcome, and lesion site in patients after rupture and repair of anterior communicating artery aneurysm. *J Neurol Neurosurg Psychiatry* (1998) **65(1):** 93–102.

7. D'Esposito M, Alexander MP, Fischer R et al. Recovery of memory and executive function following anterior communicating artery aneurysm rupture. *J Int Neuropsychol Soc* (1996) **2(6):** 565–70.

8. Ogden JA, Mee EW, Henning M. A prospective study of impairment of cognition and memory and recovery after subarachnoid hemorrhage. *Neurosurgery* (1993) **33(4):** 572–87.

9. Tidswell P, Dias PS, Sagar HJ et al. Cognitive outcome after aneurysm rupture: relationship to aneurysm site and perioperative complications. *Neurology* (1995) **45(5):** 875–82.

10. McCormick WF. Pathology and pathogenesis of intracranial saccular aneurysms. *Semin Neurol* (1984) **4(3):** 291–303.

11. Rinkel G, Djibuti M, Algra A, van Gijn J. Prevalence and risk of rupture of intracranial aneurysms: a systematic review. *Stroke* (1998) **29:** 251–6.

12. Adams HP, Biller J. Hemorrhagic intracranial vascular disease. *Clin Neurol* (1992) **2:** 1–64.

13. Alexander MP, Freedman M. Amnesia after anterior communicating artery aneurysm rupture. *Neurology* (1984) **34(6):** 752–7.

14. Tatu L, Moulin T, Bogousslavsky J, Duvernoy H. Arterial territories of the human brain: cerebral hemispheres. *Neurology* (1998) **50(6):** 1699–708.

15. Haley EC Jr, Kassell NF, Torner JC. The International Cooperative Study on the Timing of Aneurysm Surgery. The North American experience. *Stroke* (1992) **23(2):** 205–14.

16. Takaku A, Tanaka S, Mori T, Suzuki J. Postoperative complications in 1000 cases of intracranial aneurysms. *Surg Neurol* (1979) **12(2):** 137–44.

17. Hutter BO, Gilsbach JM. Early neuropsychological sequelae of aneurysm surgery and subarachnoid hemorrhage. *Acta Neurochir (Wien)* (1996) **138(12):** 1370–9.

18. Artiola i Fortuny L, Prieto-Valiente L. Long-term prognosis in surgically treated intracranial aneurysms. Part 1: Mortality. *J Neurosurg* (1981) **54(1):** 26–34.

19. Kassell NF, Torner JC, Haley EC Jr et al. The International Cooperative Study on the Timing of Aneurysm Surgery. Part 1: Overall management results. *J Neurosurg* (1990) **73(1):** 18–36.

20. Richardson JT. Cognitive performance following rupture and repair of intracranial aneurysm. *Acta Neurol Scand* (1991) **83(2):** 110–22.

21. Lindqvist G, Norlen G. Korsakoff's syndrome after operation on ruptured aneurysm of the anterior communicating artery. *Acta Psychiatr Scand* (1966) **42(1):** 24–34.

22. Talland GA, Sweet WH, Ballantine HT Jr. Amnesic syndrome with anterior communicating artery

aneurysm. *J Nerv Ment Dis* (1967) **145(3):** 179–92.

23. Luria AR, Konovalov AN, Podgornaja AY. *Memory Disturbances in Anterior Communicating Artery Aneurysms* (Moscow: Moscow University Press, 1970).

24. Crowell RM, Morawetz RB. The anterior communicating artery has significant branches. *Stroke* (1977) **8(2):** 272–3.

25. Volpe BT, Hirst W. Amnesia following the rupture and repair of an anterior communicating artery aneurysm. *J Neurol Neurosurg Psychiatry* (1983) **46(8):** 704–9.

26. Vilkki J. Amnesic syndromes after surgery of anterior communicating artery aneurysms. *Cortex* (1985) **21(3):** 431–44.

27. Damasio AR, Graff-Radford NR, Eslinger PJ et al. Amnesia following basal forebrain lesions. *Arch Neurol* (1985) **42(3):** 263–71.

28. Phillips S, Sangalang V, Sterns G. Basal forebrain infarction. A clinicopathologic correlation. *Arch Neurol* (1987) **44(11):** 1134–8.

29. Parkin AJ, Leng NR, Stanhope N, Smith AP. Memory impairment following ruptured aneurysm of the anterior communicating artery. *Brain Cogn* (1988) **7(2):** 231–43.

30. DeLuca J, Cicerone KD. Cognitive impairments following anterior communicating artery aneurysm. *J Clin Exp Neuropsychol* (1989) **11:** 47.

31. Leng NR, Parkin AJ. Amnesic patients can benefit from instructions to use imagery: evidence against the cognitive mediation hypothesis. *Cortex* (1988) **24(1):** 33–9.

32. Corkin S, Cohen NJ, Sullivan EV et al. Analyses of global memory impairments of different etiologies. *Ann NY Acad Sci* (1985) **444:** 10–40.

33. Laiacona M, De Santis A, Barotto R et al. Neuropsychological follow-up of patients operated for aneurysms of anterior communicating artery. *Cortex* (1989) **25(2):** 261–73.

34. Okawa M, Maeda S, Nukui H, Kawafuchi J. Psychiatric symptoms in ruptured anterior communicating aneurysms: social prognosis. *Acta Psychiatr Scand* (1980) **61(4):** 306–12.

35. Teissier du Cros J, Lhermitte F. Neuropsychological analysis of ruptured saccular aneurysms of the anterior communicating artery after radical therapy (32 cases). *Surg Neurol* (1984) **22(4):** 353–9.

36. Stenhouse LM, Knight RG, Longmore BE, Bishara SN. Long-term cognitive deficits in patients after surgery on aneurysms of the anterior communicating artery. *J Neurol Neurosurg Psychiatry* (1991) **54(10):** 909–14.

37. Tarel V, Pellat J, Naegele B et al. Memory disorders following rupture of anterior communicating artery aneurysm. 22 cases. *Rev Neurol* (1990) **146(12):** 746–51.

38. Irle E, Wowra B, Kunert HJ et al. Memory disturbances following anterior communicating artery rupture. *Ann Neurol* (1992) **31(5):** 473–80.

39. Eslinger PJ, Grattan LM. Frontal lobe and frontal–striatal substrates for different forms of human cognitive flexibility. *Neuropsychologia* (1993) **31(1):** 17–28.

40. Abe K, Inokawa M, Kashiwagi A, Yanagihara T. Amnesia after a discrete basal forebrain lesion. *J Neurol Neurosurg Psychiatry* (1998) **65:** 126–30.

41. Moscovitch M, Melo B. Strategic retrieval and the frontal lobes: evidence from confabulation and amnesia. *Neuropsychologia* (1997) **35(7):** 1017–34.

42. Joseph R. Confabulation and delusional denial: frontal lobe and

lateralized influences. *J Clin Psychol* (1986) **42(3):** 507–20.

43. Stuss DT, Alexander MP, Lieberman A, Levine H. An extraordinary form of confabulation. *Neurology* (1978) **28(11):** 1166–72.

44. Luria AR. *The Working Brain.* (New York: Basic Books, 1973).

45. Luria AR. *Higher Cortical Functions in Man.* (New York: Basic Books, 1980).

46. DeLuca J. Predicting neurobehavioral patterns following anterior communicating artery aneurysm. *Cortex* (1993) **29(4):** 639–47.

47. Morris MK, Bowers D, Chatterjee A, Heilman KM. Amnesia following a discrete basal forebrain lesion. *Brain* (1992) **115(Pt 6):** 1827–47.

48. Squire LR, Shimamura AP, Graf P. Strength and duration of priming effects in normal subjects and amnesic patients. *Neuropsychologia* (1987) **25(1B):** 195–210.

49. Fischer RS, Alexander MP, D'Esposito M, Otto R. Neuropsychological and neuroanatomical correlates of confabulation. *J Clin Exp Neuropsychol* (1995) **17(1):** 20–8.

50. Schnider A, von Daniken C, Gutbrod K. The mechanisms of spontaneous and provoked confabulations. *Brain* (1996) **119:** 1365–75.

51. Johnson MK, O'Connor M, Cantor J. Confabulation, memory deficits, and frontal dysfunction. *Brain Cogn* (1997) **34:** 189–206.

52. Blumer D, Benson DF. *Psychiatric Aspects of Neurological Disease.* (New York: Grune and Stratton, 1975).

53. Steinman SE, Bigler ED. Neuropsychological sequelae of ruptured anterior communicating artery aneurysm. *Int J of Clin Neuropsychol* (1986) **8:** 135–40.

54. Sengupta RP, Chiu JSP, Brierley H. Quality of survival following direct surgery for anterior communicating artery aneurysms. *J Neurosurg* (1975) **43(1):** 58–64.

55. DeLuca J, Locker R. Cognitive rehabilitation following anterior communicating artery aneurysm bleeding: a case report. *Disabil Rehabil* (1996) **18(5):** 265–72.

56. Luria AR. *The Neuropsychology of Memory* (Washington DC: V.H. Winston, 1976).

57. Van der Linden M, Bruyer R, Roland J, Schils JP. Proactive interference in patients with amnesia resulting from anterior communicating artery aneurysm. *J Clin Exp Neuropsychol* (1993) **15(4):** 525–36.

58. Gade A, Mortensen EL. Temporal gradient in the remote memory impairment of amnesic patients with lesions in the basal forebrain. *Neuropsychologia* (1990) **28(9):** 985–1001.

59. Ljunggren B, Sonesson B, Saveland H, Brandt L. Cognitive impairment and adjustment in patients without neurological deficits after aneurysmal SAH and early operation. *J Neurosurg* (1985) **62(5):** 673–9.

60. Sonesson B, Ljunggren B, Saveland H, Brandt L. Cognition and adjustment after late and early operation for ruptured aneurysm. *Neurosurgery* (1987) **21(3):** 279–87.

61. Shoqeirat MA, Mayes A, MacDonald C et al. Performance on tests sensitive to frontal lobe lesions by patients with organic amnesia: Leng & Parkin revisited. *Br J Clin Psychol* (1990) **29(Pt 4):** 401–8.

62. Kapur N, Coughlan AK. Confabulation and frontal lobe dysfunction. *J Neurol Neurosurg Psychiatry* (1980) **43(5):** 461–3.

63. Diamond BJ, DeLuca J, Kelley SM. Memory and executive functions in amnesic and non-amnesic patients with aneurysms of the

anterior communicating artery. *Brain* (1997) **120(Pt 6):** 1015–25.

64. Shallice T, Evans ME. The involvement of the frontal lobes in cognitive estimation. *Cortex* (1978) **14(2):** 294–303.

65. Banks G, Short P, Martinez J et al. The alien hand syndrome. Clinical and postmortem findings. *Arch Neurol* (1989) **46(4):** 456–9.

66. Starkstein SE, Berthier ML, Leiguarda R. Disconnection syndrome in a right-handed patient with right hemispheric speech dominance. *Eur Neurol* (1988) **28(4):** 187–90.

67. Beukelman DR, Flowers CR, Swanson PD. Cerebral disconnection associated with anterior communicating artery aneurysm: implications for evaluation of symptoms. *Arch Phys Med Rehabil* (1980) **61(1):** 18–23.

68. Tanaka Y, Bachman DL, Miyazaki M. Pharmacotherapy for akinesia following anterior communicating artery aneurysm hemorrhage. *Jpn J Med* (1991) **30(6):** 542–4.

69. Maiuri F, Gangemi M, Corriero G, D'Andrea F. Anterior communicating artery aneurysm presenting with sudden paraplegia. *Surg Neurol* (1986) **25(4):** 397–8.

70. Ohno K, Masaoka H, Suzuki R et al. Symptomatic cerebral vasospasm of unusually late onset after aneurysm rupture. *Acta Neurochir (Wien)* (1991) **108(3–4):** 163–6.

71. Hori S, Suzuki J. Early and late results of intracranial direct surgery of anterior communicating artery aneurysms. *J Neurosurg* (1979) **50(4):** 433–40.

72. Fasanaro AM, Valiani R, Russo G et al. Memory performances after anterior communicating artery aneurysm surgery. *Acta Neurologica* (1989) **11:** 272–8.

73. Locksley HB. Natural history of subarachnoid hemorrhage, intracranial aneurysms and arteriovenous malformations. Based on 6368 cases in the cooperative study. *J Neurosurg* (1996) **25(2):** 219–39.

74. Storey PB. Psychiatric sequelae of subarachnoid haemorrhage. *BMJ* (1967) **3(560):** 261–6.

75. Storey PB. Brain damage and personality change after subarachnoid haemorrhage. *Br J Psychiatry* (1970) **117(537):** 129–42.

76. Vilkki J, Holst P, Ohman J et al. Social outcome related to cognitive performance and computed tomographic findings after surgery for a ruptured intracranial aneurysm. *Neurosurgery* (1990) **26(4):** 579–84.

77. Fukunaga A, Uchida K, Hashimoto J, Kawase T. Neuropsychological evaluation and cerebral blood flow study of 30 patients with unruptured cerebral aneurysms before and after surgery. *Surg Neurol* (1999) **51(2):** 132–8.

78. Wilson BW. Long-term prognosis of patients with severe memory disorders. *Neuropsychol Rehabil* (1991) **1:** 117–34.

79. DeLuca J. Rehabilitation of confabulation: the issue of unawareness of the deficit. *NeuroRehabilitation* (1992) **2:** 23–30.

80. Schacter DL. Memory, amnesia and frontal lobe dysfunction. *Psychobiology* (1987) **15:** 21–36.

3
The neuropsychological consequences of temporal lobe lesions

Ingrid S Johnsrude

Summary

The temporal lobe is structurally and functionally the most diverse of the human brain, and is the most studied from a neuropsychological perspective. Its varied anatomical structures are intimately connected with extratemporal regions that together form systems necessary for auditory, visual and olfactory perception, memory, language, and emotional processing. This chapter is an attempt to synthesize the results of much of the research, conducted over the last 50 years, on the consequences of temporal lobe lesions. Memory defects constitute the best known and most intensively studied symptom of temporal lobe damage, and the phenomenology of temporal lobe memory syndromes will be discussed. The temporal lobe also contains primary auditory and olfactory cortices, and damage to these areas can result in auditory and olfactory perceptual and processing deficits. The amygdala, structurally and hodologically one of the most complex regions of the entire brain, is also located in the temporal lobe, and the most obvious effects of amygdalar damage will be presented. Visual perceptual deficits can result from damage to geniculostriate afferents in the posterior temporal lobe, or to the higher-order visual processing stream that courses anteriorly along the temporal lobe from the occipital cortex. Language deficits constitute another well-known result of temporal lobe cortical lesions and are often seen in clinical syndromes involving temporal lobe degeneration, such as semantic dementia. An understanding of the consequences of temporal lobe damage requires both knowledge of underlying anatomy and respect for the degree to which cortical developmental plasticity can compensate for early damage.

Introduction

The temporal lobes of the human brain encompass a wide variety of anatomical areas that subserve a host of different functions. Primary auditory and olfactory regions are found in this lobe, as are structures critical for long-term memory, language and emotional behavior. This functional heterogeneity is reflected in the great variety of neuropsychological deficits that are observed after damage, either unilateral or bilateral, to this region.

The temporal lobe lies below the Sylvian fissure in both hemispheres, and has traditionally been defined using gross morphological criteria.[1,2] Although these vary somewhat depending on the source consulted, the approximate extent of the temporal lobe is shown in Figure 3.1. It com-

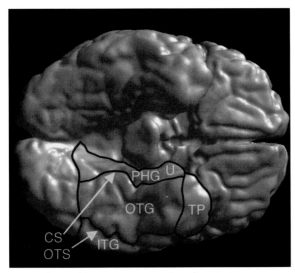

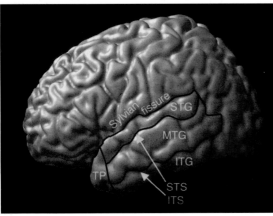

Figure 3.1

The temporal lobe. The posterior border of the temporal lobe is ambiguous, but is roughly determined on the lateral surface by drawing an imaginary line between the preoccipital notch and the parieto-occipital sulcus, and then approximately bisecting this with another line extending from the point at which the Sylvian fissure begins to curve dorsally. This imaginary boundary is roughly coextensive with the dorsal and posterior border of Brodmann area 22, on the superior temporal gyrus, and Brodmann area 37. On the inferior surface, the posterior extent is defined by an imaginary line running from the preoccipital notch to the anterior termination of the calcarine sulcus. CS, collateral sulcus; ITG, inferior temporal gyrus; ITS, inferior temporal sulcus; MTG, middle temporal gyrus; OTG, occipitotemporal gyrus; OTS, occipitotemporal sulcus; PHG, parahippocampal gyrus; STG, superior temporal gyrus; STS, superior temporal sulcus; TP, temporal pole; U: uncus.

prises not only the neocortex of the lateral and basolateral surfaces, but also the phylogenetically older cortex (archicortex and paleocortex) of the medial surface. This includes the parahippocampal gyrus (PHG) and its medial protrusion (the uncus), the hippocampal formation (HC), and the amygdaloid nuclear complex (ANC). The temporal lobe is intimately connected with extratemporal regions such as the orbitofrontal cortex, the striatum and basal forebrain, and parietal and occipital cortex, so examining the effects of temporal lobe damage 'in isolation' is necessarily artificial. In general, however, only disorders that are thought to be consequent upon damage to a critical temporal area will be discussed: those resulting from disconnection of critical extratemporal areas will not.

Damage to the temporal lobes can occur in a variety of ways and at any age. Although etiology and age at onset are important determinants of the precise constellation of deficits exhibited by a particular patient, and this is an important clinical issue, I will restrict the discussion to more general effects of damage. Furthermore, although the consequences of naturally occurring damage, such as that resulting from perinatal trauma, developmental abnormalities, tumors, stroke and dementia will be mentioned, I will focus on deficits observed in patients with surgical excisions whenever possible. Anterior temporal lobe resection is an effective treatment for seizures of temporal lobe origin that are resistant to drug therapy: it has been demonstrated to produce a marked reduction in seizure frequency or even complete abolition of seizures.[3] Since these excisions are discrete and focal, involving temporal lobe structures in one hemisphere only, such patients can provide valuable information concerning functional specialization within the temporal lobes. The resection in such patients typically includes the amygdala and surrounding cortex, a variable amount of the hippocampus and PHG, and a variable amount of anterior temporal neocortex (Figure 3.2). Some normal, as well as abnormal, tissue is usually removed. These resections typically do not extend posterior to the level of the central gyrus on the lateral surface of the temporal lobe, and so do not generally encroach upon primary or immediately adjacent secondary auditory cortex or the posterior speech zone of the dominant hemisphere (Wernicke's area). The most striking feature of these patients, providing that the epileptogenic lesion is confined to the operated side, is how cognitively intact they are. No lasting impairment in general intelligence is evident after temporal lobe excision,[4] and patients are generally able to carry on a normal and productive life postoperatively. Nevertheless, specific, often subtle, cognitive impairments can be detected against this background of preserved intellectual function. Furthermore, the pattern of deficits in any patient is dependent upon the side and extent of the excision, reflecting the specialization of the two hemispheres and of discrete anatomical structures within them.

Clinical manifestations of temporal lobe damage can include defects of long-term memory, disturbances in auditory and visual perception,

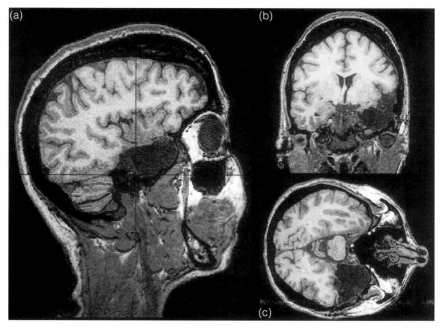

Figure 3.2

T1-weighted MR scan of a patient treated for epilepsy with anterior temporal lobe resection (right hemisphere): (a) sagittal, (b) coronal and (c) axial views. Heschl's gyri are intact, but the resection includes a considerable portion of hippocampus and parahippocampal gyrus.

disorders of the sense of smell, alterations in affective and motivated behaviors, and deficits in linguistic perception and production. In patients who are left-hemisphere dominant for language, left temporal lobe resection is generally associated with verbal deficits,[4–10] whereas right-sided lesions usually impair processing of and memory for material that is not readily associated with verbal labels.[10–15] Hemispheric specialization for stimuli that fall outside of this verbal/visual–spatial dichotomy is still being explored.

A model that represents these processes in a more interactive way has replaced the traditional distinction drawn between perception and processing on the one hand, and learning and memory on the other. For example, recent neuroimaging studies indicate that memory encoding crucially involves cortices previously regarded as involved in perception alone.[16] In the following sections, the phenomenology of cognitive impairment after temporal lobe damage will be divided into functional categories for convenience, but the reader should keep in mind that the boundaries between different categories are often blurred.

Memory

The importance of temporal regions, particularly the medial structures, to aspects of memory was made clear in the 1950s. Earlier studies suggested that damage to the hippocampal region (including the hippocampus and PHG) in humans could produce memory defects,[17] but it was the research of Milner and her colleagues on several patients with bilateral medial temporal lobe damage that conclusively demonstrated the importance of this region.[18,19]

The most well-known and intensively studied of these patients is HM, a 29-year-old mechanic who suffered from severely debilitating seizures that were uncontrolled by medication. His surgeon, Scoville, carried out a radical bilateral resection of the medial temporal lobe region in 1953. This was a last resort, and was successful in controlling his seizures. However, HM was left with a profound anterograde amnesia that persists to this day: he is almost completely unable to retain anything of events that happened since his operation. His moment-to-moment experience is, in his own words, 'as though I am just waking up from a dream'.[18] Any form of distraction appears to obliterate his memory of what had happened seconds before. Despite this catastrophic memory impairment, HM demonstrates remarkably intact learning on tasks that do not require conscious recollection of facts or events for their successful performance. The kinds of tasks HM *can* perform emphasize skill acquisition and perceptual learning. For example, several years after his operation HM was tested on a mirror-drawing task, in which visual feedback is given only via a mirror reflection. Normal subjects learn gradually to trace a complex outline accurately: they show an incremental improvement of performance over many trials. HM also showed a normal learning curve on this task, and, like that of normal subjects, his learning carried over from day to day. In sharp contrast, he did not recall ever performing the task before: this was learning without any sense of familiarity.[18]

HM's preserved learning abilities were an important early demonstration that memory relies on multiple anatomically distinct and process-specific systems in the brain. Since that time, a detailed and extensive body of literature has amassed on the role of the medial temporal lobe in memory. This literature, on both amnesic patients and animal models, has confirmed a critical role for medial temporal lobe structures in aspects of memory, particularly memory for consciously accessible information such as facts and events.[20] Nevertheless, this is a controversial area: the precise characteristics of medial temporal lobe-dependent memory,[21–23] and the cognitive processes subserved by the various structures within this heterogeneous region,[24–26] remain topics of involved debate.

In contrast to the catastrophic memory impairments observed after bilateral medial temporal lobe damage, unilateral temporal lobe resection generally results in only mild memory impairments that are material-specific depending on the side of excision. Damage to the hemisphere dominant for language selectively impairs learning and retention of verbal material such as single words and short prose passages. This deficit affects both recall and recognition, and does not depend on whether the material to be learned is heard or read.[4,9,27,28] Patients with such lesions have trouble with the initial learning of verbal paired associates,[4,9,27] word lists[5,7] and definitions of unfamiliar words,[9] and their retention of this material over a delay is also poor.[4,9] The impoverished recall of short prose passages, four or five sentences in length, is the most conspicuous deficit exhibited by such patients. Their recall of these passages is unusually scanty immediately after presentation,[4,6] with further loss evident after a delay.[4] Thus, both encoding and consolidation mechanisms appear to be impaired.

In order to clarify the cognitive deficits underlying this verbal memory impairment, Frisk and Milner[6] examined the ability of patients with temporal lobe excisions to learn and retain a short prose passage. The passage was read aloud repeatedly until participants were able to correctly answer a set of questions on its content. Compared to normal subjects, patients with left temporal lobe resections required more trials to criterion, indicating a slower rate of acquisition. This effect did not depend on the extent of hippocampal excision. When tested for retention after a 20-min delay, however, only patients with left temporal lobe resections that included a large portion of the hippocampus were impaired. This suggests that the hippocampus and/or adjacent structures are important for the consolidation and long-term maintenance of learned verbal material, whereas both neocortical and medial structures are involved in the initial encoding of such material.

Rausch[29] analyzed the types of recognition error made by patients with left temporal lobectomies on a word-list learning test. She found that patients falsely recognized significantly more words than normal subjects did, and, furthermore, these errors only occurred for foils that bore some relationship (semantic or acoustic) to a target word, particularly for foils that represented a category name for a target item (e.g. toy, given the target doll). This indicates that forgetting is not an all-or-nothing phenomenon in patients with left temporal lobe lesions: some identifying characteristics are retained while others are lost.

Right temporal lobe resection is associated with a marked impairment in the recognition and recall of complex patterns that cannot easily be verbally encoded. In the visual modality, this takes the form of a deficient memory for faces, geometric or abstract designs, features of objects, and object location.[12-15,30-33] In the auditory modality, the deficit takes the form of an impairment in memory for tonal patterns, both melodic and rhythmic, and tonal quality (pitch and timbre).[34-38]

In an elegant series of studies, Smith and Milner[32] tested patients on their ability to remember the locations of toy objects within a two-dimensional spatial array. Patients with right temporal lobe lesions were as able as normal subjects to replace the objects in their correct positions immediately after presentation, indicating that they perceived the array accurately. They were, however, significantly impaired after a delay, even when this was as short as 4 min. Rapid forgetting was contingent upon an extensive removal of the medial structures: patients with removals largely sparing the region of the hippocampus were unimpaired. Crane (unpublished data) has recently extended this work, modifying the Smith and Milner procedure to include a trials-to-criterion measure of acquisition. She found that patients with right-sided removals required significantly more trials to learn to replace the objects in their correct positions within the array. Furthermore, the magnitude of this deficit correlated with the extent of hippocampal excision but not with the extent of parahippocampal or entorhinal excision, suggesting that the hippocampus itself is critically involved in object-location memory. This conclusion is given ecological validity by the non-human literature. For example, several neuroethological studies in birds demonstrate a correlation between hippocampal size and behaviors reliant upon object-location memory, such as brood parasitism and food caching.[39]

Patients with right, but not left, temporal lobe resections also have difficulty learning to navigate through a maze with a stylus, regardless of whether feedback is visual or tactile.[10,31] This deficit is clearly sensitive to the degree of excision of medial structures. Patients with large removals of the hippocampus and PHG had particular difficulty, compared to those with small removals, even if these latter patients had large neocortical excisions. Maguire et al[40] found that patients with either left or right temporal lobe removal were impaired on a real-world navigation task. Performance on this task may have relied on verbal as well as spatial strategies, and there may have been undiagnosed contralateral damage in the left temporal lobe group.[28] These factors may explain why patients with left temporal lobe damage were impaired.

Memory for musical items is also impaired after temporal lobe damage, although laterality effects are not as clear-cut as for verbal or visual–spatial material. In an early study, Milner and colleagues (cited in Zatorre[38]) asked subjects to listen to a series of birdsongs, and, in a continuous recognition paradigm, to indicate those that they had heard before. Temporal lobectomy patients were significantly impaired relative to control subjects, but there was no effect of side of removal. Several studies have demonstrated that patients with right temporal lobe lesions are impaired on tasks requiring the comparison of auditory tonal stimuli,[34,36] but since temporal lobe lesions also affect auditory perception (see below), it remains unclear whether this impairment is primarily due to a memory defect, to a perceptual one, or to a mixture of the two.

The left anterior temporal neocortex may play a role in processing and retaining the sounds of recently heard words.[10] Read (unpublished data) required normal participants and those with left or right temporal lobe excisions to generate supraspan word lists according to one of two rules. In one condition, participants were given a synonym and the first letter of the target word, and were thus required to generate the target words on the basis of semantic cues. In the other condition, participants were given a rhyming word and the first letter, and thus generated the target words on the basis of phonological cues. Shortly afterwards, retention of the word lists was tested. Words generated to semantic cues are normally better remembered than those generated to phonological ones,[41] and this was observed in all subject groups. However, Read found that although patients with left temporal lesions recalled as many semantically generated words as control subjects did, their immediate recall of words generated on the basis of rhymes was markedly inferior. This result was obtained for patients in whom the hippocampus had been largely or entirely spared, which may indicate that the neocortex is important for maintaining the 'sound image' of a word. A similar effect was found by Rains and Milner,[42] and further converging evidence comes from two studies of recognition errors committed by temporal lobe patients on tests of memory for single words.[29,42] Rains and Milner[42] found that whereas left temporal lobe patients committed more recognition errors than normal subjects and right temporal lobe patients, a significantly lower percentage of these were phonemic, compared to semantic. A similar finding was obtained by Rausch.[29] If patients with left temporal lobe excisions do not have an 'image' in their minds of what the word sounds like, then they would not be tempted, as normal subjects are, to mistake a phonemically similar foil for the target, and this phenomenon would produce the observed patterns of performance.

A possible right-hemisphere homolog to this verbal auditory memory deficit was noted by Zatorre and Samson.[37] They tested patients with unilateral temporal lobe lesions on a pitch discrimination task, in which the two tones to be compared were presented either in succession or separated by distracting material. Performance by the patient groups was indistinguishable from that of normal controls when the discriminanda were presented one after the other, but interposing six tones between the test stimuli (total inter-stimulus interval of just over 1 s), produced a marked impairment in the right temporal lobe group relative to normal subjects and patients with left temporal lobe excisions. In a recent study, patients with right, but not left, anterior temporal lobe resections that included some auditory cortex were shown to be impaired at reproducing auditory, but not visual, rhythmic patterns.[35] They were able to indicate correctly the order of long and short elements within a sequence, but were unable to mimic the actual durations of the elements. These two studies indicate that auditory short-term memory for non-verbal stimuli (pitch on the one hand, and stimulus duration on the other) can be impaired by right temporal lobe damage.

Subjects with temporal lobe damage often report memory defects, and memory is, by a considerable margin, the most investigated function in such people. However, other impairments, not as apparent in everyday life as a deficient memory, are also evident in patients with temporal lobe damage, and these will now be reviewed.

Olfaction

The part of the PHG anterior to the HC (including the uncus and the peri-amygdaloid area), together with the lateral olfactory stria on the adjoining orbital surface of the frontal lobe, constitute the primary olfactory cortex. It is therefore not surprising to find that patients with anterior temporal lobe damage, even confined to one hemisphere, have olfactory deficits. Although olfactory detection thresholds are generally intact after temporal lobe resection,[43–45] impairments have been noted in the ability to identify familiar odors,[45] and the ability to discriminate and remember initially unfamiliar odors.[46,47] Furthermore, Jones-Gotman and Zatorre[45] have demonstrated that the impairment in odor identification is partially dependent on the side of resection: the deficit is greatest when odors are presented to the nostril ipsilateral to the resection, consistent with the dominant anatomical projections. This deficit in odor identification does not appear to depend on the extent of amygdaloid, hippocampal, parahippocampal or neocortical excision. In other words, damage to the anterior temporal region, perhaps the periamygdaloid area, is sufficient to cause an impairment.

Affect and motivation

The ANC is a highly differentiated gray-matter region located just anterior to the hippocampus, at the tip of the inferior horn of the lateral ventricle. The ANC receives an enormous array of input from multiple, high-order, unimodal sensory cortices and multimodal and limbic association areas, and it projects to numerous subcortical areas, including the hypothalamus, ventral striatum, basal forebrain, and autonomic centers in the midbrain.[48] It is therefore in a good position to influence affective behavior on the basis of external events. Most of what is known about the function of this area comes from studies of rats and non-human primates. Bilateral lesions of this area have long been known to disrupt emotional and social behavior in primates,[49,50] and studies of patients with lesions to the ANC region confirm a role for this area in emotional responsiveness, emotional learning, and the regulation of memory and attention relative to affective stimuli.

The most dramatic consequence of amygdalectomy in monkeys is a lack of emotional reactivity, and reports of previously aggressive human patients being rendered 'placid', 'indifferent' and 'calm' by ANC lesions are consistent with postoperative hypoemotionality.[49] Unlike in monkeys, unilateral lesions in humans appear sufficient to produce an attenuation in emotional responsiveness. Furthermore, the effects of left and right amygdala lesions appear similar,[49] although hemispheric specialization of function within this area has not been investigated in detail.

Lesions of the ANC also seem to disrupt the recognition of the emotional states of others. For example, patients with bilateral lesions of this area have difficulty in identifying facial expressions of emotion, such as fear and anger.[51] A recent study demonstrates that the amygdala's role in the recognition of emotional expression is not limited to the visual modality: a patient with bilateral amygdalar damage is also impaired in the recognition of vocal affect.[52]

The ability to evaluate and remember the motivational significance of items in the environment has obvious survival value. A very large number of studies in animals point to a role for the ANC in the process by which stimuli acquire significance (either positive or negative) through association with rewarding or aversive events. Consistent with the animal literature on fear conditioning, the association of a novel and neutral stimulus with an aversive event, such as a loud noise, is impaired in humans after bilateral amygdala damage,[53] and after unilateral temporal lobe resection that includes the ANC.[54] The ANC is also important for stimulus–reward learning in humans, just as it is in other animals. In a recent study, three abstract monochrome patterns were incidentally presented in the context of a working memory task to neurosurgical patients and normal control subjects.[55] Unknown to the subjects, the patterns were paired with food reward at different contingencies. Subsequently, normal participants preferred the pattern paired with reward on 90% of trials to that paired with reward on 10% of trials, but patients with unilateral temporal lobe resections that included the ANC (15 left, 18 right) did not (Figure 3.3a). Together with the study by LaBar et al,[54] these data suggest that unilateral excision of the amygdaloid region is sufficient to impair the normal associative mechanisms of affective learning.

Considerable evidence from animals also suggests that the ANC is critically involved in a memory-modulating system that regulates the strength of a memory trace based on its importance.[56] Consistent with the animal literature, recent evidence from humans with selective amygdalar damage indicates that the facilitating effects of emotional arousal on conscious memory depend on the ANC.[56,57]

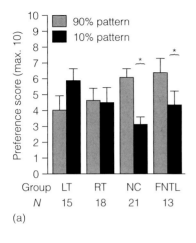

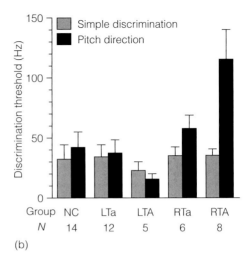

Figure 3.3

(a) Mean preference scores (maximum = 10) and standard errors for the 90% and 10% patterns in patients with left or right temporal lobe damage (LT; RT), normal control participants (NC) and patients with unilateral excisions from frontal cortex (FNTL). Bars show standard error of the mean. LT and RT participants fail to show conditioned preference, unlike subjects in the other two groups.[55] (b) Mean frequency-difference discrimination thresholds (+SE) observed in normal control volunteers (NC), patients with anterior left temporal resection sparing primary auditory cortex (LTa), patients with similar lesions that encroached upon primary auditory cortex (LTA) and analogous groups with right temporal lobe resections (RTa and RTA). Simple discrimination thresholds were not different across the groups, but thresholds in the pitch-direction task were significantly higher in the RTA group than in any of the other groups.[76]

Visual perception

The most obvious visual perceptual impairment resulting from anterior temporal lobe resection is an upper visual field defect resulting from the transection of Meyer's loop, a subset of geniculostriate fibers that course around the lateral ventricle in the temporal lobe. Patients typically present a 'pie in the sky' homonymous defect in the contralateral upper visual field, of which they are not aware.[58] More subtle, higher-order, visual perceptual impairments are also evident, particularly in patients with right temporal lobe excisions. These are both milder and more variable than the memory deficits resulting from such lesions. Deficits are observed on tests requiring the interpretation of complex visual material,[4,12,59–61] particularly when fragmented material needs to be integrated in some way.[59,62]

The first visual deficits to be noted in patients with right temporal lobe lesions were elicited by tasks in which the normal stimulus redundancy was reduced, either by tachistoscopic presentation or by reduction in figural detail.[4,12,13,60] For example, such patients are impaired in identifying overlapping nonsense figures.[12] The visual deficits observed in humans appear analogous to the visual-discrimination deficits produced by bilateral inferotemporal lesions in the monkey[63] and are consistent with the large body of work demonstrating that the inferotemporal cortex is part of an extrastriate visual system.

Auditory perception

The transverse gyri of Heschl are found on the superior temporal plane within the Sylvian fissure. These are sometimes single and sometimes multiple, and primary auditory cortex has been reliably identified as being located on the anterior-most of these gyri when there is more than one.[64] The primary cortex and the surrounding 'belt' of architectonically distinguishable auditory fields receive direct input from the medial geniculate body of the thalamus, and project to a lateral parabelt region.[65] This 'tertiary' area connects with cortex in the superior temporal gyrus and sulcus.

Basic auditory discrimination thresholds are not usually permanently affected by even large bilateral auditory cortex lesions,[66] but a variety of perceptual deficits have been reported following auditory cortical damage. Furthermore, although anterior temporal lobe resection usually spares primary auditory cortex, it generally includes anterior belt and parabelt areas, as well as the association cortex of the anterior temporal lobe. It is therefore not surprising to find auditory perceptual deficits in patients after unilateral temporal lobe resection.

Stroke lesions close to primary auditory regions (either bilaterally, or in the left hemisphere) can produce the condition referred to as 'word deafness' or 'verbal auditory agnosia'.[67] Although such damage never appears to affect speech uniquely, a dominant feature of this disorder is the occurrence of a severe comprehension deficit for spoken words, with relatively intact abilities in other areas of language. In particular, word-deaf patients consistently show disordered perception and discrimination of stimuli containing stop-consonants, while showing relatively intact processing of vowel stimuli. One possible reason for this dissociation relates to the different spectral and temporal characteristics of stop-consonants and vowels. Consistent with the idea that damage to auditory cortex interferes with the ability to resolve acoustic events of a fine temporal grain, patients with such lesions require longer silent durations than normal subjects to detect a gap between two bursts of noise and to perceive two discrete click events instead of a fused single one.[67] Furthermore, Sherwin and Efron[68] found elevated thresholds for performing temporal-order judgments on pairs of 10-ms pure tones in patients who had sustained either right or left temporal lobectomy (sparing primary auditory cortex), when stimulation was to the ear contralateral to the lesion.

Temporal lobe damage, particularly on the right, can impair at least some aspects of pitch processing.[34,37,69] For example, Zatorre[70] found that patients with surgical excisions of right, but not left, auditory cortex are impaired at perceiving the pitch of complex tones when the fundamental is absent, but not when it is present. Similarly, patients with right- but not left-hemisphere vascular lesions are impaired at tasks requiring processing of complex spectral structure.[71,72] Timbre-discrimination tasks, in which discrimination must be based on harmonic structure, are also sensitive to right temporal lobe damage.[34,73,74]

Patients with right superior temporal resections are also impaired at using pitch contour information to discriminate between two short melodies,[34,36,75] although much more severe deficits are observed after bilateral damage.[66] At least some of these deficits probably reflect the auditory memory impairment discussed earlier. Melodies are necessarily extended in time, and elements must be presented one after another. This means that perception and retention over time cannot be dissociated easily. A recent study examined the simplest case of pitch contour perception, namely the determination of the pitch trajectory from one note to the next in a pair.[76] Patients with right anterior temporal lobe excisions that included some auditory cortex were impaired at this up–down discrimination task, relative to other patient groups and normal controls, but they were only impaired when the pitch difference between the two elements was small. Furthermore, these patients behaved like normal subjects on a task requiring same–different judgments which had the same time course as the up–down task and used the same stimuli (Figure 3.3b). The deficit in trajectory discrimination is therefore not likely to result from a memory defect. Instead, damage to the right auditory cortex may cause impairments in the representation of relative pitch, which is necessary for accurate melodic perception.

Language

The investigations by Penfield and colleagues, using electrical stimulation to map function on the exposed cortex of surgical patients, were the first to demonstrate the extent of the neocortical speech zones.[77] They observed that speech arrest could be produced by electrical stimulation in a region that includes the left posterior superior and middle temporal gyri, as well as adjacent parietal cortex: this is a region that had long been implicated in the condition of fluent aphasia.[77] Fluent aphasia is a syndrome in which patients' speech, although articulate, is garbled and almost devoid of meaning, and comprehension is also severely compromised. The deficit pertains to both oral and written language. The aphasic syndromes, including this 'posterior' or 'Wernicke's' aphasia, have been intensively studied, in order to characterize patterns of impairment and, in so doing, clarify the processes of normal language.

Patients who have undergone left temporal lobe resection, sparing this posterior region, also show some linguistic impairment, although not generally frank aphasia.[5,78] Many researchers have noted that patients with such excisions are particularly impaired at oral confrontation naming: when presented with a familiar object, they are less accurate and take longer to produce the name, relative to normal subjects.[5,78] This anomia can be accompanied by other linguistic impairments, such as mild comprehension difficulty or poor word fluency. In recent years, stimulation mapping has revealed eloquent cortex in the anterior temporal lobe of some patients, using the less stringent criterion of speech errors instead of speech arrest.[79,80] These areas are often within the area excised in a standard temporal lobe resection. It has been suggested that if anterior temporal language sites are damaged in surgery, language deficits are likely to result.[81,82] Thus, the deficits that are observed on tasks such as confrontation naming in groups of patients with left temporal lobe excisions may reflect poor performance by a subgroup of patients in whom anterior temporal language areas have been damaged.

A recent series of papers on semantic dementia highlights another possible consequence of temporal lobe abnormality. Semantic dementia is characterized by a progressive deterioration in expressive and receptive vocabulary and factual knowledge, while syntactic and phonological processes are relatively preserved in the early stages of the disorder. Likewise, other cognitive abilities, such as episodic memory, visual–spatial skills, and problem-solving, appear to be unaffected initially.[83] Early-stage semantic dementia has recently been linked to severe atrophy in the anterolateral temporal lobe, particularly the temporal pole and middle and inferior temporal gyri.[83] In a subset of patients, the atrophy is much greater in, and indeed sometimes confined to, the left temporal lobe.[83] Semantic dementia is both anatomically and clinically dissociable from early dementia of the Alzheimer's type, which is generally associated with severe medial–temporal lobe atrophy and pronounced episodic memory impairment. The neuropsychology (location of lesion and cognitive sequelae) of Alzheimer's dementia is consistent with studies of patients with epileptic lesions, such as HM, whereas the neuropsychology of semantic dementia is not: patients with surgical lesions encompassing the areas involved in the pathology of semantic dementia do not generally show catastrophic language impairments. The similarities and differences in the clinical manifestations of damage among these patient populations may underline the importance of considering developmental history when drawing conclusions about functional organization from lesion studies.

Developmental issues

Functional organization can be altered by brain damage, particularly if it occurs before the nervous system is completely mature. Anatomical data suggest that structures within the human temporal lobe mature at different rates, with the older structures (such as the hippocampus) maturing relatively early, around the age of 3 years,[84] whereas neuronal connections within the lateral neocortex are still being established at the age of 11.[85] Brain injury incurred while these systems are still maturing may change neurocognitive development, resulting in altered functional organization. Support for this idea comes from a study in monkeys by Bachevalier and Mishkin.[86] They showed that the dramatic visual–recognition–memory impairment evident in animals with inferotemporal cortical ablations received in adulthood was almost absent when the lesion was received in infancy. The authors concluded that the hippocampal–neocortical interactions subserving this kind of memory must have reorganized in the infant monkeys. This reorganization was specific to neocortical mechanisms: early and late medial temporal lobe ablations produced very similar recognition–memory defects. A recent study of 100 patients with epilepsy undergoing left anterior temporal lobectomy demonstrates a similar finding: namely, that surgery in childhood results in a sparing of cortically mediated cognitive functions, relative to surgery in adulthood.[11] As in the monkey study, cognitive functions reliant upon medial temporal lobe structures were impaired regardless of the age at surgery. In a recent series of papers, Mishkin, Vargha-Khadem and colleagues have shown that the pattern of impairment evident in three patients with bilateral hippocampal damage acquired early is consistent with an anatomical dissociation between episodic and semantic memory.[26] These patients all show a global anterograde amnesia for personal information and events in their lives, but have nevertheless been able to acquire an adequate store of information about the world, including vocabulary and factual knowledge. A possible explanation for this dissociation is that the neural systems underlying semantic learning and memory were either preserved, or were damaged early enough for reorganization to occur. Episodic memory, relying on the early-maturing hippocampus, cannot reorganize and is consequently impaired.

The developmental factor may help to explain, at least in part, the dramatic cognitive differences between patients with semantic dementia, in whom there is quite focal (sometimes even left-lateralized) anterior temporal lobe damage, and epileptic patients, who generally exhibit only subtle language defects after left anterior temporal lobe resection. This difference may result from the different disease histories of the two patient groups: late-onset cortical damage in the case of the semantic dementia patients, and early-onset damage with subsequent altered functional organization in the epileptic patients. The possibility of functional reorganization after neocortical brain damage raises questions about the generalizability of results from studies of patients with childhood lesions, and has implications for the surgical treatment of patients with epilepsy.

Conclusions

I have been able to discuss only briefly the defects observed in cognitive systems after temporal lobe damage. The temporal lobes support a large array of functions, and the left and right hemispheres show differential specialization. The precise syndrome observed after damage is unique to each patient, and reflects the anatomical/functional systems that have been disrupted. However, certain consistent patterns have emerged which make it clear that aspects of language and memory, vision, audition, olfaction and emotional processing rely critically upon temporal lobe structures. This chapter has necessarily ignored the functional imaging literature, which is a valuable adjunct to the traditional lesion approach in studying functional organization within the brain.[87] For each of the conclusions about anatomical specialization that I have drawn in this chapter, at least one, and often several, supporting neuroimaging papers could have been cited, if space had allowed. The new imaging tools are also ideal for investigating brain and cognitive development and plasticity, which are increasingly being recognized as critical factors in determining functional organization.

Acknowledgments

I wish to thank AL Giraud, TD Griffiths, EA Maguire, JB Rowe and KE Watkins for helpful discussions. I am particularly grateful to B Milner for all she has taught me.

References

1. Damasio H. *Human Brain Anatomy in Computerized Images.* (Oxford: Oxford University Press, 1995).

2. Rademacher J, Galaburda AM, Kennedy DN et al. Human cerebral cortex: localization, parcellation, and morphometry with magnetic resonance imaging. *J Cog Neurosci* (1992) **4:** 352–74.

3. Eliashiv SD, Dewar S, Wainwright I et al. Long-term follow-up after temporal lobe resection for lesions associated with chronic seizures. *Neurology* (1997) **48:** 1383–8.

4. Milner BA. Psychological defects produced by temporal lobe excision. In *The brain and human behaviour,* Proceedings of the Association for Research in Nervous and Mental Disease (1958) **36:** 244–57.

5. Bell BD, Davies KG. Anterior temporal lobectomy, hippocampal

sclerosis, and memory: recent neuropsychological findings. *Neuropsychol Rev* (1998) **8:** 25–41.

6. Frisk V, Milner B. The role of the left hippocampal region in the acquisition and retention of story content. *Neuropsychologia* (1990) **28:** 349–59.

7. Helmstaedter C, Elger CE. Cognitive consequences of two-thirds anterior temporal lobectomy on verbal memory in 144 patients: a three-month follow-up study. *Epilepsia* (1996) **37:** 171–80.

8. Hermann BP, Wyler AR, Somes G et al. Declarative memory following anterior temporal lobectomy in humans. *Behav Neurosci* (1994) **108:** 3–10.

9. Meyer V, Yates AJ. Intellectual changes following temporal lobectomy for psychomotor epilepsy: preliminary communication. *J Neurol Neurosurg Psychiatry* (1955) **18:** 44–52.

10. Milner B. Memory and the human brain. In Shafto M. (ed.) *How We Know: Nobel Conference XX* (San Francisco: Harper & Row, 1985) 31–59.

11. Helmstaedter C, Elger CE. Functional plasticity after left anterior temporal lobectomy: reconstitution and compensation of verbal memory functions. *Epilepsia* (1998) **39:** 399–406.

12. Kimura D. Right temporal lobe damage: perception of unfamiliar stimuli after damage. *Arch Neurol* (1963) **8:** 264–71.

13. Milner B. Right temporal lobe contribution to visual perception and visual memory. In Iwai E, Mishkin M (eds) *Vision, Memory, and the Temporal Lobe* (New York: Elsevier Science, 1990): 43–53.

14. Pigott S, Milner B. Memory for different aspects of complex visual scenes after unilateral temporal- or frontal-lobe resection. *Neuropsychologia* (1993) **31:** 1–15.

15. Abrahams S, Morris RG, Polkey CE et al. Hippocampal involvement in spatial and working memory: a structural MRI analysis of patients with unilateral mesial temporal lobe sclerosis. *Brain Cogn* (1999) **41:** 39–65.

16. Köhler S, McIntosh AR, Moscovitch M, Winocur G. Functional interactions between the medial temporal lobes and posterior neocortex related to episodic memory retrieval. *Cerebral Cortex* (1998) **8:** 451–61.

17. Glees P, Griffith HB. Bilateral destruction of the hippocampus (Cornu Ammonis) in a case of dementia. *Psychiatrie Neurol* (1952) **123:** 193–204.

18. Milner B. Amnesia following operation on the temporal lobes. In Whitty CWM, Zangwill OL (eds), *Amnesia* (London: Butterworths, 1966): 109–33.

19. Rempel-Clower NL, Zola SM, Squire LR, Amaral DG. Three cases of enduring memory impairment after bilateral damage limited to the hippocampal formation. *J Neurosci* (1996) **16:** 5233–5.

20. Milner B, Squire LR, Kandel ER. Cognitive neuroscience and the study of memory. *Neuron* (1998) **20:** 445–68.

21. Eichenbaum H, Dudchenko P, Wood E et al. The hippocampus, memory, and place cells: is it spatial memory or a memory space? *Neuron* (1999) **23:** 209–26.

22. Squire LR, Zola SM. Episodic memory, semantic memory, and amnesia. *Hippocampus* (1998) **8:** 205–11.

23. Tulving E, Markowitsch H. Episodic and declarative memory: role of the hippocampus. *Hippocampus* (1998) **8:** 198–204.

24. Aggleton JP, Brown MW. Episodic memory, amnesia and the hippocampal–anterior thalamic axis.

Behav Brain Sci (1999) **22:** 425–500.

25. Miller LA, Lai R, Munoz DG. Contributions of the entorhinal cortex, amygdala and hippocampus to human memory. *Neuropsychologia* (1998) **36:** 1247–56.

26. Vargha-Khadem F, Gadian DG, Watkins KE et al. Differential effects of early hippocampal pathology on episodic and semantic memory. *Science* (1997) **277:** 376–80.

27. Blakemore CB, Falconer MA. Long-term effects of anterior temporal lobectomy on certain cognitive functions. *J Neurol Neurosurg Psychiatry* (1967) **30:** 364–7.

28. Incisa della Rocchetta A, Gadian DG, Connelly A et al. Verbal memory impairment after right temporal lobe surgery: role of contralateral damage as revealed by 1H magnetic resonance spectroscopy and T2 relaxometry. *Neurology* (1995) **45:** 797–802.

29. Rausch R. Lateralization of temporal lobe dysfunction and verbal encoding. *Brain Lang* (1981) **12:** 92–100.

30. Jones-Gotman M. Right hippocampal excision impairs learning and recall of a list of abstract designs. *Neuropsychologia* (1986) **24:** 659–70.

31. Corkin S. Tactually-guided maze learning in man: effects of unilateral cortical excisions and bilateral hippocampal lesions. *Neuropsychologia* (1965) **3:** 339–51.

32. Smith ML, Milner B. Right hippocampal impairment in the recall of spatial location: encoding deficit or rapid forgetting? *Neuropsychologia* (1989) **27:** 71–81.

33. Warrington EK, James M. An experimental investigation of facial recognition in patients with unilateral cerebral lesions. *Cortex* (1967) **3:** 317–26.

34. Milner BA. Laterality effects in audition. In Mountcastle VB (ed.) *Interhemispheric Relations and Cerebral Dominance.* (Baltimore: Johns Hopkins Press, 1962): 177–98.

35. Penhune VB, Zatorre RJ, Feindel W. The role of auditory cortex in retention of rhythmic patterns in patients with temporal lobe removals including Heschl's gyrus. *Neuropsychologia* (1999) **37:** 315–31.

36. Samson S, Zatorre RJ. Melodic and harmonic discrimination following unilateral cerebral excision. *Brain Cogn* (1988) **7:** 348–60.

37. Zatorre RJ, Samson S. Role of the right temporal neocortex in retention of pitch in auditory short-term memory. *Brain* (1991) **114:** 2403–17.

38. Zatorre RJ. Discrimination and recognition of tonal melodies after unilateral cerebral excisions. *Neuropsychologia* (1985) **23:** 31–41.

39. Lee DW, Miyasato LE, Clayton NS. Neurobiological bases of spatial learning in the natural environment: neurogenesis and growth in the avian and mammalian hippocampus. *Neuroreport* (1998) **9:** R15–27.

40. Maguire EA, Burke T, Phillips J, Staunton H. Topographical disorientation following unilateral temporal lobe lesions in humans. *Neuropsychologia* (1996) **34:** 993–1001.

41. Craik FI, Lockhart RS. Levels of processing: a framework for memory research. *J Verbal Learning Verbal Behav* (1972) **11:** 671–84.

42. Rains GD, Milner B. Verbal recall and recognition as a function of depth of encoding in patients with unilateral temporal lobectomy. *Neuropsychologia* (1994) **32:** 1243–56.

43. Jones-Gotman M, Zatorre RJ.

Olfactory identification deficit in patients with focal cerebral excision. *Neuropsychologia* (1988) **26:** 387–400.

44. Jones-Gotman M, Zatorre RJ. Odor recognition memory in humans: role of right temporal and orbitofrontal regions. *Brain Cogn* (1993) **22:** 182–98.

45. Jones-Gotman M, Zatorre RJ, Cendes F et al. Contribution of medial versus lateral temporal lobe structures to human odour identification. *Brain* (1997) **120:** 1845–56.

46. Eskenazi B, Cain WS, Novelly RA, Mattson R. Odor perception in temporal lobe epilepsy patients with and without temporal lobectomy. *Neuropsychologia* (1986) **24:** 553–62.

47. Rausch R, Serafetinides EA, Crandall PH, Olfactory memory in patients with anterior temporal lobectomy. *Cortex* (1977) **13:** 445–52.

48. Aggleton JP. The contribution of the amygdala to normal and abnormal emotional states. *TINS* (1993) **16:** 328–33.

49. Aggleton JP. *The Amygdala: Neurobiological Aspects of Emotion, Memory, and Mental Dysfunction.* (Chichester: Wiley-Liss, 1992).

50. Gallagher M, Chiba AA. The amygdala and emotion. *Curr Opin Neurobiol* (1996) **6:** 221–7.

51. Calder AJ, Young AW, Rowland D et al. Facial emotion recognition after bilateral amygdala damage: differentially severe impairment of fear. *Cognitive Neuropsychol* (1996) **13:** 699–745.

52. Scott SK, Young AW, Calder AJ et al. Impaired auditory recognition of fear and anger following bilateral amygdala lesions. *Nature* (1997) **385:** 254–7.

53. Bechara A, Tranel D, Damasio H et al. Double dissociation of conditioning and declarative knowledge relative to the amygdala and hippocampus in humans. *Science* (1995) **269:** 1115–18.

54. LaBar KS, LeDoux JE, Spencer DO, Phelps EA. Impaired fear conditioning following unilateral temporal lobectomy in humans. *J Neurosci* (1995) **15:** 6846–55.

55. Johnsrude IS, Owen AM, White NM et al. Impaired preference conditioning after anterior temporal lobe resection in humans. *J Neurosci* (2000) **20:** 2649–56.

56. Cahill L, McGaugh JL. Mechanisms of emotional arousal and lasting declarative memory. *Trends Neurosci* (1998) **21:** 294–9.

57. Adolphs R, Cahill L, Schul R, Babinsky R. Impaired declarative memory for emotional material following bilateral amygdala damage in humans. *Learn Memory* (1997) **4:** 291–300.

58. Hughes TS, Abou-Khalil B, Lavin PJ et al. Visual field defects after temporal lobe resection: a prospective quantitative analysis. *Neurology* (1999) **13:** 167–72.

59. Doyon J, Milner B. Right temporal lobe contribution to global visual processing. *Neuropsychologia* (1991) **29:** 343–60.

60. Lansdell H. Effect of extent of temporal lobe ablations on two lateralized deficits. *Physiology Behav* (1968) **3:** 271–3.

61. Mendola JD, Rizzo JF, Cosgrove GR et al. Visual discrimination after anterior temporal lobectomy in humans. *Neurology* (1999) **52:** 1028–37.

62. Newcombe F, Ratcliff G, Damasio H. Dissociable visual and spatial impairments following right posterior cerebral lesions: clinical, neuropsychological and anatomical evidence. *Neuropsychologia* (1987) **25:** 149–61.

63. Iwai E, Mishkin M. Two visual foci in the temporal lobe of monkeys. In Yochi N, Buchwald NA (eds)

Neurophysiological Basis of Learning and Behavior (Osaka: Osaka University Press, 1968): 7–11.

64. Rademacher J, Werner C, Morosan P et al. Localization and variability of cytoarchitectonic areas in the human superior temporal cortex. *NeuroImage* (1996) **3:** S456.

65. Kaas JH, Hackett TA. Subdivisions of auditory cortex and levels of processing in primates. *Audiol Neuro Otol* (1998) **3:** 73–85.

66. Peretz I, Kolinsky R, Tramo M et al. Functional dissociations following bilateral lesions of auditory cortex. *Brain* (1994) **117:** 1283–301.

67. Phillips DP, Farmer ME. Acquired word deafness, and the temporal grain of sound representation in the primary auditory cortex. *Behav Brain Res* (1990) **40:** 85–94.

68. Sherwin I, Efron R. Temporal ordering deficits following anterior temporal lobectomy. *Brain Lang* (1980) **11:** 195–203.

69. Peretz I. Processing of local and global musical information by unilateral brain-damaged patients. *Brain* (1990) **113:** 1185–205.

70. Zatorre RJ. Pitch perception of complex tones and human temporal lobe function. *J Acoust Soc Am* (1988) **84:** 566–72.

71. Robin DA, Tranel D, Damasio H. Auditory perception of temporal and spectral events in patients with focal left and right cerebral lesions. *Brain Lang* (1990) **39:** 539–55.

72. Sidtis JJ, Volpe BT. Selective loss of complex-pitch or speech discrimination after unilateral lesion. *Brain Lang* (1988) **34:** 235–45.

73. Paquette C, Peretz I. Role of familiarity in auditory discrimination of musical instruments: a laterality study. *Cortex* (1997) **33:** 689–96.

74. Samson S, Zatorre RJ. Contribution of the right temporal lobe to musical timbre discrimination. *Neuropsychologia* (1994) **32:** 231–40.

75. Liégeois-Chauvel C, Peretz I, Babaï M et al. Contribution of different cortical areas in the temporal lobes to music processing. *Brain* (1998) **121:** 1853–67.

76. Johnsrude IS, Penhune VB, Zatorre RJ. Functional specificity in right human auditory cortex for perceiving pitch direction. *Brain* (2000) **123:** 155–63.

77. Penfield W, Roberts L. *Speech and Brain Mechanisms* (Princeton: Princeton University Press, 1959).

78. Saykin AJ, Stafiniak P, Robinson LJ et al. Language before and after temporal lobectomy: specificity of acute changes and relation to early risk factors. *Epilepsia* (1995) **36:** 1071–7.

79. Devinsky O, Perrine K, Llinas R et al. Anterior temporal language areas in patients with early onset of temporal lobe epilepsy. *Ann Neurol* (1993) **34:** 727–32.

80. Haglund MM, Berger MS, Shamseldin M et al. Cortical localization of temporal lobe language sites in patients with gliomas. *Neurosurgery* (1994) **34:** 567–76.

81. Davies KG, Maxwell RE, Jennum P et al. Language function following subdural grid-directed temporal lobectomy. *Acta Neurol Scand* (1994) **90:** 201–6.

82. Krauss GL, Fisher R, Plate C et al. Cognitive effects of resecting basal temporal language areas. *Epilepsia* (1996) **37:** 476–83.

83. Mummery CJ, Patterson K, Wise RJS et al. Disrupted temporal lobe connections in semantic dementia. *Brain* (1999) **122:** 61–73.

84. Diamond A. Rate of maturation of the hippocampus and the developmental progression of children's performance on the

delayed non-matching to sample and visual paired comparison tasks. *Ann NY Acad Sci* (1990) **608:** 394–433.

85. Sininger YS, Doyle KJ, Moore JK. The case for early identification of hearing loss in children. Auditory system development, experimental auditory deprivation, and development of speech perception and hearing. *Pediatr Clin North Am* (1999) **46:** 1–14.

86. Bachevalier J, Mishkin M. Effects of selective neonatal temporal lobe lesions on visual recognition memory in rhesus monkeys. *J Neurosci* (1994) **14:** 2128–39.

87. Frackowiak RSJ, Friston KJ, Frith CD et al. *Human Brain Function* (London: Academic Press, 1997).

4
Parietal lobe syndromes

Masud Husain

Anatomy

Damage to the parietal lobe may lead to a number of impairments of perception and motor control. It is possible to discuss all of these without any reference to the anatomy of the parietal lobe. However, general principles of parietal structure and connectivity shed important light on its function. For this reason, this chapter begins with a brief anatomical introduction.

On its lateral surface, the parietal lobe consists of an anterior and a posterior portion. The anterior parietal lobe is bounded by the central sulcus anteriorly and the postcentral sulcus posteriorly. The posterior parietal lobe lies between the postcentral sulcus and the occipital and temporal lobes. It is further subdivided into two segments (Figure 4.1a) by the intraparietal sulcus (IPS): above the IPS lies the superior parietal lobule (SPL) and below it lies the inferior parietal lobule (IPL). The IPL consists of the supramarginal and angular gyrus. The portion of the lateral parietal cortex that lies deep to the temporal lobe within the insula is referred to as the parietal operculum and posterior insula. On its medial surface (Figure 4.1b), the parietal lobe consists of a large cortical area, including the precuneus and part of the cingulate gyrus.

Our understanding of the connectivity of parietal cortex (its inputs and outputs) is based on studies in monkeys.[1] However, there is considerable debate about whether the parietal lobes in human and monkey are homologous structures. The IPL is proportionately much larger in humans, and it has been argued that it may have a completely different structure and function to the IPL in monkey. Conversely, there is much evidence also to suggest that the region may be homologous across the two species. This long-standing debate is unlikely to be settled in the near future, but for the purposes of this chapter it is not important to have detailed knowledge of parietal connectivity in the monkey. However, a general overview is useful if one is to attempt to place the disorders following parietal damage into a coherent framework.

The main projections to the monkey parietal cortex come from areas involved in sensory processing (e.g. visual, somatosensory and

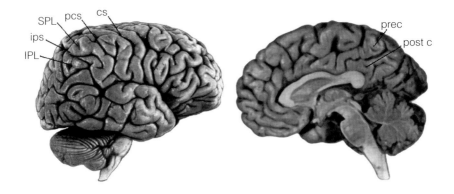

Figure 4.1

Lateral and medial views of the brain. (a) Lateral view showing the central sulcus (cs) and postcentral sulcus (pcs) between which lies the anterior parietal lobe. The posterior parietal lobe consists of the superior parietal lobule (SPL) and inferior parietal loblue (IPL) which is divided by the intraparietal sulcus (ips). (b) Medial view showing the precuneus (prec) and posterior cingulate (post c) gyrus.

vestibular), while the major outputs are to premotor regions (frontal eye fields and superior colliculus, which control saccadic eye movements, and premotor cortex, which controls reaching and grasping). In turn, these premotor areas project back to parietal cortex, which also projects back to brain regions involved in sensory processing. Thus, the parietal lobe is an important location for the convergence of information from different sensory modalities, as well as for the association of sensory and motor signals.[1]

In the monkey, the anterior parietal lobe is the site of primary somatosensory processing. This region projects heavily to the SPL, whereas visual signals project from occipital cortex predominantly to the IPL. The visual projection to the IPL in the monkey is considered to be part of a 'dorsal stream' of pathways involved in spatial perception[2] or visual control of movement.[3] The IPS appears to be an extremely important site for the convergence of information from the SPL and IPL, as well as from premotor centers. The medial parietal cortex is not well understood but it appears to receive both visual and somatosensory inputs and also projects forward to premotor cortex.

From these anatomical considerations, one would expect that damage to the parietal lobe may lead to disorders of sensation as well as sensorimotor control, ranging from simple impairments of perception to complex disorders of eye and hand control. Although it would be useful to classify syndromes according to the precise location of damage, our knowledge of regional specialization within human parietal cortex is far from complete. Detailed functional–pathological correlates of patients with discrete lesions are few, and much of the non-invasive data regarding localization in the modern era has come from relatively low-resolution computed tomography (CT) imaging. Structural and functional magnetic resonance imaging (MRI) studies may contribute to improve this situation, but it is not yet possible to give detailed accounts of all human parietal disorders according to lesion site. Therefore, this chapter is organized according to the nature of the functional impairment. However, wherever possible, the best current understanding of localization is also given.

Disorders of touch and proprioception

Cortical sensory loss

Classically, parietal lesions lead to 'discriminative' sensory loss.[4] Two-point discrimination, position sense, texture discrimination, stereognosis (impaired tactile spatial perception, manifested by an inability to identify by touch objects placed in the hand, due to severe basic somatosensory imperception) and graphesthesia (inability to recognize numbers written on the hand) may all be impaired. Usually, this 'cortical sensory loss' is limited to one or two body parts, is more prominent in the arm than the leg, and follows damage to the anterior parietal lobe or its connections.[5] However, there are also reports of astereognosis following damage to the SPL or IPL. One patient with a large SPL cyst sought medical attention because she kept 'losing' her arm if she did not look at it. Impairments of light touch, pain, temperature and vibration have classically been considered to be associated with damage to the thalamus, but recent investigations have demonstrated that these modalities may also be lost following damage to the inferior anterior parietal lobe.[6]

Tactile agnosia

In contrast to astereognosis, tactile agnosia refers to selective impairment of tactile object recognition in the absence of a clinically demonstrable basic somaesthetic impairment (light touch, pin-prick, temperature, vibration sense and proprioception are preserved). With their eyes closed, patients with tactile agnosia are unable to recognize familiar objects placed in the hand contralateral to the lesion. Thus one patient remarked that she would have to bring her keys out of her pocket to be sure what they were, despite the fact that she did not appear to have any discriminative sensory loss. In general, tactile agnosia is not very disabling, presumably because vision compensates so well. It appears to be related to lesions of the contralateral IPL, although damage to the posterior insula may also be important.[7] It has been suggested that the disorder reflects impaired high-level perceptual processing of somaesthetic information.

Tactile extinction and neglect

Some patients with parietal lesions demonstrate what is considered to be a disorder of directing attention—tactile extinction. The examiner asks the patient to close their eyes. When a brief touch is applied to the hand either ipsilateral or contralateral to the lesion, the patient has no difficulty in reporting its presence, indicating preserved sensation. However, if both hands are simultaneously touched, the patient fails to report the contralesional touch. In other words, it appears effectively to be 'extinguished' by the ipsilesional stimulus. Tactile extinction, like its visual counterpart (see below), is considered to result from competition between representations of the ipsilesional and contralesional stimulus within parietal cortex. Unilateral parietal damage may also lead to tactile neglect—failure to report tactile stimuli administered to the contralesional hand (even when a competing stimulus is not applied to the ipsilesional hand) which cannot be explained by a 'cortical sensory loss'. As one might imagine, this is a difficult syndrome to distinguish on clinical testing from a primary disorder of sensation.

Disorders of vision

A vast range of disorders of vision follow damage to the posterior parietal lobe. Most of them are characterized by a spatial component. At one end of the spectrum are field defects (classically inferior quadrantanopias), which arise because of damage to part of the optic radiations as they pass through the parietal white matter from lateral geniculate nucleus to the calcarine sulcus. These primary sensory deficits will not be considered further here. At the other end of the spectrum are complex disorders of visual attention which can have devastating consequences for a patient and present an enormous challenge for rehabilitation.[8]

Visual mislocalization and visual disorientation

Holmes[9] described in great detail a syndrome he termed 'visual disorientation' in cases of bilateral posterior parietal damage following gunshot wounds in World War I. Holmes' descriptions have since become classics of both the neurological and neuropsychological literature.[9,10] Typically, when asked to touch an object in front of him, a patient would reach in the wrong direction and grope hopelessly until his hand or arm came into contact with it, almost as if he was searching for a small object in the dark. He would have great difficulty in walking through a room without bumping into objects, so that a casual onlooker might think he was blind. But, through careful observation, Holmes came to the conclusion that this disorder was primarily one of judging visual location. He noted that his patients had no difficulty in judging the position of their arms but suffered from a remarkable inability to judge the position of objects in the world around them.

Less dramatic impairments of visual localization have been demonstrated in patients with unilateral lesions. For example, patients with parietal lesions have been found to misreach when pointing to visual targets presented on a perimeter.[11] However, a potential confound is that parietal damage may lead to a disorder of visually guided reaching in addition to problems of visual localization. In order to demonstrate impaired visual localization, therefore, it is better to use tests which do not require reaching. Several investigators have used such perceptual tests, e.g. by first briefly presenting a dot and then a card on which appeared numbers at different locations and then asking subjects to report the number which best approximated the location of the dot. The results of these studies have suggested that visual localization is more impaired following lesions of the right hemisphere than the left. Furthermore, posterior lesions appear to be particularly associated with mislocalization.[12,13] Depth perception and judgment of line orientation may also be impaired after unilateral parietal lesions.[14]

Remarkably, Holmes[9] suggested that the mislocalization seen in his patients was not simply a visual problem. He thought that retinal signals alone are insufficient for absolute localization of objects in space in relation to the body. For such egocentric localization, he argued, we need information about the position of our eyes, the attitude of our heads and the orientation of our bodies in space. He felt that association of retinal signals with eye-, head- and body-position signals was required. Electrophysiological studies in monkeys have since confirmed that exactly such associations occur in the posterior parietal cortex.[15] Functional imaging studies in humans confirm a special role for the parietal lobe in visual localization.[16]

Constructional apraxia

A common way to demonstrate visuospatial impairments following parietal damage is to ask patients to copy a drawing or a three-dimensional block design. Typically, patients encounter difficulty in understanding the spatial relationships of the drawing or block design and produce poor reproductions. Such an inability to use visual information to guide acts which require an understanding of the spatial relationship of objects is referred to as constructional apraxia, a syndrome associated with inferior parietal lobe damage.[17] Paterson and Zangwill[18] gave a particularly clear account of a young patient with a very focal lesion of the right IPL. They observed that the patient drew complex objects or scenes detail by detail, and appeared to lack any real grasp of the object as a whole. They characterized this problem as a 'piecemeal approach'—a fragmentation of the visual contents with deficient synthesis.

The issue of whether constructional apraxia is a disorder of visual perception or control of hand movements has since been intensively debated. In theory, of course, it could result from either, or indeed both. Allied to this debate has been the question of whether the syndrome is more frequently associated with right- than left-hemisphere damage. The evidence to date suggests that overall there might be a slight preponderance of constructional apraxia following right parietal lesions. However, it has been suggested that there are qualitative differences, with limb apraxia being the important underlying cause following left parietal damage, and impairments in visuospatial perception dominating after right-sided lesions. There was some evidence in favor of this proposal when patients were studied using tasks which place minimal demands upon hand control.[19,20]

If the problem in constructional apraxia is visual, the question arises as to why perception is 'piecemeal'. One possibility is that these patients have difficulty combining visual signals with signals regarding where the eyes are looking—the mechanism invoked by Holmes[9] to account for impaired spatial localization. As the eyes scan across an object, vision is effectively limited to a small region around the fovea each time the eye fixates part of the object. Perception of the object is built up by integrating information across saccades. An impairment in the process of combining retinal signals with eye position signals could account for the failure to synthesize the 'snapshots' obtained at each fixation into a coherent and spatially accurate representation of the entire object.

Disorders of visual attention

Three disorders of attention follow damage to the posterior parietal lobes: extinction, neglect and (dorsal) simultanagnosia. The first two often occur after unilateral damage, whereas the last is less common and is observed in its full-blown form after bilateral parietal lesions. None of them can be adequately explained as simple sensory impairments. Interestingly, neglect is most severe and most long-lasting following right parietal lesions, although it can also occur after right frontal, basal ganglia and thalamic damage.[21] Rather than considering these three disorders separately, there is some merit in discussing them together, since they may well share common mechanisms.

Visual extinction is the failure to report a contralesional stimulus in the presence of a competing ipsilesional stimulus. Patients acknowledge the presence of a single visual stimulus (e.g. the examiner's finger) when it is presented briefly in either left or right visual hemifields. However, when both stimuli are simultaneously presented transiently, one in each hemifield, patients report seeing only the ipsilesional one. Thus, they fail to acknowledge the presence of the contralesional stimulus when there is a competing stimulus in the ipsilesional hemifield.

Visual neglect is a failure to acknowledge a stimulus presented in space opposite the side of the brain lesion, regardless of the presence or absence of a competing stimulus in ipsilesional space.[22,23] The same definition could apply to hemianopia. Indeed, if neglect is very dense it can be difficult to distinguish from hemianopia, and some patients with large lesions suffer from both a hemianopia and neglect. However, the clinician is often alerted to the presence of neglect by the patient's persistent turning of eyes and head towards the ipsilesional side (without an associated gaze palsy), by finding that unawareness of contralesional stimuli can vary and is not absolute, by observing that the apparent visual field loss does not obey the vertical meridian (unlike homonymous hemianopia), and by the patient's failure to orient fully into contralesional space on simple pen and paper tasks such as line bisection and cancellation (Figure 4.2). Some patients also fail to draw the contralesional side of objects. A patient with hemianopia (without neglect) may be slow in performing these tasks but will usually explore contralesional space. Finally, an important clinical clue comes from the patient's history. Most patients with neglect are not aware they have a problem, whereas those with a

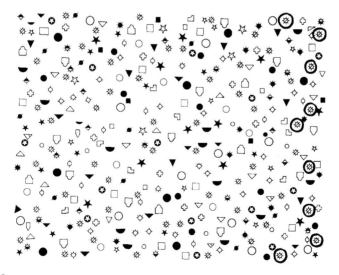

Figure 4.2

Cancellation performance of a patient with left neglect. Notice how the patient has found targets on only the extreme right of the search display.

hemianopia (without neglect) complain bitterly that they have difficulty seeing on one side of space.

Simultanagnosia is, at least overtly, rather different from the spatial deficits in extinction and neglect. In general, this term refers to a disorder of vision in which the individual parts of a display are better perceived than the entire scene. The classical demonstration is that of getting patients to describe what they see in a complex picture. They may describe some of the details meticulously but still not appreciate what is happening overall in the picture. Farah[24] has proposed that there are two types of simultanagnosia, associated respectively with lesions of the dorsal (occipitoparietal) or ventral (occipitotemporal) visual pathways. Dorsal simultanagnosia is characterized by an inability to perceive more than one object at a time, regardless of its spatial extent. In this regard, the condition appears, at least overtly, to be strikingly different from either extinction or neglect, where the clinical presentation is dominated by a spatial deficit.

Consider first the two spatial disorders. There is an important distinction to be made between them. Whereas the phenomenon of extinction is observed using brief stimuli at the bedside or in experimental testing, patients with neglect may fail to report contralesional stimuli regardless of the time given to them. In everyday situations, they ignore food placed on the contralesional side of the plate and fail to be aware of people approaching them from that side. Thus, extinction appears to be a mild spatial disorder brought out by testing, whereas neglect is a more severe disabling syndrome which is usually readily evident to the observer. Some have argued that extinction may actually be a milder version of neglect, whereas others consider it to be caused by a completely different mechanism, or that, in addition to extinction, there are several other components of the neglect syndrome. Several different types of mechanism have been proposed to account for these disorders.[23] Previously, these have been described separately as attentional, representational or motor impairments. However, it is possible that these different types of mechanism are not mutually incompatible; all three types of disorder may co-exist (with other impairments) in the neglect.[23,25]

A very influential approach to extinction and neglect has been to consider them to be disorders of directing spatial attention. In particular, experimental evidence has suggested that these patients encounter difficulty in disengaging attention from the ipsilesional side and shifting it contralesionally.[26,27] This experimentally defined deficit is correlated best with damage to the temporoparietal junction,[28] the area that is classically associated with clinically defined neglect.[29] Problems for the disengage and shift deficit theory proposed by Posner et al[26] have been presented by at least two recent studies of patients with left-sided extinction. These demonstrate that a left-sided stimulus can be extinguished by a right-sided one, even if the left-sided stimulus is presented several hundred milliseconds before the right one.[30,31] Thus the left stimulus is extinguished even when there is no initial right-sided stimulus for attention to engage upon. A further difficulty for the Posner hypothesis is that the putative disengage and shift deficit does not explain why, when presented with bilateral stimuli, attention would always first engage the ipsilesional one.

A slightly different attentional approach to extinction and neglect is to consider them to be the result of an imbalance of attentional mechanisms across the two cerebral hemispheres following unilateral damage. Kinsbourne[32] proposed that each hemisphere normally directs attention to the contralateral side of space; when one is damaged, there will be an imbalance in this mechanism and attention will be directed towards the side of the damaged hemisphere. Such a mechanism would account for many of the impairments found in the neglect syndrome. It has been suggested that the higher prevalence of neglect following right-hemisphere lesions may be due to an attentional mechanism that operates on both sides of visual space in the right parietal lobe, compared to one which directs attention to only right space in the left parietal lobe.[33]

An alternative proposal has been that neglect is due to a failure to represent contralesional space. Perhaps the most remarkable evidence in favor of such a view has been presented by Bisiach and Luzzatti,[34] who asked Milanese patients to describe from memory the large cathedral square in the city from one particular side of the square. The patients described locations which were predominantly on the left of the square from their imagined vantage point. However, when they were asked to imagine that they were at the other end of the square, they described details on the left from that perspective. In other words, they now recounted details that had been on the right from the opposite imagined viewpoint. Thus, from either vantage point, they appeared to report predominantly places located on the left in a viewer-centered representation of the square.

Both a gradient of visual attention biased to the right and a deficit of representing left space would account for many perceptual aspects of left neglect. However, they do not easily explain an impairment in directing leftward hand movements which has recently been described in parietal neglect.[35] Previously it had been suggested that such an 'intentional' impairment (a disorder of initiating movements toward the neglected side) may occur in neglect following right frontal lesions. Mattingley et al[35] have found a direction-specific impairment of initiating leftward movements in right parietal neglect patients which cannot be accounted for by impaired visual processing of left-sided stimuli. This would be consistent with electrophysiological studies in monkey parietal cortex, which have demonstrated reach-related neurons encoding the intended direction of an upcoming movement.[36]

Finally, there has been growing interest in the possibility that the deficits in the neglect syndrome may not all be spatially lateralized. There have been demonstrations of so-called object-centered neglect, in which patients appear to ignore the left side of individual objects, regardless of where they are located in space.[37] In addition, there is evidence that the level of arousal may be reduced[38] and that there is an impairment of directing attention over time in spatial neglect, with the processing of small stimuli presented at fixation being prolonged.[39] Such non-spatial impairment may also be an underlying factor in dorsal simultanagnosia following bilateral parietal damage.

Bálint[40] observed that his patient with bilateral occipitoparietal infarcts could attend to only one object at a time, regardless of the size of the object or the number of objects placed in front of him. Subsequently, Luria[41] demonstrated an important non-spatial impairment in simultanagnosia. He showed his patient two overlapping triangles in the configuration of a Star of David. The patient had no difficulty in reporting a star. However, when one of the triangles was drawn in red and the other in blue ink, the patient reported only one or other of the triangles and never said he saw two triangles or a star. Thus, when two forms (triangles of different colors) overlapped in space, only one was perceived. Simultaneous perception of two forms was not possible at the same location, even though the patient could apparently see both these forms when they were drawn in the same ink to form one object (the star). This may be a non-spatial form of extinction.[42] Other studies have demonstrated an impairment of feature binding—putting together features such as color and form of an object to obtain a coherent percept.[43] It remains unclear whether the underlying mechanisms in simultanagnosia and neglect are similar.

Disorders of spatial working memory

Visuospatial memory has classically been tested using the Corsi block-tapping task, in which patients view an array of nine cubes and are asked to reproduce, after a delay, the sequence of cubes tapped by the examiner. In experiments conducted before the advent of CT imaging, patients with posterior right-hemisphere lesions were found to be particularly impaired on this test of spatial span.[44] Right-parietal patients are impaired also in estimating the number of dots presented in tachistoscopic displays,[45] a task which may also require spatial working memory. Finally, functional imaging demonstrates parietal, as well as dorsolateral prefrontal, activation in neurologically normal individuals performing tasks considered to test spatial working memory.[46]

Topographical disorientation

A number of different types of underlying disorder, associated with lesions of different brain regions, may lead to topographical disorientation or difficulty in finding one's way in large-scale environments.[47] One such syndrome appears to follow damage to the parietal lobe, particularly on the right side.[14] These patients frequently get lost in previously familiar or new environments. Their verbal descriptions of routes from one place to another or sketch-maps of familiar places are poor. But in addition to their topographical problems, they also suffer from visual disorientation with impaired visual localization of objects in their immediate surroundings. It has been proposed that this parietal form of topographical disorientation results from a basic deficit in apprehending the egocentric spatial relationships of places.[47]

Disorders of visuomotor and motor control

Optic ataxia

Bálint[40] first used the term 'optic ataxia' to refer to an impairment of visually guided reaching that he observed following bilateral parietal damage. Since then, many reports have followed of patients with unilateral or bilateral parietal lesions.[14] The term 'Bálint's syndrome' is used to refer to a combination of optic ataxia, simultanagnosia and neglect of objects in the visual surroundings. However, many patients have been reported with optic ataxia alone. The most commonly described defect appears to be a 'field effect', i.e. inaccurate reaching with either hand to visual targets poitioned in the visual hemifield contralateral to the lesion. However, an 'arm effect' has also been observed, i.e. misreaching with the contralesional arm to targets in either visual field. Such an 'arm effect' may occur with or without a 'field effect', and various combinations of arm and field deficits have been reported in the clinical literature.[48,49]

At the bedside, the disorder is best demonstrated by asking the patient to fixate centrally (e.g. on the examiner's nose) and point to a target presented peripherally (e.g. the examiner's finger). If the patient is allowed to move his eyes and look at the target, the misreaching may not be evident. In experimental testing, the misreaching is worse when patients have to make movements without visual inspection of the position of the hand, i.e. when they make so-called 'open-loop' or ballistic reaches.[49] As well as misdirecting their reaches, optic ataxic patients may also encounter difficulty in planning the appropriate grasp required to pick up an object.[49]

The critical lesion site for optic ataxia appears to be the SPL and adjacent IPS.[49] Lesions in either hemisphere appear to cause the syndrome, although right parietal lesions may be more likely to produce a 'field effect', whereas injury to the left parietal lobe produces, in addition, an 'arm effect'. It has been suggested that various combinations of field and arm effects arise if there is a disconnection from motor centers in the frontal lobes.[48] Such a view echoes traditional anatomical models of limb apraxia (see below).

An alternative possibility is that optic ataxia results from an impairment in the parietal mechanisms which localize a visual target with respect to the body and compute the spatial motor signals required to direct the hand accurately onto the target. The egocentric spatial representation which Holmes[9] invoked to explain the visual disorientation in his patients may also be required to direct limb movements, because retinal signals alone cannot localize a target with respect to the body or limb. In monkeys, electrophysiological recordings have demonstrated reach-related neurons in posterior parietal cortex[50] which appear to encode the intended direction of an upcoming reach.[36] Functional imaging studies in humans have begun to define the cortical network, including parietal structures, involved in reaching.[51] In both monkeys and humans, there is also evidence for a parietal representation of grasp, as well as reach, control. This appears to reside within the IPS in both species.[51,52]

Impairments of gaze control or ocular apraxia

The patient Bálint[40] described with bilateral parietal lesions suffered, in addition to optic ataxia, from 'a psychic paralysis of gaze': difficulty in looking at objects other than the one he was fixating. On cursory examination it might have been thought that he had paralysis of eye movements. More careful observation showed that the patient could in fact move his eyes, his apparent paralysis of gaze being due to an inability to notice spontaneously visual objects other than the one fixated. Bálint had to direct him to seeing other objects in the visual surround, even though on careful testing the patient's visual fields appeared to be intact. Bálint therefore described the fixation of gaze as due to a constriction of the 'psychic field-of-view'. It is as if the patient's vision was locked into the object at fixation because he was simply not aware of other objects in the visual surround—a constriction of visual attention.

Holmes[9] described a similar problem in his patients with visual disorientation, but in addition he observed other disorders of oculomotor control. Typically, when one of his patients was asked to look at something or spoken to, he would stare in the wrong direction and then move his eyes awkwardly until he found, often as if by chance, the object he was looking for. Some of Holmes' cases also failed to accommodate and converge their eyes correctly, and smooth pursuit could also be impaired.[10] Some authors consider the patients described by Bálint and Holmes to be representative of the same core disorder and prefer to refer to this as Bálint–Holmes syndrome.

Holmes considered the oculomotor problems in his patients (now termed ocular apraxia) to be secondary to the visual perceptual derangement. However, it is possible that these disorders may be accounted for by loss of neurons associated with maintaining fixation, directing saccades or pursuit eye movements, all of which have been demonstrated in studies of monkey posterior parietal cortical neurons.[1,15,50,53] The fixation of gaze observed by both Bálint and Holmes is perhaps explained by the homologues of loss of light-sensitive neurons which appear to be important in detecting novel events in the visual periphery.[54,55] Functional imaging studies in humans suggest that the parietal eye field is located within the IPS.[56]

Limb apraxia

The term 'apraxia' refers to an impairment in the ability to perform skilled movements which cannot be attributed to weakness, sensory disturbance or involuntary movements such as tremor. It may occur in up to 50% of unselected patients with left-hemisphere damage;[57] but frequently goes unrecognized either because patients may not be aware of a problem in daily life, or because praxis is commonly not tested, or because many left-hemisphere patients are dysphasic. For a clinically useful battery of praxis tests, consult De Renzi et al[57] and De Renzi and Faglioni.[58]

Liepmann, at the turn of the last century, originally proposed that there are three types of apraxia: ideational, ideomotor and limb-kinetic (or melokinetic). He considered that inadequate formulation of a motor program would result in ideational apraxia. Traditionally, this has been considered to be best observed when a patient is asked to produce a sequence of gestures on command, rather than when the examiner performs a gesture for him to imitate. By contrast, in ideomotor apraxia, a patient may know what to do but cannot produce the correct actions either on verbal request or when asked to imitate gestures. He is aware of his poor performance and tries to correct it, so the problem is one of defective execution rather than ideation. Finally, limb-kinetic apraxia consists of loss of control of fine finger movements and often follows damage to the corticospinal pathways. It will not be considered further in this discussion.

The use of the term ideational apraxia has been extremely confusing. Indeed, some have wondered whether it is simply a more severe form of ideomotor apraxia. Ideational apraxia is often used to refer to an impairment in the ability to perform a series of motor acts. For example, when asked to make a cup of tea, a patient may perform each element of the sequence but in an incorrect order. Originally, this was observed most commonly in the context of a generalized dementing illness. Perhaps this explains the view taken by some investigators that ideational apraxia may not be a useful concept.

However, De Renzi has argued against this view. According to him, ideational apraxia refers to an inability to recall previously well-established actions, e.g. object use. Furthermore, although a series of actions may bring out this deficit most clearly in some individuals, difficulty in producing a sequence of motor acts is not critical to this disorder. Rather, he considers ideational apraxia to be an 'amnesia of usage'—impaired recall of how objects must be used.[59] There are certainly examples of patients who have difficulty using a single object without having to perform a sequence of acts using multiple objects; for example, Pick reported a case who used a razor as a comb![60] Moreover, there is evidence that difficulty in using multiple or single objects does not correlate with movement imitation performance, which is considered a test of ideomotor apraxia.[59] However, ideational apraxia continues to be controversial subject.

Heilman and colleagues favor the introduction of a new term—conceptual apraxia—to specify a defect in the knowledge required to select and use tools and objects.[61] They note that whereas traditionally most patients with ideational apraxia improve with tool usage, those studied by De Renzi and his colleagues actually made errors with objects. Heilman appears to reserve the term 'ideational apraxia' for an inability to carry out a sequence of actions, and 'conceptual apraxia' to refer to a defect in the knowledge required to use objects or tools.

In contrast to ideational apraxia, there is more general agreement regarding ideomotor apraxia, although we still understand very little about the mechanisms underlying either condition. In ideomotor apraxia, the representation of the gesture to be performed is considered to be intact but its execution is defective. Traditionally, an important piece of evidence in favor of this distinction is the failure of patients to produce correct gestures even when asked to imitate the examiner's movements. Thus these patients, unlike those with ideational apraxia, perform poorly regardless of whether they have to produce a gesture on verbal command (by recalling a movement representation) or imitate it. Typically, however, their performance is better when imitating movements or using objects than when they are asked to pantomime transitive acts, i.e. mime the use a tool or instrument. Intransitive movements (communicative gestures such as waving goodbye) may be relatively preserved. Thus, ideomotor apraxia appears to spare movements that are automatic (habitual such as waving, or repetitive as in finger-tapping).

According to some investigators, ideomotor apraxics may make two general types of movement production errors—spatial and temporal. The spatial impairments may be further sub-divided. For example, patients may make postural errors, using a body part as a tool, such as using their fingers to act like scissor blades when asked to pantomime using scissors.[62] This type of error may have been overemphasized, since even neurologically normal subjects will sometimes do this. Another type of spatial error is the production of incorrect trajectories which may be associated with inappropriate movements about multiple joints.[63,64] For example, when asked to pantomime the use of a screwdriver, a patient may rotate his arm at the shoulder rather than at the elbow. A recent investigation has demonstrated that spatial errors can occur when ideomotor apraxics make even simple aiming movements.[65] Finally, temporal errors in movement execution have also been observed, e.g. either delays in initiation or transient stops during movement producing a stuttering gesture.[66] Unfortunately, these investigations, although a useful first step, have not to date convincingly uncovered the basic disorder underlying ideomotor apraxia.

The localization of apraxia appears to be the mirror image of the neglect syndrome. It has long been appreciated that apraxia is far more common after damage to the left hemisphere than to the right. Liepmann considered ideomotor apraxia to be a disconnection of sensory visual and audioverbal representations (in the posterior left hemisphere) and kinesthetic-motor engrams in the sensorimotor cortex around the central sulcus. The critical anatomical site of the disconnection, he suggested, was the white matter underlying the left inferior parietal cortex. Ideational apraxia, he suggested, arose from damage posterior to this site at the junction of the temporal, parietal and occipital lobes.

Liepmann was quite clear that his model did not envisage a center for gesture control within the IPL, but subsequent investigators have challenged this scheme. Heilman et al,[61] in particular, have proposed that movement representations ('praxicons' in their jargon) are stored within the left IPL. They consider these representations to encode the spatial and temporal patterns of skilled movements, and that damage to these representations leads to ideomotor apraxia. In addition, damage to connections between the left parietal lobe and regions involved in the execution of motor programs will also lead to ideomotor apraxia. Conceptual apraxia in their terminology and ideational apraxia as envisaged by De Renzi appears most frequently to follow lesions of the posterior parietal lobe near its boundary with the occipital and temporal lobes. Functional imaging studies are beginning to delineate the network of brain regions involved in generating movements and perceiving the actions of others.[67]

Alexia, agraphia and Gerstmann's syndrome

Disorders of reading and writing following parietal lobe damage are considered in the chapter concerning lesions of the perisylvian cortex. Gerstmann's syndrome refers to a combination of finger agnosia (an impairment in identifying the different fingers of a hand), agraphia, acalculia and right–left disorientation which was considered to follow lesions of the left IPL, specifically of the angular gyrus. Doubt has been cast on the validity of this syndrome.

Anosoagnosia

Unawareness of illness is referred to as anosoagnosia. Patients may steadfastly deny they have suffered a stroke or hemiparesis, even if the examiner demonstrates that one limb is weak. The condition is often but not invariably associated with unilateral neglect, and appears most commonly after right-hemisphere lesions. Although it is traditionally associated with right-parietal damage, it appears to be most common after large lesions involving cortex and subcortical structures in the frontal and temporal lobe.[17]

Conclusions

A variety of sensory, motor and attentional deficits follow damage to the parietal lobe. Our understanding of the mechanisms underlying these syndromes is improving with novel experimental testing of patients with these disorders, as well as functional imaging studies in neurologically normal individuals and electrophysiological studies in monkeys.

References

1. Andersen RA. Inferior parietal lobule function in spatial perception and visuomotor integration. In Plum F, Mountcastle VB (eds) *Handbook of Physiology, Vol V, Part II* (Rockville, MD: American Physiological Society 1987): 483–518.

2. Ungerleider L, Mishkin M. Two cortical visual systems. In Ingle DJ, Mansfield RJW, Goodale MS (eds). *The Analysis of Visual Behavior* (Cambridge, MA: MIT Press, 1985): 21–33.

3. Milner AD, Goodale MA. *The Visual Brain in Action* (Oxford: Oxford University Press, 1995).

4. Head H, Holmes G. Sensory disturbances from cerebral lesions. *Brain* (1911) **34:** 102–254.

5. Roland E. Astereognosis. Tactile discrimination after localized hemispheric lesions in man. *Arch Neurol* (1976) **33:** 543–50.

6. Bassetti C, Bogousslavsky J, Regli F. Sensory syndromes in parietal stroke. *Neurology* (1993) **43:** 1942–9.

7. Caselli RJ. Ventrolateral and dorsomedial somatosensory association cortex damage produces distinct somaesthetic syndromes in humans. *Neurology* (1993) **43:** 762–71.

8. Robertson IH. Cognitive rehabilitation: attention and neglect. *Trends Cogn Sci* (1999) **3:** 385–93.

9. Holmes G. Disturbances of visual orientation. *Br J Ophthalmol* (1918) **2:** 449–506.

10. Holmes G, Horrax G. Distur-

bances of spatial orientation and visual attention with loss of stereoscopic vision. *Arch Neurol Psychiatry* (1919) **1:** 385–407.

11. Ratcliff G, Davies-Jones GAB. Defective visual localisation in focal brain wounds. *Brain* (1972) **95:** 46–60.

12. Warrington EK, Rabin P. Perceptual matching in patients with cerebral lesions. *Neuropsychologia* (1970) **8:** 475–87.

13. Hannay HJ, Varney N, Benton AL. Visual localisation in patients with unilateral brain disease. *J Neurol Neurosurg Psychiatry* (1976) **39:** 307–13.

14. De Renzi E. *Disorders of Space Exploration and Cognition* (New York: Wiley, 1982).

15. Andersen RA. Multimodal integration for the representation of space in the posterior parietal cortex. *Philos Trans R Soc Lond B* (1997) **352:** 1421–8.

16. Haxby JV, Grady CL, Horwitz B et al. Dissociation of object and spatial visual processing pathways in human extrastriate cortex. *Proc Nat Acad Sci USA* (1991) **88:** 1621–5.

17. Hier DB, Mondlock J, Caplan LR. Behavioural abnormalities after right hemisphere stroke. *Neurology* (1983) **33:** 337–44.

18. Patterson A, Zangwill OL. Disorders of visual space perception associated with lesions of the right cerebral hemisphere. *Brain* (1944) **67:** 331–58.

19. Mack JL, Levine RN. The basis of constructional disability in patients with unilateral cerebral lesions. *Cortex* (1981) **17:** 515–32.

20. Griffiths K, Cook M. Attribute processing in patients with graphical copying disability. *Neuropsychologia* (1986) **24:** 371–83.

21. Heilman KM, Valenstein E, Watson RT. Localization of lesions in neglect and related disorders. In Kertesz A (ed.) *Localization and Neuroimaging in Neuropsychology* (San Diego: Academic Press, 1994): 495–524.

22. Robertson IH, Marshall JC. (1993). *Unilateral Neglect: Clinical and Experimental Studies* (Hove: Lawrence Erlbaum, 1993).

23. Vallar G. Spatial hemineglect in humans. *Trends Cogn Sci* (1998) **2:** 87–97.

24. Farah M. *Visual Agnosia: Disorders of Object Recognition and What They Tell Us About Normal Vision* (Cambridge, MA: MIT Press, 1990).

25. Bisiach E. Mental representation in unilateral neglect and related disorders: The twentieth Bartlett Memorial Lecture. *Q J Exp Psychol* (1993) **46A:** 435–61.

26. Posner MI, Walker JA, Friedrich FJ, Rafal R. Effects of parietal injury on covert orienting of attention. *J Neurosci* (1984) **4:** 1863–74.

27. Morrow LA, Ratcliff G. The disengagement of covert attention and the neglect syndrome. *Psychobiology* (1988) **16:** 261–9.

28. Friedrich FJ, Egly R, Rafal RD, Beck D. Spatial attention deficits in humans: a comparison of superior parietal and temporo-parietal junction lesions. *Neuropsychology* (1998) **12:** 193–207.

29. Vallar G, Perani D. The anatomy of unilateral neglect after right hemisphere stroke lesions: a clinical CT correlation study in man. *Neuropsychologia* (1986) **24:** 609–22.

30. Rorden C, Mattingley JB, Karnath H-O, Driver J. Visual extinction and prior entry: impaired perception of temporal order with intact motion perception after parietal injury. *Neuropsychologia* (1997) **35:** 421–33.

31. di Pellegrino G, Basso G,

Frassinetti F. Spatial extinction on double asynchronous stimulation. *Neuropsychologia* (1997) **9:** 1215–23.

32. Kinsbourne M. Mechanisms of unilateral neglect. In Jeannerod M (ed.) *Neurophysiological and Neuropsychological Aspects of Spatial Neglect*, 69th edn (Amsterdam: Elsevier, 1987): 69–86.

33. Mesulam M-M. A cortical network for directed attention and unilateral neglect. *Ann Neurol* (1981) **10:** 309–25.

34. Bisiach E, Luzzatti C. Unilateral neglect of representational space. *Cortex* (1978) **14:** 129–33.

35. Mattingley J, Husain M, Rorden C et al. Motor role of human inferior parietal lobe revealed in unilateral neglect patients. *Nature* (1998) **392:** 179–82.

36. Snyder LH, Batista AP, Andersen RA. Coding of intention in the posterior parietal cortex. *Nature* (1997) **386:** 167–70.

37. Driver J. Egocentric and object-based visual neglect. In Burgess N, Jeffery KJ, O'Keefe JO (eds) *The Hippocampal and Parietal Foundations of Spatial Cognition* (Oxford: Oxford University Press, 1999): 66–89.

38. Robertson IH, Mattingley JBM, Rorden C, Driver J. Phasic alerting of neglect patients overcomes their spatial deficit in visual awareness. *Nature* (1998) **395:** 169–72.

39. Husain M, Shapiro K, Martin J, Kennard C. Abnormal temporal dynamics of visual attention in spatial neglect patients. *Nature* (1997) **385:** 154–6.

40. Bálint R. Seelenlähmung des 'Schauens', optische Ataxie, räumliche Störung der Aufmerksamkeit. *Monatschr Psychiatr Neurol* (1909) **25:** 51–81.

41. Luria AR. Disorders of 'simultaneous perception' in a case of bilat-

eral occipitoparietal brain injury. *Brain* (1959) **83:** 437–49.

42. Humphreys GW, Romani C, Olson A et al. Non-spatial extinction following lesions of the parietal lobe in humans. *Nature* (1994) **372:** 357–9.

43. Friedman-Hill SR, Robertson LC, Treisman A. Parietal contributions to visual feature binding: evidence from a patient with bilateral lesions. *Science* (1995) **269:** 853–5.

44. De Renzi E, Faglioni P, Previdi P. Spatial memory and hemispheric locus of lesion. *Cortex* (1977) **13:** 424–33.

45. Warrington E, James M. Tachistoscopic number estimation in patients with unilateral cerebral lesions. *J Neurol Neurosurg Psychiatry* (1967) **30:** 468–74.

46. Owen AM, Evans AC, Petrides M. Evidence for a two-stage model of spatial working memory processing within the lateral frontal cortex. A positron emission tomography study. *Cerebral Cortex* (1996) **6:** 31–8.

47. Aguirre GK, D'Esposito M. Topographical disorientation: a synthesis and taxonomy. *Brain* (1999) **122:** 1613–28.

48. Rondot P, de Recondo J, Ribadeau Dumas JL. Visuomotor ataxia. *Brain* (1977) **100:** 355–76.

49. Perenin MT, Vighetto A. Optic ataxia: a specific disorder in visuomotor mechanisms. I. Different aspects of the deficit in reaching for objects. *Brain* (1988) **111:** 643–74.

50. Mountcastle VB, Lynch JC, Georgopoulos A et al. Posterior parietal association cortex of the monkey: command function for operations within extrapersonal space. *J Neurophysiol* (1975) **38:** 871–908.

51. Rizzolatti G, Fogassi L, Gallese V. Parietal cortex: from sight to action. *Curr Opin Neurobiol* (1997) **7:** 562–7.

52. Binkofski F, Dohle C, Hefter H et al. Human anterior intraparietal area subserves prehension. A combined lesion and functional MRI activation study. *Neurology* (1998) **50:** 1253–9.

53. Lynch JC, Mountcastle VB, Talbot WH, Yin TCT. Parietal lobe mechanisms for directed visual attention. *J Neurophysiol* (1977) **40:** 362–89.

54. Yin TCT, Mountcastle VB. Visual input to the visuomotor mechanisms of the monkey's parietal lobe. *Science* (1977) **197:** 1381–3.

55. Yin TCT, Mountcastle VB. Mechanisms of neural integration in the parietal lobe for visual attention. *Fed Proc* (1978) **37:** 2251–7.

56. Corbetta M, Akbudak E, Conturo TE et al. A common network of functional areas for attention and eye movements. *Neuron* (1998) **21:** 761–73.

57. De Renzi E, Motti F, Nichelli P. Imitating gestures: a quantitative approach to ideomotor apraxia. *Arch Neurol* (1980) **37:** 6–10.

58. De Renzi E, Faglioni P. Apraxia. In Denes G, Pizzamiglio L (eds) *Handbook of Clinical and Experimental Neuropsychology* (Hove: Psychology Press, 1999): 421–40.

59. De Renzi E, Lucchelli F. Ideational apraxia. *Brain* (1988) **111:** 1173–85.

60. De Renzi E. Methods of limb apraxia examination and their bearing on the interpretation of the disorder. In Roy EA (ed.) *Neuropsychological Studies of Apraxia and Related Disorders* (Amsterdam: Elsevier, 1985): 45–64.

61. Heilman KM, Watson RT, Gonzalez Rothi L. Disorders of skilled movements: limb apraxia. In Farah M, Feinberg T (eds) *Behavioural Neuropsychology* (1999).

62. Goodglass H, Kaplan E. Disturbance of gesture and pantomime in aphasia. *Brain* (1963) **86:** 703–20.

63. Clark M, Merians AS, Kothari A et al. Spatial planning deficits in limb apraxia. *Brain* (1994) **117:** 1093–106.

64. Poizner H, Clark M, Merians AS et al. Joint coordination deficits in limb apraxia. *Brain* (1995) **118:** 227–42.

65. Haaland KY, Harrington DL, Knight RT. Spatial deficits in ideomotor limb apraxia. A kinematic analysis of aiming movements. *Brain* (1999) **122:** 1169–82.

66. Poizner H, Mack L, Verfaellie M et al. Three-dimensional computergraphic analysis of apraxia. Neural representations of learned movement. *Brain* (1990) **113:** 85–101.

67. Decety J, Grèzes J. Neural mechanisms subserving the perception of human actions. *Trends Cogn Sci* (1999) **3:** 172–8.

5
The neuropsychological sequelae of frontal lobe damage

Adrian M Owen

Summary

Historically, the prefrontal cortex has been symbolically described using a multitude of vivid metaphors, 'uncharted provinces of the brain', being a typical example. Recently, however, cognitive and brain scientists have begun to unravel the mysteries of the frontal lobe, yielding what must now be one of the most exciting and important areas of research in contemporary neuroscience. The fact that the functional anatomy of this region has remained unclear for so long can be attributed to two general principles. First, while the frontal lobe undoubtedly contributes to many aspects of cognition and behavior, it does so via reciprocal connections with many other cortical and subcortical regions. Thus, while studies of patients with frontal lobe damage have implicated this region in functions as diverse as attention, memory, language, planning, social cognition and motor control, the specificity of this contribution often remains in some doubt; patients with damage to posterior cortical regions, for example, often exhibit behavioral changes reminiscent of those observed after frontal lobe damage. Second, the frontal cortex is not a homogeneous region of the brain but comprises several cytoarchitectonic areas that differ in terms of their connections with other cortical and subcortical areas. Relative to the enormous amount of information that is available about the structural and functional organization of the monkey brain, very little is known of the connections between specific cortical areas in humans. Even with the advent of high-resolution structural imaging, in patient studies it is often not possible to relate any particular area of the frontal cortex to a given cognitive process with any degree of anatomical precision, since the excisions are rarely confined to specific cytoarchitectonic areas. Rather than attempting a broad-brush overview of this complex field, this chapter focuses on three interrelated neuropsychological themes that have emerged as consistent hallmarks of the so-called 'frontal lobe syndrome'; namely, deficits of planning, attentional 'set' and memory. In each case, the specificity of the frontal lobe impairment will be considered, together with related evidence from functional neuro-imaging.

Introduction

Much has been written about the functions of the frontal lobes and the effects of lesions to this region in humans. A summary of this body of work, however succinct, is well beyond the scope of this chapter and will not be attempted here. In short, disturbances of attentional function,[1-3] reasoning and planning,[4-5] the ability to utilize past experience or regulate behavior according to instructions,[4,6,7] initiative, spontaneity and verbal and constructional fluency,[4,8] spatial orientation,[9,10] social affect and global features of personality[3,7] have all been reported after frontal lobe damage in humans. Parallel lesion studies in primates and other mammals have demonstrated deficits in cognitive,[11,12] motivational[13] and social[14-17] behavior that essentially mirror the results of these human studies.

Against this background, it is perhaps not surprising that no clear consensus has been reached as to whether any or all of these deficits can be understood in terms of the disruption of a common underlying mechanism. Broadly speaking, the frontal lobes appear to be essential for tasks that require anticipation, reasoning, goal establishment, planning, the organization of behavior in time and space and monitoring of feedback; terms that are often subsumed under the heading 'executive functions'. The executive functions therefore control the temporal organization of behavior, whether expressed through a motor or a mental act.[18]

Planning

Historically, patients with 'executive dysfunction' were often described as lacking initiative and the organizational abilities required for everyday situations.[19] For example, Penfield and Evans[20] described a young housewife with a right frontal lobe tumor who was unable to plan and prepare a family meal but was, nevertheless, perfectly capable of cooking the individual dishes. Experimentally, such patterns of behavior are usually accounted for in terms of deficits in the cognitive processes involved in planning, and several studies have addressed this issue directly. An early investigation by Porteus and Kepner[21] established that, following prefrontal leucotomy, patients were impaired in maze learning, a deficit attributed to a loss of 'planning skill'. A more direct approach was taken by Klosowska,[22] who developed a novel task that specifically required the development of a plan for successful performance. Subjects were shown a number of objects on a table and were given a specific goal (to cork a bottle). This goal could only be reached by combining a number of discrete steps into a comprehensive plan of action, and then executing each step in the correct order. Fifty patients with unilateral or bilateral frontal lobe damage of mixed etiology exhibited a marked deficit on the task relative to a group of 25 patients with more posterior lesions.

While the tasks developed by Klosowska,[22] and earlier by Porteus and Kepner,[21] certainly appear to require cognitive planning, they also have strong visuospatial components which may have independently contributed to the deficits described. To overcome this difficulty, Shallice and McCarthy (described in Shallice[5]), developed the 'Tower of London' test, a series of problems thought to depend more heavily on planning than on spatial-processing abilities. In this test, subjects are required to move colored disks or balls between three vertical rods[5] or 'pockets'[23,24] of different lengths in order to match a goal arrangement. The difficulty of the problem can be manipulated by varying the starting position of the initial arrangement with respect to the goal arrangement. Shallice[5] demonstrated that patients with left anterior cortical pathology required more moves to complete the Tower of London problems. This finding could not be explained in terms of visuospatial factors, since the results were unchanged when performance was covaried against performance on the spatially demanding Block Design subtest of the Wechsler Adult Intelligence Scale (WAIS). More recently, Owen et al[23] employed a computerized version of the Tower of London task (Figure 5.1) to assess 26 neurosurgical patients with unilateral or bilateral frontal lobe excisions, and later[24] a group of 20 patients with unilateral temporal lobe excisions and 11 patients in whom the more selective amygdalohippocampectomy had been performed. Compared to age- and IQ-matched controls, the frontal lobe group required more moves to complete the problems and, overall, produced fewer perfect solutions. Initial 'thinking' or 'planning' time was unimpaired in these patients, although the amount of time spent thinking on line (i.e. subsequent to the first move) was significantly prolonged. This pattern of impairment appears to be relatively specific at the cortical level, since no deficits were observed in a group of neurosurgical patients with damage to the medial temporal lobe region (Figure 5.2).[24]

In a follow-up study,[25] the Tower of London task was modified to examine the relationship between thinking (planning) time, problem difficulty and solution accuracy in the group of patients with frontal lobe excisions. Subjects were required to study each of the original Tower of London problems and then to decide how many moves would be required to reach an ideal solution (i.e. with the minimum number of moves), without actually moving any of the balls. Because this modification required subjects to evaluate and solve the problems in full, without executing any of the necessary sub goals (i.e. moving the balls), it was no longer possible to compromise 'initial planning time' (i.e. the time before a response was made) in favor of 'on-line' consideration of the problem during the execu-

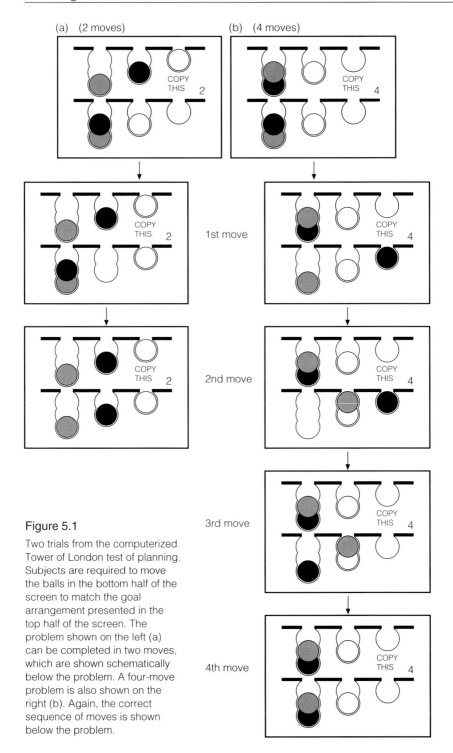

Figure 5.1

Two trials from the computerized Tower of London test of planning. Subjects are required to move the balls in the bottom half of the screen to match the goal arrangement presented in the top half of the screen. The problem shown on the left (a) can be completed in two moves, which are shown schematically below the problem. A four-move problem is also shown on the right (b). Again, the correct sequence of moves is shown below the problem.

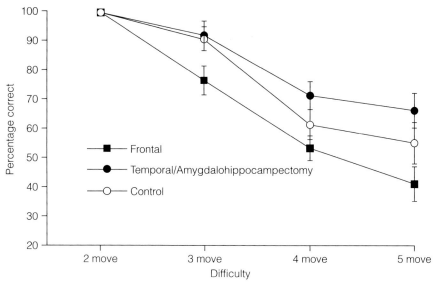

Figure 5.2

The performance of patients with frontal lobe damage and a combined group of patients with temporal lobe removals or amygdalohippocampectomy on the Tower of London task. Data represent the percentage of problems solved perfectly (within the minimum number of moves). Bars represent standard error of the mean (SEM). (Adapted from Owen et al.[23,24])

tion of the solution (i.e. 'subsequent thinking time'). This modification served to encourage subjects to plan the solution in full, before they initiated a response. In the frontal lobe patients, the results of the previous study were essentially confirmed; that is, compared to the matched control group, the frontal lobe patients were significantly impaired in terms of solution accuracy, while solution latency (or 'initial thinking time'), was relatively preserved. One might have expected to see prolonged thinking times in the frontal lobe group, given those patients' profound difficulty with solving these problems and the fact that prolonged 'subsequent thinking' times on the earlier version of this task were reported previously.[23] In the previous study, however, prolonged *subsequent* thinking time in frontal lobe patients was assumed to reflect the additional time required to revise and refine a solution following an inadequately planned, or impulsive, attempt to solve the problem. Because performance on the modified Tower of London task used in the later study was measured by a single response, the results further suggest that the behavior of frontal lobe patients in tests that require forward thinking or planning is indeed impulsive; that is, these patients initiate a response, or make the first move, before they have successfully generated an appropriate solution to the problem, a view consistent with the conclusions of other investigators (e.g. Stuss and Benson[26]).

In summary, the results of the studies described above make a convincing case for a significant association between cognitive planning and the frontal cortex in humans.

Attentional 'set'

Although clinically the inability to plan is perhaps the most consistently reported prefrontal symptom, the deficit is rarely observed in isolation. For example, Ackerley and Benton[27] described a typical patient who had suffered bilateral frontal lobe damage during the perinatal period or at birth. While IQ, memory, perceptual speed and visuomotor coordination were unaffected, two very striking behavioral abnormalities were reported. First, the patient's interest was confined almost exclusively to the immediate present; he was unconcerned about the past and made few, if any, plans for the future. Second, he appeared to be unable to maintain or shift mental set. Thus, if performing one task, he was unable to perform another. Such 'behavioral rigidity' is one of the most clearly defined characteristics of frontal lobe patients and is often investigated using tests that involve 'sorting' or 'concept formation'.[4,28–33] The Wisconsin Card Sorting Test (WCST)[34,35] is the most widely used, and simply requires that subjects sort a deck of cards according to a number of dimensions. Each card varies in three dimensions — number, color and shape — and as each card is presented, the subject is required to match it according to a specified dimension. After a certain number of correct 'sorts', the principle is changed and the subject is required to begin sorting according to an alternative dimension. Most studies have suggested that frontal lobe patients complete fewer categories and make more perseverative errors than controls on this task, continuing to sort cards according to a previous rule, even when the rule has been explicitly changed (e.g. from color to shape). For example, Milner[4] reported that these patients make significantly more 'perseverative' than 'non-perseverative' errors. Subsequent studies[29–31] have suggested that perseveration on the WCST is a relatively specific indicator of frontal lobe dysfunction and usually interpret the deficit as one of impaired attentional set-shifting ability. The term 'set', used in this context, refers to a predisposition to attend selectively to a particular stimulus dimension (such as 'color' or 'shape'), established on the basis of reinforcing feedback (i.e. 'correct' or 'incorrect' cues). In fact, the WCST also tests the ability to *form* a response set and to *maintain* it in the face of distraction from competing stimulus dimensions.

On the basis of clinical data alone, it has not been possible to define a specific area within the frontal cortex which is critically involved in this task, since dorsolateral,[35,36] orbitofrontal,[33] and medial[29] regions have all been implicated in separate studies. In fact, it has been argued that the

WCST is not differentially sensitive to frontal lobe damage at all, since generalized or diffuse brain injury can produce similar cognitive deficits.[31,37,38] Moreover, in several studies, no impairment has been found in cases of known frontal lobe pathology,[29,35,39] while in others, significant effects have been demonstrated following localized damage to specific non-frontal regions.[40,41]

The WCST involves a number of distinct cognitive operations, only some of which may be dependent on the integrity of the frontal lobes. Several recent studies[23,42–44] have argued that pure 'set-shifting ability' may be more accurately assessed using the intra- and extradimensional shifting paradigms described frequently in the animal-learning literature.[45,46] An 'intradimensional shift' (IDS) occurs when a subject is required to cease responding to one exemplar of a particular stimulus dimension (e.g. 'blue' from the dimension 'color') and must begin responding to a new exemplar of that same dimension (e.g. 'red'). An 'extradimensional shift' (EDS) occurs when a subject is required to switch responding to a novel exemplar of a previously irrelevant dimension (e.g. from 'blue' to 'squares' from the dimension 'shape'). In one study, a group of neurosurgical patients with frontal lobe lesions were shown to be specifically impaired in their ability to shift response set to the previously irrelevant stimulus dimension (i.e. at the EDS stage of learning) but not to shift attention to new exemplars of a previously relevant dimension (i.e. at the IDS stage of learning[47]). By comparison, patients with medial temporal lobe excisions were not impaired in their ability to perform either shift. In a follow-up study,[44] the EDS effect was decomposed further, and patients with frontal lobe damage were shown to be selectively impaired in their ability to shift attention away *from* a previously relevant stimulus dimension and not *to* a previously irrelevant dimension (Figure 5.3). This finding essentially confirms previous suggestions that the behavior of these patients on test which require a shift of attentional set is indeed specifically perseverative.[28–31,35]

Memory

While deficits in planning and set-shifting have been central concepts in the description of patients with frontal lobe damage, recent evidence suggests that these symptoms form only part of a more complex neuropsychological profile which may involve many other aspects of cognition. For example, although the prefrontal cortex was implicated in memory processes as early as 1936, with the pioneering work of Jacobsen,[12] in recent years this region has emerged as a primary contributor to many aspects of mnemonic processing. There are two reasons for this. First, recent electrophysiological recording studies in the monkey have identified neurons within the prefrontal cortex that respond preferentially

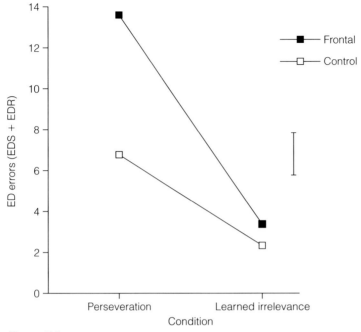

Figure 5.3

The performance of patients with frontal lobe damage on the extradimensional shift task described by Owen et al.[44] Data represent the mean total errors to reach criterion for the perseveration and learned irrelevance conditions. Bars represent one standard error of the difference between the means. (ED: Extra dimensional; EDS: Extra dimensional shift; EDR: Extra dimensional shift reversal.)

during the delay period of memory tasks[48,49] (see Rushworth and Owen[50] for a review). Second, with the emergence of positron emission tomography (PET) and functional magnetic resonance imaging (fMRI) as viable tools for investigating cortical functioning in vivo in humans, numerous memory-related 'activations' have been reported in regions of the frontal lobe previously assumed to be uninvolved in mnemonic processing.

Recent studies in patients with neurosurgical excisions of the frontal cortex[23,24,51] have demonstrated that damage to this area can impair performance on certain types of memory tasks, although it is important to emphasize that, on many tests, performance remains unaffected. For example, Owen et al[24] compared three groups of patients (with frontal lobe excisions, temporal lobe removals or unilateral amygdalohippocampectomy) on a computerized battery of tasks designed to assess visuospatial short-term recognition memory and learning. In one task, the patients were required to remember a complex visual pattern for up to 12 s and then to select that pattern from among three distractors. In the two posterior lesion groups, significant deficits were observed, while the frontal lobe group performed at an equivalent level to controls. Unlike the temporal lobe and amygdalohippocampectomy groups, the frontal lobe patients were also unimpaired at a pattern recognition memory task which required that they remember a series of 12 abstract color patterns and then select from sequentially presented pairs of stimuli those that had been seen previously.

The results of this study[24] are typical of many neuropsychological investigations which have shown that patients with frontal lobe lesions are often largely unimpaired on standard tests of memory.[52,53] For example, Wheeler et al[54] recently investigated the relationship between frontal lobe lesions and performance on episodic memory retrieval tasks through a review of neuropsychological studies carried out since 1984. Less than half of these studies (44%) reported a significant impairment in pre-frontal-lesioned patients when compared to normal subjects. This pattern stands in stark contrast to the plethora of functional neuroimaging studies that have reported frontal lobe activation foci in healthy control subjects performing various memory tasks (see Lee et al[55]). This discrepancy between the results of classic neuropsychological investigations and more recent functional neuroimaging studies suggests that while the frontal lobes may be actively involved in many memory tasks, they may not be critical for normal performance to occur. Importantly, this relation-ship appears not to be related in any direct way to the classic distinction between declarative ('episodic' and 'semantic') memory and short-term or 'working' memory, since preserved performance may be observed in frontal lobe patients on both types of task.[24,51,54]

With this in mind, it is clear that further insights into the role of human frontal cortex in memory are likely to emerge from careful comparisons between studies such as those described above (in which preserved performance is observed in patients with frontal lobe damage) and stud-ies of other types of mnemonic processes which can be shown to be more critically dependent on the frontal lobe. In one recent study, 32 neu-rosurgical patients with unilateral or bilateral frontal lobe excisions, 41 patients with unilateral temporal lobe lesions and 19 patients who had undergone unilateral amygdalohippocampectomy were compared to matched controls on a computerized spatial searching task which taps aspects of working memory.[51] This task is essentially a modification of a test used by Passingham[56] to examine the effects of prefrontal cortex lesions in primates, and conceptually similar to the 'radial arm maze' which has been successfully used to assess working memory in rats.[57] Subjects were required to 'search through' a number of colored boxes presented on the computer screen (by touching each one) in order to find blue 'tokens' which were hidden inside. The object was to avoid those boxes in which a token had already been found. Clearly, like the recognition memory tasks described above, this test places a significant load on memory, although, unlike those tests, it also requires the active reorganization and manipulation of information within memory, factors which interact closely with the more fundamental mnemonic requirements to affect performance. For example, control subjects often adopt a search strategy which involves retracing a systematic 'route' and 'editing' or 'monitoring' those locations where tokens have been found previously. This search strategy can be captured by an index which is demonstrably uncontaminated by overall mnemonic performance[23,51] and yet which correlates highly with such performance.[58] Neurosurgical patients with frontal lobe damage are significantly impaired on this 'strategic' searching task and make more returns to boxes in which a token has previously been found ('between-search' errors) even at the simplest levels of task difficulty (Figure 5.4).[23,24,51] In addition, these patients are less efficient in the use of the repetitive searching strategy described above, confirming that at least some of their memory impairment may arise secondarily from a more fundamental deficit in the use of organizational strategies. In contrast, deficits in the temporal lobe group and the amygdalohippocampectomy group were only observed at the most difficult level of the task, and in neither group could the deficit be related to the inefficient use of any particular searching strategy (Figure 5.4).

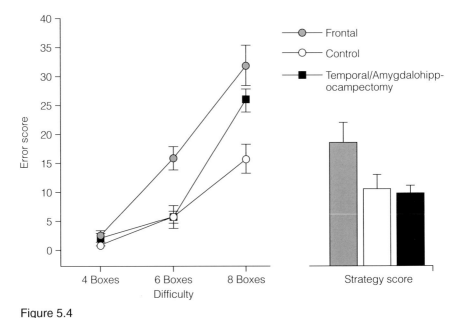

Figure 5.4

The performance of patients with frontal lobe damage and a combined group of patients with temporal lobe removals or amygdalohippocampectomy on the strategic spatial working memory task reported by Owen et al.[23,51] On the left, the mean number of 'between-search errors' is shown for each level of problem difficulty. On the right, the estimated strategy score is shown. In both cases, bars represent the standard error of the mean (SEM).

In a follow-up study, the three patient groups were compared on analogous computerized tests, including one of visual working memory involving a self-ordered search of abstract visual patterns. Although both the temporal lobe patients and the amygdalohippocampectomy group were significantly impaired in the visual working memory test, as they were in the spatial working memory analog of that task, no deficits were observed in the frontal lobe group. Importantly, the impairment in the two posterior groups in terms of errors was not related to any detectable impairment in the extent to which any search strategy was employed to solve the task. In fact, unlike in the spatial search task, no systematic searching strategy could be identified which could be employed to effectively improve overall performance (for discussion see Owen et al[51]).

The results described above suggest that frontal lobe patients may be specifically impaired on tasks for which a strategy exists that may be employed to alleviate the load on working memory imposed by the task. This conclusion substantiates previous suggestions by other investigators that the behavior of frontal lobe patients on certain memory tasks on which they are impaired reflects 'poor organizational strategies, poor monitoring of responses or both.[59] Poor 'cognitive strategies' have also been described in relation to the deficits that are observed in frontal lobe patients performing tasks which require 'estimates' or 'logical reasoning'.[53,60] Organizational 'strategies', when applied to self-ordered searching tasks of the type described here, may serve to reduce the overall load on working memory, and would, presumably, improve performance at all levels of task difficulty.

One general theoretical framework for understanding the role played by the prefrontal cortex in mnemonic processing and its relationship to more posterior cortical association systems is that proposed by Petrides,[61] based originally on lesion studies in the monkey. According to that model, basic memory functions, including storage and immediate processing of incoming and recalled information, are carried out within sensory specific and multimodal posterior association areas in the parietal and temporal cortices. Thus, these areas are principally concerned not only with perceptual processing and long-term storage of information, but also short-term retention and integration of new or recently recalled information. One obvious advantage of this model is that the frontal lobes are not necessarily required in all forms of memory encoding and retrieval, particularly where relatively 'automatic' (i.e. passive) processing of information is involved. Thus, in situations that involve incidental learning or the encoding of relatively simple stimuli or short uninterrupted retention intervals, successful retrieval may occur on the basis of stimulus familiarity alone and may require no additional higher-order memory processing. Thus, the common observation discussed above that patients with frontal lobe lesions can perform perfectly well on certain tasks which undoubtedly tap episodic and working memory processes (e.g. Owen et al[24]) does not contravene the assumptions of the model. The frontal lobes may, however, receive and act upon this information via bidirectional connections between the posterior cortical association areas and the ventrolateral frontal cortex, which, in turn, is closely connected to the mid-dorsolateral frontal cortex, or via direct connections between dorsal regions of the frontal cortex and the medial temporal lobe. Thus the ventrolateral frontal cortex constitutes the first level of interaction between posterior cortical regions and the entire lateral frontal cortex and, in this capacity, this ventral area is assumed to be critical for various 'second-order' memory processes, such as comparisons between, or judgments about, the occurrence or non-occurrence of remembered stimuli. In this sense, the ventrolateral frontal cortex may trigger active low-level encoding strategies such as rehearsal and may initiate explicit (i.e. intentional) retrieval of information from long-term memory. In the case of working memory, this would correspond to the relatively straightforward mapping of stimuli to responses such as that which is assumed to occur in spatial and digit span tasks[23,62] or even simple delayed matching to sample paradigms.[63] In the case of long-term episodic memory (e.g. verbal paired associate learning), these more active encoding and retrieval processes might correspond to the active mapping and implementation of a somewhat arbitrary learned response (e.g. a category exemplar) to a specific stimulus (e.g. a category name). In contrast, the mid-dorsolateral frontal cortex is assumed to provide a third level of processing within memory and is recruited when active manipulation or 'monitoring' of remembered information is required. For example, as described above, in the more complex self-ordered spatial working memory tasks that are sensitive to frontal lobe damage,[23,51] an encoding strategy for determining the optimal sequence of choices is required which must be constantly updated or 'monitored' during its execution (for further discussion see Owen et al[51]).

In neural terms, one critical aspect of this and similar contemporary models is that memory is assumed to depend upon a close functional interaction between sensory specific and multimodal posterior association areas and more dynamically flexible 'executive' regions within the frontal lobe. Thus, while conscious recall of remembered information may be preferentially mediated by the prefrontal cortex,[61,64] passive recognition and familiarity judgments may be accomplished by more posterior medial temporal lobe regions. In this light, this apparent incongruity between results from brain-damaged patients and functional neuroimaging can be more clearly understood. Thus, many episodic memory tasks can be performed adequately in a number of different ways; for example, on the basis of judgments of relative familiarity or through the active (conscious) recollection of encoded information.[65,66] On seeing a test stimulus, a subject may decide that it appears familiar but be unable specifically to recall having seen the stimulus before or any information about the stimulus. Wheeler et al[54] reported that while only 8% and 50%

of neuropsychological studies since 1984 demonstrated that prefrontal patients are significantly impaired on recognition and cued recall tasks, respectively, 80% of these studies reported significant impairments in frontal lobe patients on tests of free recall. Similarly, prefrontal patients have been shown to be impaired on tests that require memory for temporal and sequential information,[36,67–69] while, as we describe above, pattern recognition memory and simple delayed matching to sample are relatively unaffected.[24] These findings suggest that, in recall, the prefrontal cortex is only essential when the retrieval of stored information is self-initiated and depends on strategies generated by the subject in the absence of external cues.[70,71]

Discussion

In the previous three sections, characteristic patterns of impairment have been described in groups of patients with localized excisions of the frontal cortex. On the basis of the studies described, one might predict that planning deficits in patients with frontal lobe damage would be accompanied by impairments on tests of working memory function and attentional set-shifting. In fact, neurosurgical patients with frontal lobe damage who are impaired on the Tower of London task are also frequently impaired on tests of attentional set-shifting and on the spatial working memory task described above, making more returns to boxes in which a token has previously been found, even at the simplest levels of task difficulty.[23,24,51] However, while aspects of planning, attention and memory may all be affected by widespread damage to this area, they may depend upon differential involvement within this structure. Importantly, the frontal cortex is not a homogeneous region of the brain, but comprises several architectonic areas that differ in terms of their connections with other cortical and subcortical areas.[72] Experimental lesions in non-human primates performing similar tasks to those used to assess the effect of frontal lobe lesions in humans suggest, for example, that working memory is especially sensitive to dorsolateral frontal lobe damage,[73] whereas aspects of attentional set-shifting may be dependent on orbitofrontal damage.[74] In patient studies, it is not possible to establish which areas of the frontal cortex are involved in a given cognitive process with any degree of anatomical precision, since the excisions are rarely confined to specific cytoarchitectonic areas. In recent years, functional neuroimaging techniques such as single photon emission tomography (SPECT), PET and fMRI have provided new opportunities for assessing the relationship between patterns of cortical and subcortical activation and different aspects of cognitive processing in healthy control volunteers. The most widely used blood-flow activation techniques use regional cerebral blood flow (rCBF) as an indirect index of neuronal (synaptic) activity. Several SPECT studies of normal subjects have demonstrated increased cerebral blood flow in the frontal cortex during versions of the Tower of London task,[75,76] further implicating this region in some of the higher-level processes involved in planning. However, the spatial resolution of neuroimaging techniques such as SPECT is inadequate for investigating functional specialization within the human frontal cortex, given the large number of distinct cytoarchitectonic areas within this region. More recent studies have measured rCBF using PET, which has improved spatial resolution, combined with structural MRI to achieve a higher degree of precision with respect to neuroanatomical localization. Several PET studies have reported activation in the mid-dorsolateral frontal region during tests of planning,[77–79] working memory (for review, see Owen[80]) and attentional set-shifting.[81] While one possible interpretation of this pattern of findings is that specific regions of the prefrontal cortex are dynamically flexible, with neurons within these regions being able to adapt their properties to the solution of diverse cognitive problems, some functional specialization within the frontal cortex seems inevitable. A more parsimonious explanation is that some degree of functional segregation may exist within the frontal cortex, although the structural organization of this system may not relate, in any straightforward way, to contemporary models of cognition. Successful planning on tests such as the Tower of London task requires working memory, for both the storage and execution of a correct sequence and also in the search processes required in any analytical problem of this type, by which possible solutions are tried and tested, and then accepted or rejected. Given that frontal lobe patients are specifically impaired in 'strategic' aspects of performance on the spatial working memory test, the inappropriate use of organizational strategies to assess the problems may also explain the deficit observed in the Tower of London planning task. The results of these behavioral studies suggest an association, therefore, between aspects of cognitive planning and working memory. Furthermore, in normal control subjects, strong inter-relationships are observed between different tasks which emphasize either planning or working memory,[82] while, as noted above, in frontal lobe patients deficits are observed in both types of task.[23,24] However, the relationship between planning and working memory on the one hand and attentional set-shifting on the other is currently rather less clear; for example, in normal control subjects, significant inter-relationships are not observed between these two types of task, suggesting that they may, in fact, rely on separate neural substrates.[82]

In future, increasingly sophisticated functional imaging techniques such as PET and fMRI will supplement such comparisons between groups of patients with different pathology of both cortico-cortical and cortico-subcortical circuitry and provide a mechanism by which the neural underpinnings of some of the deficits described can be more clearly defined. Such investigations, when combined with information derived from cognitive psychology, neuropsychology and neurobiology, can only improve our understanding of the relationship between brain and behavior and help to further refine the way we think about planning, working memory and other complex cognitive processes in terms of the precise mechanisms involved.

References

1. Knight RT. Decreased response to novel stimuli after prefrontal lesions in man. *Electroencephalogr Clin Neurophysiol* (1984) **59:** 9–20.

2. Luria AR, Karpov BA, Yarbuss AL. Disturbances of active visual perception with lesions of frontal lobes. *Cortex*, (1966) **2:** 202–12.

3. Rylander G. *Personality Changes after Operations on the Frontal Lobes.* (Copenhagen: Munksgaard, 1939).

4. Milner B. Some effects of frontal lobectomy in man. In Warren JM, Akert K (eds) *The Frontal Granular Cortex and Behaviour.* (New York: McGraw-Hill, 1964): 313–31.

5. Shallice T. Specific impairments of planning. *Philos Trans R Soc Lond B* (1982) **298:** 199–209.

6. Denny-Brown D. The frontal lobes and their function. In Feiling A. (ed.) *Modern Trends in Neurology* (New York: Hoeber, 1951): 13–89.

7. Luria AR. *Higher Cortical Functions in Man.* (New York: Basic, 1966).

8. Jones-Gottman M, Milner B. Design fluency: the invention of nonsense drawings after focal lesions. *Neuropsychologia* (1977) **15:** 653–74.

9. Corkin S. Tactually-guided maze learning in man: effects of unilateral cortical excisions and bilateral hippocampal lesions. *Neuropsychologia* (1965) **3:** 339–51.

10. Semmes J, Weinstein S, Ghent L, Tueber H-L. Correlates of impaired orientation in personal and extrapersonal space. *Brain* (1963) **86:** 747–72.

11. Harlow HF, Davis RT, Settlage PH, Meyer DR. Analysis of frontal and posterior association syndromes in brain-damaged monkeys. *J Comp Physiol Psychol* (1952) **45:** 419–29.

12. Jacobsen CF. Studies of cerebral function in primates. *Comparative Psychol Monogr* (1936) **13:** 1–68.

13. Fulton JF. *Frontal Lobotomy and Affective Behavior* (New York: Norton, 1950).

14. Butter CM, Snyder DR. Alterations in aversive and aggressive behaviours following orbital frontal lesions in rhesus monkeys. *Acta Neurobiol Exp (Warsz)* (1972) **32:** 525–65.

15. Butters N, Pandya N, Stein D, Rosen J. A search for the spatial engram within the frontal lobes of monkeys. *Acta Neurobiol Exp (Warsz)* (1972) **32:** 305–29.

16. Franzen EA, Myers RE. Neural control of social behavior: prefrontal and anterior temporal cortex. *Neuropsychologia* (1973) **11:** 141–57.

17. Myers RE, Swett C, Miller M. Loss of social group affinity following prefrontal lesions in free-ranging macaques. *Brain Res* (1973) **64:** 257–69.

18. Fuster JM. *The Prefrontal Cortex:*

Anatomy, Physiology, and Neuropsychology of the Frontal Lobe, 3rd edn (Philadelphia: Lippincott-Raven Publishers, 1997).

19. Luria AR. Frontal-lobe syndromes. In Vinken PJ, Bruyn GW (eds) *Handbook of Clinical Neurology, 2* (Amsterdam: North Holland, 1969): 725–57.

20. Penfield W, Evans J. The frontal lobe in man: a clinical study of maximum removals. *Brain* (1935) **58:** 115–33.

21. Porteus SD, Kepner RD. Mental changes after bilateral prefrontal lobotomy. *Genetic Psychol Monogr* (1944) **29:** 3–115.

22. Klosowska D. Relation between ability to program actions and location of brain damage. *Polish Psychol Bull* (1976) **7:** 245–55.

23. Owen AM, Downes JD, Sahakian BJ et al. Planning and spatial working memory following frontal lobe lesions in man. *Neuropsychologia* (1990) **28:** 1021–34.

24. Owen AM, Sahakian BJ, Semple J et al. Visuo-spatial short-term recognition memory and learning after temporal lobe excisions, frontal lobe excisions or amygdalohippocampectomy in man. *Neuropsychologia* (1995) **33:** 1–24.

25. Owen AM, Sahakian BJ, Hodges JR et al. Dopamine-dependent fronto-striatal planning deficits in early Parkinson's disease. *Neuropsychology* (1995) **9:** 126–40.

26. Stuss DT, Benson DF. Neuropsychological studies of the frontal lobes. *Psychol Bull* (1984) **95:** 3–28.

27. Ackerly SS, Benton AL. Report of a case of bilateral frontal lobe neglect. *Res Publ Assoc Res Nerv Ment Dis* (1947) **27:** 479–504.

28. Cicerone KD, Lazar RM, Shapiro WR. Effects of frontal lobe lesions on hypothesis sampling during concept formation. *Neuropsychologia* (1983) **21:** 513–24.

29. Drewe EA. The effect of type and area of brain lesion on Wisconsin Card Sorting Test performance. *Cortex* (1974) **10:** 159–70.

30. Nelson HE. A modified card sorting test sensitive to frontal lobe defects. *Cortex* (1976) **12:** 313–24.

31. Robinson AL, Heaton RK, Lehman RAW, Stilson DW. The utility of the Wisconsin Card Sorting Test in detecting and localising frontal lobe lesions. *Neuropsychologia* (1980) **48:** 605–14.

32. Rosvold HE, Miskin M. Evaluation of the effects of prefrontal lobotomy on intelligence. *Can J Psychol* (1950) **4:** 122–6.

33. Stuss DT, Benson DF, Kaplan EF et al. The involvement of orbito frontal cerebrum in cognitive tasks. *Neuropsychologia* (1983) **21:** 235–48.

34. Grant DA, Berg EA. A behavioural analysis of degree of reinforcement and ease of shifting to new responses in a Weigl-type card sorting problem. *J Exp Psychol* (1948) **38:** 404–11.

35. Milner B. Effects of different brain lesions on card sorting: the role of the frontal lobes. *Arch Neurol* (1963) **9:** 100–10.

36. Milner B. Interhemispheric differences in the localisation of psychological processes in man. *Br Med Bull* (1971) **27:** 272–7.

37. De Renzi E, Faglioni P, Savoiardo M, Vignolo LA. The influence of aphasia and of the hemispheric side of the cerebral lesion on abstract thinking. *Cortex* (1966) **2:** 399–420.

38. McFie J, Piercy MF. The relation of laterality of lesion to performance on Weigl's sorting test. *J Ment Sci.* (1952) **98:** 299–305.

39. Eslinger PJ, Damasio AR. Severe

disturbance of higher cognition after bilateral frontal lobe ablation: patient EVR. *Neurology* (1985) **35:** 1731–41.

40. Canavan AGM, Passingham RE, Marsden CD et al. The performance on learning tasks of patients in the early stages of Parkinson's disease. *Neuropsychologia* (1989) **27:** 141–56.

41. Teuber H-L, Battersby WS, Bender MB. Performance of complex visual tasks after cerebral lesions. *J Nerv Ment Dis* (1951) **114:** 413–29.

42. Downes JJ, Roberts AC, Sahakian BJ et al. Impaired extra-dimensional shift performance in medicated and unmedicated Parkinson's disease: evidence for a specific attentional dysfunction. *Neuropsychologia* (1989) **27:** 1329–43.

43. Sahakian BJ, Downes JJ, Eagger S et al. Sparing of attentional relative to mnemonic function in a subgroup of patients with dementia of the Alzheimer type. *Neuropsychologia* (1990) **28:** 1197–213.

44. Owen AM, Roberts AC, Hodges JR et al. Contrasting mechanisms of impaired attentional set-shifting in patients with frontal lobe damage or Parkinson's disease. *Brain* (1993) **116:** 1159–79.

45. Mackintosh NJ. *Conditioning and Associative Learning* (Oxford: The Clarendon Press, 1983).

46. Slamecka N. A methodological analysis of shift paradigms in human discrimination learning. *Psychol Bull* (1968) **69:** 423–8.

47. Owen AM, Roberts AC, Polkey CE et al. Extra-dimensional versus intra-dimensional set shifting performance following frontal lobe excisions, temporal lobe excisions or amygdalo-hippocampectomy in man. *Neuropsychologia* (1991) **29:** 993–1006.

48. Rao SC, Rainer G, Miller EK. Integration of what and where in the primate prefrontal cortex. *Science* (1997) **276:** 821–4.

49. Wilson FAW, Scalaidhe SPO, Goldman-Rakic PS. Dissociations of object and spatial processing domains in primate prefrontal cortex. *Science* (1993) **260:** 1955–8.

50. Rushworth MFS, Owen AM. The functional organization of the lateral frontal cortex: conjecture or conjuncture in the electrophysiology literature. *Trends Cogn Sci* (1998) **2:** 46–53.

51. Owen AM, Morris RG, Sahakian BJ et al. Double dissociations of memory and executive functions in working memory tasks following frontal lobe excisions, temporal lobe excisions or amygdalo-hippocampectomy in man. *Brain* (1996) **119:** 1597–615.

52. Smith ML, Milner B. Differential effects of frontal-lobe lesions on cognitive estimation and spatial memory. *Neuropsychologia* (1984) **22:** 697–705.

53. Janowsky JS, Shimamura AP, Squire LR. Source memory impairment in patients with frontal lobe lesions. *Neuropsychologia* (1989) **27:** 1043–56.

54. Wheeler MA, Stuss DT, Tulving E. Frontal lobe damage produces episodic memory impairment. *J Int Neuropsychol Soc* (1995) **1:** 525–36.

55. Lee ACH, Robbins TW, Pickard JD, Owen AM. Asymmetric frontal activation during episodic memory: The effects of stimulus type on encoding and retrieval. *Neuropsychologia* (2000) **38:** 677–92.

56. Passingham RE. Memory of monkeys (Macaca mulatta) with lesions in prefrontal cortex. *Behav Neurosci* (1985) **99:** 3–21.

57. Olton DS, Spatially organised behaviours of animals: behavioural and neurological studies. In

Potegal M (ed.) *Spatial Abilities* (New York: Academic Press, 1982): 325–60.

58. Robbins TW. Dissociating executive functions of the prefrontal cortex. *Philos Trans R Soc Lond B* (1996) **351:** 1463–71.

59. Petrides M, Milner B. Deficits on subject-ordered tasks after frontal and temporal lobe lesions in man. *Neuropsychologia* (1982) **20:** 249–62.

60. Shallice T, Evans ME. The involvement of the frontal lobes in cognitive estimation. *Cortex* (1978) **14:** 294–303.

61. Petrides M. Frontal lobes and working memory: evidence from investigations of the effects of cortical excisions in nonhuman primates. In Boller F, Grafman J (eds) *Handbook of Neuropsychology,* Vol. 9 (Amsterdam: Elsevier, 1994): 59–82.

62. Owen AM, Herrod NJ, Menon DK et al. Redefining the functional organisation of working memory processes within human lateral prefrontal cortex. *Eur J Neurosci* (1999) **11:** 567–74.

63. Elliot R, Dolan RJ. Differential neural responses during performance of matching and non-matching to sample tasks at two delay intervals. *J Neurosci* (1999) **19(12):** 5066–73.

64. Petrides M. Functional organization of the human frontal cortex for mnemonic processing. *Ann NY Acad Sci* (1995) **769:** 85–96.

65. Jacoby LL, Dallas M. On the relationship between autobiographical memory and perceptual learning. *J Exp Psychol Gen* (1981) **110:** 306–40.

66. Mandler G. Recognising: the judgement of previous occurrence. *Psychol Rev* (1980) **87:** 252–71.

67. Milner B, Petrides M, Smith ML. Frontal lobes and the temporal organisation of memory. *Human Neurobiol* (1985) **4:** 137–42.

68. Milner B, Corsi P, Leonard G. Frontal-lobe contribution to recency judgements. *Neuropsychologia* (1991) **29:** 601–18.

69. Shimamura AP, Janowsky JS, Squire LR. Memory for the temporal order of events in patients with frontal lobe lesions and amnesic patients. *Neuropsychologia* (1990) **28:** 803–13.

70. Della Rocchetta AI, Milner B. Strategic search and retrieval inhibition: the role of the frontal lobes. *Neuropsychologia* (1993) **31:** 503–24.

71. Moscovitch M. Cognitive resources and dual-task interference effects at retrieval in normal people: the role of the frontal lobes and medial temporal cortex. *Neuropsychology* (1994) **8:** 524–34.

72. Pandya DN, Barnes CL. Architecture and connections of the frontal lobe. In Perecman E (ed.) *The Frontal Lobes Revisited.* (New York: The IRBN Press, 1987): 41–72.

73. Brozoski TJ, Brown RM, Rosvold HE, Goldman PS. Cognitive deficit caused by regional depletion of dopamine in prefrontal cortex of rhesus monkey. *Science* (1979) **205:** 929–31.

74. Passingham RE. Non-reversal shifts after selective pre-frontal ablation in monkeys (Macaca mulatta). *Neuropsychol* (1972) **10:** 41–6.

75. Morris RG, Ahmed S, Syed GM, Toone BK. Neural correlates of planning ability: frontal lobe activation during the Tower of London test. *Neuropsychol* (1993) **31:** 1367–78.

76. Rezai K, Andreasen NC, Allinger R et al. The neuropsychology of

the prefrontal cortex. *Arch Neurol* (1993) **50:** 636–42.

77. Owen AM, Evans AC, Petrides M. Evidence for a two-stage model of spatial working memory processing within the lateral frontal cortex: a positron emission tomography study. *Cerebral Cortex* (1996) **6:** 31–8.

78. Baker SC, Frith CD, Frackowiak RSJ, Dolan RJ. Active representation of shape and location in man. *Cerebral Cortex* (1996) **6:** 612–19.

79. Dagher A, Owen AM, Brooks DJ. The cortico-subcortical network for planning: a PET activation study with the 'Tower of London'. *Brain* (1999) **122:** 1973–87.

80. Owen AM. The functional organization of working memory processes within human lateral frontal cortex: the contribution of functional neuroimaging. *Eur J Neurosci* (1997) **9:** 1329–39.

81. Rogers RD, Andrews TC, Grasby PM et al. Contrasting cortical and sub-cortical activations produced by attentional set-shifting and reversal learning in humans. *J Cog Neurosci* (2000) **12:** 142–62.

82. Robbins TW, James M, Owen AM et al. A study of performance on tests from the CANTAB battery sensitive to frontal lobe dysfunction in a large sample of normal volunteers: implications for theories of executive function and cognitive ageing. *J Int Neuropsychol Soc* (1998) **4:** 474–90.

83. Owen AM, Doyon J, Petrides M, Evans AC, Planning and spatial working memory examined with positron emission tomography (PET). *Eur J Neurosci* 1996; **8:** 353–364.

84. Goldman-Rakic PS. The frontal lobes: unchartered provinces of the brain. *Trends Neurosci* (1984) **7:** 425–9.

6
Visual defects as a result of occipital lesions

Alidz LM Pambakian and Christopher Kennard

Introduction

The occipital lobes are of fundamental importance in vision. All visual information enters the eye in an undiscriminated form, and is systematically processed so that different attributes, namely form, color, motion orientation and depth, are processed at distinct locations within functionally specialized regions in the visual cortex. These fragments of information are meaningfully integrated so that perceptual and cognitive representations of objects being viewed and their spatial relations to each other are constructed. Since the visual cortex lies within the occipital lobes, characteristic visual syndromes can be recognized as a result of occipital lesions which, if small enough, can cause blindness for a single class of vision. As a result of studies of patients with such focal cortical lesions and artificial lesion work in non-human primates, recent years have seen a great expansion of knowledge about the mechanisms by which the visual world is re-created in the brain.

In this chapter we will broadly describe the relevant anatomy of the visual pathway, to clarify how different modalities of vision become segregated at the level of the cortex. We will then discuss visual syndromes caused by central disorders of vision associated with lesions at specific sites within the occipital lobes.

Anatomy and function of the visual pathway

The visual pathway consists of a series of separate but parallel pathways which relay different types of visual information in two stages: first to subcortical areas in the midbrain and thalamus, and second to functionally specialized cortical regions that are dedicated to processing vision. There are interactions between these pathways at numerous levels from the retina to the cortex, producing an intricate network with feedback and feedforward connections.

Subcortical processing

Visual information reaches the retina, where it is processed before passing along the optic nerves to the chiasm. At the chiasm, fibers from the nasal retina cross to the contralateral side and continue, still in a retinotopic grouping, to join the uncrossed fibers from the temporal retina as the optic tracts, thereby containing visual information for the contralateral visual field. The optic tracts project to two subcortical targets; predominantly to the lateral geniculate nucleus (LGN) of the thalamus, with a much smaller projection to the superior colliculus (SC) of the midbrain. There is an additional sparse projection directly to the extrastriate cortex. Four types of retinal ganglion cells are described in primates, P_α, P_β, P_γ and P_ϵ; these are specialized to transduce different types of visual signals and project to different visual areas. P_β cells are the most numerous and project exclusively to the LGN. They have small receptive fields, which are organized in a center-surround manner. In terms of their function, they are spectrally opponent, with high spatial resolution, and are involved in color and form perception. P_α ganglion cells project to both the LGN and the midbrain. They are also organized in a center-surround manner, but are spatially and not chromatically opponent. They respond transiently to stimulation and are functionally involved in the detection of borders of different luminance, stereopsis and motion perception. P_γ and P_ϵ ganglion cells project primarily to the SC, from where a small number project back to the LGN, and possibly also directly to the LGN. These cells have large receptive fields and are particularly sensitive to motion, but are poorly sensitive to color and form.

Retinal ganglion cells project to points in the LGN in an orderly manner, so that each LGN contains a visuotopic representation of the contralateral half of the visual field. The LGN is made up of six layers of cell bodies interleaved with separating layers of axons and dendrites. The layers are numbered 1–6, from ventral to dorsal. P_α ganglion cells relay in the two most ventral layers (1 and 2), which contain relatively large cells and are called the magnocellular layers, forming the magnocellular pathway. P_β ganglion cells relay in the four dorsal layers (3–6), called the parvocellular layers, forming the parvocellular pathway. Cells projecting to the LGN from the SC terminate in the interlaminar zones. Each of the six layers of the LGN receives its inputs from only one eye. Fibers from the contralateral nasal hemiretina project to layers 1, 4 and 6, whereas fibers from the ipsilateral temporal hemiretina project to layers 2, 3 and 5. The layers of the nucleus are stacked on top of one another, so that it constructs a representation of the contralateral visual hemifield in precise vertical register.

Structure and function of the primary striate visual cortex

Visual information continues through the optic radiations to the next relay point in the visual pathway which is the primary visual cortex, also known as Brodmann's area 17, visual area 1, V1 or the striate cortex. It is composed of six layers of cells (1–6). Layer 4 is further subdivided into four sublayers, 4A, 4B, $4C_\alpha$ and $4C_\beta$. Axons in the magnocellular pathway terminate mainly in sublamina $4C_\alpha$, axons of a group of cells in the parvocellular pathway terminate mainly in sublamina $4C_\beta$, whereas axons from a group of cells in the interlaminar regions of the LGN terminate in layers 2 and 3. Local interneurons integrate activity within the layers of V1 by creating local facilitatory and inhibitory feedback loops.

Unlike cells mentioned previously, cortical cells do not have circular receptive fields and respond to more sophisticated linear stimuli. There are two categories of cells: simple cells have rectangular receptive fields, built up from many circular fields, with a specific axis of orientation. They demonstrate center-surround on–off antagonism. This allows every axis of rotation to be represented for all retinal positions. Complex cells have somewhat larger receptive fields with a critical axis of rotation, but the precise position of a stimulus within the receptive field is less crucial because there are no clearly defined on or off zones. Movement across the receptive field is a particularly effective stimulus for certain complex cells. Both simple and complex cells of V1 receive inputs from the functionally distinct magnocellular and parvocellular pathways. Whereas the magnocellular pathway is mainly concerned with movement and with the rough outlines of visual stimuli, the parvocellular pathway is concerned with color, texture and pattern.

In addition to its horizontal layered structure, V1 is also organized into narrow columns called orientation columns, where layer 4C simple and complex cells with the same axis of orientation are grouped together. In neighboring columns, the axis of orientation shifts by around 10°. In this way, the primary visual cortex deconstructs the visual world into short-line segments of various orientations; this is a primary step in the discrimination of form and movement. The system of orientation columns is interrupted at intervals by blobs, which are patches of cells in layers 2 and 3 of V1 that receive direct connections from the LGN with information about color. A third system is present, comprising alternating columns devoted to either the right or the left eye. They are termed ocular dominance columns, and their purpose is to combine visual information from both eyes, a process which will eventually allow binocular vision and depth perception.

These three systems are combined functionally within the visual cortex to form units called hypercolumns. Each hypercolumn contains the components necessary to analyze a small portion of the visual field, namely, a complete set of orientation columns representing 360°, a set of left and right ocular dominance columns, and several blobs specific for color. These columns are arranged so that a retinotopic map of the contralateral half of the visual field is formed.[1]

In addition to the striate cortex, visual processing takes place in the prestriate cortex (visual association or extrastriate cortex), which, as its name suggests, lies anterior to the striate cortex. The striate cortex is the larger of the two regions and contains a single visual area, V1, in contrast to the smaller prestriate cortex which contains several visual areas. Numerous other visual areas are scattered throughout the parietal and temporal cortex which are of crucial significance in vision, but these are beyond the scope of this chapter and therefore will not be included.

Structure and function of the extrastriate visual cortex

The non-human primate extrastriate cortex is represented in Figure 6.1. Visual information projects initially to V1. V2 occupies the medial surface of the brain surrounding V1. V1 and V2 are physiologically distinct from other visual areas, because they receive information regarding all attributes of vision and segregate it into individual modalities, which are conveyed to appropriate specialized visual areas. Axons project retinotopically from V1 to V2, so that both areas contain a detailed topographical map of the retina. The result is that the upper retina (lower visual field) is represented in the part of V2 which borders the upper lip of the calcarine sulcus, known as the cuneus, whereas the lower retina (upper visual field) is represented in the part of V2 within the lingual gyrus, which borders the lower lip of the calcarine sulcus. V3 is thought

Figure 6.1

(a) Location of human visual cortical areas. (A) and (C) show the location of visual cortical areas, defined by fMRI and specific visual stimulation, in one representative subject (NH). The areas were defined by tests for motion and retinotopy, and painted onto the brain of the same subject, as reconstructed from anatomical MR images. (A) is a view of the medial bank, from a slightly inferior vantage point; the posterior brain axis is shown to the left, and anterior to the right. (C) is a view of the same brain, from a posterior–lateral vantage point. (B) and (D) show identical views of the same brain. The cortical 'areas' painted onto it have been extrapolated from the drawings of Brodmann. Except in the location of area V1, there is very little correspondence between the Brodmann-based and fMRI-based maps. (b) Two-dimensional maps of the cortical visual areas in different subjects. Each map is based on visual tests and fMRI activity acquired from the same subjects. Areas V1, V2, V3, VP, V3a and V4v are classically retinotopic areas. Areas V7, V8 and LOC/LOP are 'fringe' retinotopic areas. We have adopted the term 'MT+', introduced by others, to include area MT and adjacent motion-selective satellite areas such as MST. In different subjects, there are some overall differences in the size of the brain and visual areas, and in the exact area topography and area–sulcal/gyral relationships. However, the areas revealed by the different area-labeling tests are remarkably similar across individual MR subjects. (From Tootell et al.[2])

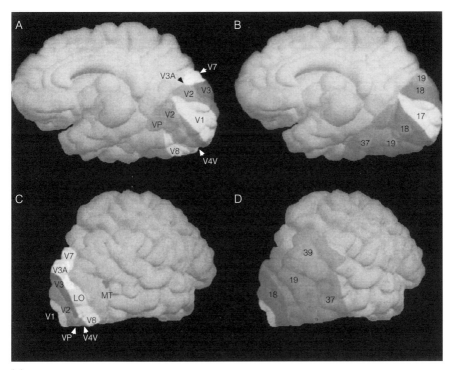

(a)

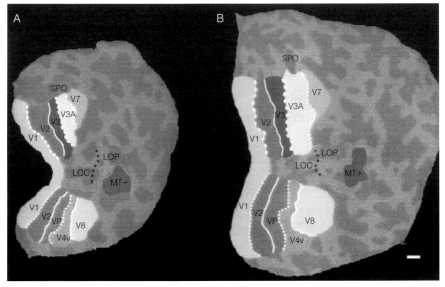

(b)

to be similarly subdivided around the calcarine sulcus. V4 receives inputs predominantly from V2, and information from the central retinal fields in V1, where fewer cones are present. The visual fields are not represented so uniformly in V4, and priority is given to color vision. Area V5 is buried within the superior temporal sulcus, on the lateral aspect of the brain. It receives information from V1 and V2 pertaining to all forms of motion. Area V6 lies on the medial aspect of the brain, within the parietal cortex. It is thought to receive information from V2 regarding depth perception. A similar structural and functional map has been characterized for the human extrastriate cortex.

The description given above is clearly a simplification of the visual pathway and does not take into account the many other subcortical and cortical connections that are known to exist in the same hemisphere and across the corpus callosum. However, it provides enough background information to explain why discrete occipital lobe lesions can cause visual field defects (V1–V3), color vision abnormalities (V4), difficulties with motion perception (V5), object agnosias and loss of stereognosis.[3] Later in the chapter, we will discuss these topics in turn.[4–6]

Dorsal and ventral processing streams

Within these multiple cortical visual areas, there appear to be two main streams of visual processing that are relatively independent (Figure 6.2). The parvocellular pathway has stronger projections to areas such as V4 located in the inferior occipital lobe and the inferior temporal cortex. These regions, along the 'ventral stream', are postulated to form the 'what' pathway, and are involved in the perception of color, luminance, stereopsis, pattern recognition and the identification of objects and faces. The magnocellular pathway has stronger projections to the posterior parietal cortex, including areas such as the middle temporal and medial superior temporal cortex, forming the 'dorsal stream'. This is considered to be the 'where' pathway, which is involved in the spatial localization and movement of objects.[7]

The notion of two separate visual streams is a useful paradigm for understanding clinical syndromes arising from damage to larger territories of the brain, since this occurs more often than damage to a single visual area. For example, damage to the inferior visual cortex, in the occipital lobe and adjacent temporal regions, affects the recognition of objects (agnosias) and faces (prosopagnosia) (Figure 6.3a), induces loss of the ability to read (alexia) and may affect color perception in the contralateral field (achromatopsia) (Figure 6.3a). Damage to the superior visual cortex, in the occipital lobe and adjacent parietal cortex, produces difficulties with judgment of the location, depth, distance, orientation, size and motion (Figure 6.3b) of objects, and affects eye–hand co-ordination.[8–10]

Although the dorsal and ventral visual cortex are associated with differ-

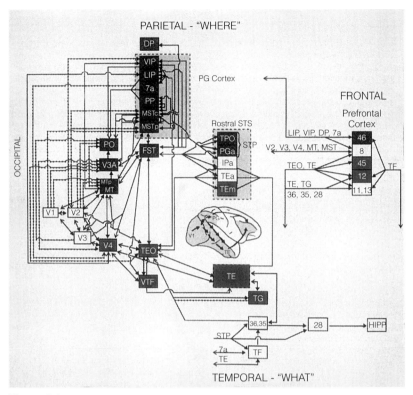

Figure 6.2

The dorsal and ventral processing streams. Abbreviations for visual areas: PO (parieto-occipital), MT (medial temporal), DP (dorsal parietal), VIP (ventral intraparietal), LIP (lateral intraparietal), PP (posterior parietal), MST (medial superior temporal), FST (floor of the superior temporal sulcus). Other abbreviations indicate various temporal areas.

ent, behaviorally separate functions, there is growing evidence that these two major divisions also have overlapping functions and are not indepen-dent of one another.[11]

Visual defects as a result of occipital lobe lesions

Visual field defects

Damage to the visual pathway, from the eye to the visual cortex, is reflected by a disturbance in the field of vision.[12] Because of the invariate ordering of nerve fibers along the visual pathway, lesions at specific sites produce field defects of specific shapes which are of diagnostic value. As a general rule, pregeniculate lesions are uni-ocular or non-congruous,

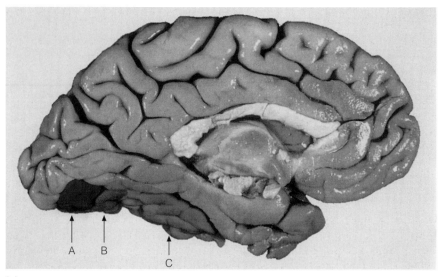

(a)

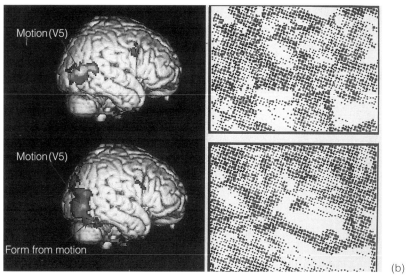

(b)

Figure 6.3

(a) A view of the human brain from the medial side. Zone A is critical for the perception of colors, and lesions here cause achromatopsia; zone B is critical for the perception of faces, and lesions affecting it lead to an incapacity to recognize faces, expecially familiar ones. Lesions in C region cause a variety of problems, including an incapacity to perceive the expression on a face. (b) The maximum changes in blood flow, which is an index of brain activity, are concentrated in area V5 (top left), when subjects see meaningless moving stimuli (top right). By contrast, the activity induced by meaningful moving forms (bottom right: a car can be clearly seen when the image is moving) is not restricted to V5 but also includes an area inferior to it (bottom left). (From Zeki[13].)

whereas retrogeniculate lesions most commonly result in the formation of homonymous hemianopias (loss of vision in one hemifield of both eyes), and less often in quadrantinopias (loss of vision in one quadrant), and scotomas (regions of blindness occurring mainly in the central visual field), which correspond retinotopically to the damaged area (Figure 6.4). Most homonymous hemianopias involve lesions in the contralateral occipital lobe, affecting areas V1–V3, and a few are bilateral, affecting both occipital lobes. Superior and inferior quadrantanopias arise from lesions below or above the calcarine fissure, respectively.

The hallmark of occipital lobe disease is that the resultant field defects are exquisitely congruous. Another feature unique to occipital lobe lesions which can be seen occasionally when the visual fields are plotted is preservation of the temporal crescent. Light emanating from most of the visual field enters both eyes, except for light in the most peripheral part of the temporal hemifield, which only strikes the ipsilateral nasal hemiretina, because it is blocked from the contralateral eye by the nose. This strip of nasal hemiretina is represented by an area of visual cortex lying anteriorly in the contralateral calcarine cortex. It is possible for this section of cortex to be spared by lesions affecting the occipital lobe, giving rise to a hemianopic field defect which spares the so-called 'temporal crescent'. Conversely, it is theoretically possible for a lesion to be restricted to the portion of the visual cortex representing the temporal crescent, resulting in loss of the temporal portion of only one hemifield but not in a hemianopic pattern. At one time, macular sparing (sparing of the most central 1–2° of vision in the hemianopic field) was thought to be a hallmark of occipital hemianopias. However, it is now accepted that the presence or absence of macular sparing is of no use in defining the site of the lesion, and there is still debate as to whether it simply represents a perimetric artefact.

Regarding etiology, 70% of lesions causing field defects are arterial infarctions, 15% tumors, and 5% hemorrhages.

Residual vision

Traditionally, geniculostriate lesions were considered to result in complete and permanent visual loss in the topographically related area of visual field. However, it has become clear that this is not necessarily the case. Work with monkeys and, later, humans demonstrated that, despite destruction of the striate cortex, or even hemispherectomy, some patients retain certain visual functions. Twenty per cent of patients retain the ability to make accurate saccades to visual targets presented tachistoscopically in their blind hemifield. This phenomenon was termed 'blindsight' to emphasize that these residual functions are not consciously perceived and depend on the use of a forced-choice technique. Its functions are thought to be primitive and concerned with the registration and localization of objects, whereas the geniculostriate system is primarily concerned

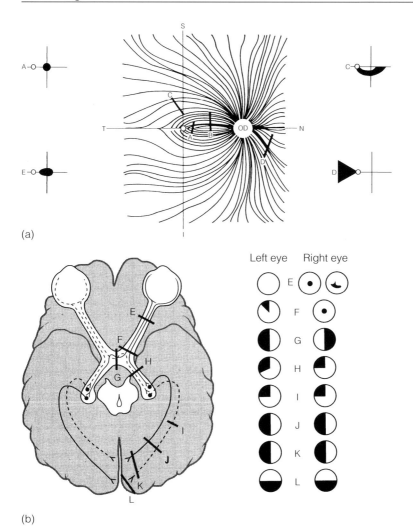

(a)

(b)

Figure 6.4

(a) Patterns of visual field loss. Diagrammatic representation of the retinal nerve fiber layer, with fibers passing towards the optic disk (OD). The resulting visual field defects due to a lesion located in different parts of the layer A–D are shown on either side. I, inferior; N, nasal; S, superior; T, temporal. (b) Patterns of visual field loss. E: optic nerve lesions result in a central scotoma or arcuate defect. F: optic nerve lesions just prior to the chiasm produce junctional scotoma due to ipsilateral nerve involvement with the inferior contralateral crossing fibers (dashed line). G: chiasm lesions produce bitemporal hemianopia. H: optic tract lesions result in incongruous hemianopic defects. I and J: lesions of the optic radiation result in either homonymous quadrantinopia or hemianopia, depending on the extent and location of the lesion (upper quadrant, temporal lobe; lower quadrant, parietal lobe). K: lesions of the striate cortex produce a homonymous hemianopia, sometimes with macular sparing, particularly with vascular disturbances. L: partial lesions of the superior or inferior bank of the striate cortex cause inferior or superior altitudinal defects, respectively.

with their identification.[14–16] A wide range of visual functions is associated with blindsight or residual vision, including spatial localization and discrimination of form, orientation, color and motion. Since these patients no longer have a functional striate cortex on the affected side, blindsight is probably mediated via subcortical structures, such as the SC, with or without projection via the LGN or the inferior pulvinar, to the prestriate cortex. Alternatively, it may involve the sparse projection from the LGN directly to the prestriate cortex (V5). The reason why so few patients with cortical field defects have blindsight remains unclear, and is not adequately explained by differences in lesion anatomy or the patient's age at its onset.[17]

Spontaneous recovery
Visual field defects show some spontaneous improvement, although the degree of resolution depends on the underlying pathology. Up to 50% show spontaneous regression of varying degrees. Vision returns to the perimetrically blind field in definite temporal stages, starting with the perception of light, motion, form, color and finally stereognosis.

Treatment of patients with hemianopia
Patients with hemianopia complain mainly of difficulties with reading and scanning scenes. Consequently, they fail to notice relevant objects or avoid obstacles on their affected side and may collide with approaching people or cars. On the other hand, a small group are unaware of their defects, which are picked up on routine ophthalmic examination.

Cognitive rehabilitation techniques
Over the last 40 years, several research groups have set out to determine whether patients with hemianopia have the ability to compensate for their field defect using eye movements, head movements and extrastriate vision. Some have integrated this information into training techniques aimed at systematically reinforcing compensatory oculomotor strategies, thereby fortifying and enlarging the field of search. Other groups, inspired by the success of animal physiologists in restoring the lost visual field of nonhuman primates, attempted to reproduce the results in humans, using similar training techniques.[18]

Spatial contrast sensitivity

Occipital lesions do not interfere with visual acuity as measured with Snellen charts or reading test types. Nevertheless, some patients with unilateral or bilateral occipital lobe lesions complain of blurred or foggy vision and that letters merge together, even though their acuities, pupil responses and eye movements are normal. Such patients may have impaired spatial contrast sensitivity.

Standard tests of acuity measure the ability to resolve small detail at high contrast, yet everyday visual experience is not a high-contrast phenomenon. Visual scenes are made up of both steep and shallow transitions of contrast. Therefore, visual acuity in its usual measured form does not truly represent the ability to discriminate form. The measurement of contrast sensitivity can demonstrate the acuity problems missed by standard tests. It determines the minimum contrast necessary for detecting test figures of various sizes. The most common test pattern used is a grating where the transition from light to dark is gradual and the luminance profile of the pattern can be represented by a sinusoidal waveform. Patients with occipital lesions have abnormal contrast sensitivities, suggesting that their visual symptoms may be caused by damage to frequency-selective neurons and their connections in the cortex.

Regarding recovery, the spatial contrast sensitivity of some patients has improved noticeably following treatment of their lesion, for example the surgical debulking of an occipital tumor, while in others it remained permanently disturbed.

Photopic and scotopic adaptation

Patients with uni- or bilateral occipital lesions can have problems with light (photopic) or dark (scotopic) adaptation. Occasionally, both light and dark adaptation can be affected in the same patient. Patients with impaired light adaptation are dazzled by normal daylight or artificial light, and reading text on a white page causes blinding and blurring of the words. Patients with impaired dark adaptation complain that the world appears so dark that they are unable to identify objects, faces or text with normal illumination. Treatment is limited to the use of sunglasses for patients with defective light adaptation, and increasing the level of ambient light for those with impaired dark adaptation.

Color vision abnormalities of central origin

Dyschromatopsia and achromatopsia
Acquired changes in color vision (dyschromatopsia) are predominantly a sign of anterior visual pathway disease. However, unilateral lesions of the occipital lobe may rarely cause previously normal color vision to be impaired in the contralateral hemifield or superior quadrant, but never the lower quadrant alone, with preservation of form vision.[19] Postmortem data and studies using three-dimensional MR localization studies, together with PET analysis in normals and patients, have implicated the lingual and fusiform gyri as the focal sites of cortical damage. These gyri lie inferiorly in the occipital lobe, an observation that explains the predominance of dyschromatopsia in the upper field quadrants.[20–22]

The degree of impairment can vary from hemidyschromatopsia, where patients retain some capacity for color discrimination, to hemiacromatopsia, where color appreciation is completely lost and patients perceive the world in shades of gray. For this reason, patients may not be aware of their defect and simply complain of a non-specific unpleasant sensation or that brightly saturated colors look pale. Their abnormalities can be detected by use of Ishiahara pseudoisochromatic plates, the Farnsworth–Munsell (FM) 100-hue test, and by plotting visual fields with colored targets. Since color is processed in both cerebral hemispheres, patients with bilateral occipital lesions may develop cerebral dyschromatopsia, where color vision is affected to some degree in the entire visual field, or cerebral achromatopsia, where color vision is completely lost, resulting in significant disability.[23,24]

Patients often have additional problems in recognizing familiar faces (prosopagnosia), recognizing previously familiar objects (agnosia), reading (alexia), topographic disorientation (topographagnosia) and impairments of visual memory. However, these deficits are not necessary accompaniments to dyschromatopsia, but are consistent with the concept of damage to areas served by the ventral processing stream.

Various groups have attempted to treat dyschromatopsias/achromatopsias with training programs of specific practice, with some degree of success, but the technique remains experimental.[25–27]

Color anomia

Patients with color anomia are unable to name colors or point to colors when given their names, in the absence of a demonstrable defect of color perception or aphasia. Such patients perform normally on the FM 100-hue test. They tend to have left occipital lesions which are associated with a right homonymous hemianopia, and the lesion usually lies mesially at the junction of the occipital and temporal lobes in the left hemisphere. It is not known whether this is due to a deficit of a specific step in color processing, which takes place in this region, or to a disconnection of color information, via the corpus callosum to the left hemisphere: because of the complete right homonymous hemianopia, visual input to language areas in the left hemisphere must arise from the right visual cortex. A coexisting lesion of the splenium of the corpus callosum interrupts this process, so that patients can percieve colors but cannot name them.[25,28]

Color-naming defect

Patients with color-naming defects are unable to name colors, but can point to the correct color when the name is given. This deficit is usually associated with other aphasic syndromes.[25]

Visual space perception

Disorders of visual space perception can be observed following unilateral or bilateral parieto-occipital injury. Various disabilities result, ranging from elementary problems with visual localization to complex disorders of spatial appreciation and visuo-construction. Following a unilateral posterior brain lesion, patients may have problems localizing accurately in the contralateral hemifield, although, rarely, both hemifields can be affected. The most severe impairments are seen in patients with bilateral posterior brain lesions. Patients may have difficulty in shifting their gaze to specific positions in space and in reaching to targets accurately. Defective depth perception may result in over- or underestimation of distances. Consequently, when standing in front of a flight of stairs, patients report seeing a number of straight lines on the floor, or complain that everything looks flat and two-dimensional, rather like a picture or photograph. Impaired depth perception is not only associated with impaired reaching in depth, but also with the appreciation of size (micropsia or macropsia) and binocular vision (stereopsis).

A further visual spatial deficit concerns difficulties with the perception of the main spatial axes. There is a strong tendency for patients to shift the main spatial axes, vertical, horizontal, and egocentric visual midline, to the side opposite to their brain injury. Shifts in the vertical and horizontal axes have been linked to right occipitoparietal lesions, whereas shifts in the straight-ahead direction have been reported in patients with either left- or right-sided damage. Patients with horizontal and vertical axis shifts may have difficulty in maintaining a line when writing, drawing and copying, whereas those with shifts in the egocentric visual midline cannot walk in a straight line. Visuospatial disorientation is sometimes seen together with hemianopia, and the resulting disability is severe. Occulomotor scanning appears spatially incoherent and disorganized.

With respect to recovery, several groups have monitored the progress of patients with impaired visual space perception and have reported variable degrees of recovery. There have also been attempts to actively rehabilitate patients with visuospatial disorders, although there are no specific proven techniques.

Visual illusions and hallucinations

Lesions at any point in the visual pathway, including the occipital lobes, can interfere with normal visual perception and predispose to the development of illusions or hallucinations. For the purposes of this chapter, we will confine the discussion to those phenomena originating from occipital lobe lesions, and not discuss anterior visual pathway disease, delirium, drug intoxication or withdrawal states. Examples of these include the Charles Bonnet syndrome, where visual hallucinations occur in association with severe bilateral visual loss, and peduncular hallucinations, which are linked to mesencephalic lesions and comprise extremely vivid and terrifying visual hallucinations that are associated with a gaze palsy, disorder of the sleep–wake rhythm, change in the level of consciousness and limb ataxia.[29]

Perceptual disorders are not uncommon, but patients often do not report their experiences, either because they are preoccupied with coexisting visual loss or because the experience is so bizarre that they question their own sanity.

Visual illusions

Visual illusions are misinterpretations or transformations of external stimuli. They arise when incoming visual information is processed abnormally. They are not necessarily pathological, and may occur in healthy individuals. They are highly transient symptoms after brain injury, and may be forgotten or go unnoticed by patients. They usually persist for seconds or minutes and disappear within a few days. In some cases, however, they may persist for several weeks or months. Several forms are recognized.

Visual perseveration

Visual perseveration is the persistence of a visual image in the absence of its original stimulus. It is an intermittent phenomenon. Patients often have a hemifield defect, which is necessarily incomplete to retain some residual visual capacity. The illusion is unilateral, with the abnormal image being placed slightly off-center between the affected and normal hemifields, rather than in the periphery. It persists despite redirection of gaze. Visual perseveration in the absence of lateralization or visual field defect is more likely to be due to the aura of a focal epileptic seizure. Visual perseveration occurs with lesions in occipital, occipitoparietal and occipitotemporal regions of the brain, especially the right hemisphere, and arises from a wide range of pathologies. Several forms of perseveration are described, depending on the interval of time that elapses between the disappearance of the original object and the appearance of its illusion.[30]

Immediate perseveration occurs when an object disappears but its image remains, and is so strikingly similar to the original object that it may initially be mistaken for reality, except that it shifts with the gaze rather like a retinal afterimage.

Palinopsia involves a longer latency period of minutes to hours between the original perception and the illusion, in which patients see a previously viewed scene being 'played back' before their eyes. The illusion usually bears a meaningful relationship with the patient's surroundings, for example the patient who was looking for a taxi who suddenly saw illuminated taxi signs on every passing car. The objects or faces which are perceived are extremely true to life, to the extent that the observer mistakes the illusion for reality.[31]

Hallucinatory perseveration involves a lengthy latency of days or weeks between the initial stimulus and its illusion. In contrast to true pallinopsia, the illusion disappears upon redirection of gaze, a feature more in keeping with complex hallucinations.

Polyopia

This describes the perception of a series of multiple images of an object that are precipitated by movement of either the patient or the object. The relationship between the secondary images and the true image may be either constant or changing, and the multiple images may or may not overlap. It often occurs during the evolution or recovery phases of central visual disorders. It is a poor localizing sign, although many anecdotal reports link it to the presence of occipital tumors.[32]

Visual illusionary spread

Here there is extension of the visual perseveration in the spatial domain. There is an extension of the visual perseveration over an area greater than that excited by the object presented to the observer.

Visual allesthesia

This involves the transposition of a perceived visual image from one quadrant or hemifield to another. Not infrequently, a distortion of the displaced image is reported.

Monocular diplopia

This is the rare perception of double vision in the hemianopic field in patients with an occipital lesion causing a relative or absolute hemianopia or quadrantinopia. The diplopia persists despite closure of one eye.

Dysmorphopsias

Unlike the repeated stereotyped visual auras of epileptic seizures and migraines, these are usually once-in-a-lifetime experiences for most patients. They involve transformations of images which may be altered in size (micropsia or macropsia), shape (metamorphopsia), position (telopsia), axis (tilted or inverted), movement (slow motion or elapsed time) or color. Patients initially see the object in question in its correct form, but it undergoes illusionary transformation as it is fixated for a longer period.

Visual hallucinations

Visual hallucinations, on the other hand, are not based on incoming visual information and arise when action potentials are pathologically generated and discharged in the brain, causing the patient to see something that is not evident to others in the same environment. Visual hallucinations can be simple or complex, but are always pathological.[33,34]

Simple visual hallucinations

These are also termed phosphenes or photopsias. They are crude unformed sensations comprising flashes of light which may be colored or white, lines and simple shapes. Photopsias commonly occur as part of migraine auras, and transiently at the onset of ischemic occipital infarctions which may cause field defects. Photopsias that persist in the blind hemifield tend to be epileptic in origin. Other causes include compression of brain substance by occipital tumors which disappears as the tumor expands to destroy the tissue.[35]

Complex visual hallucinations

These are highly organized hallucinations of faces, people, numbers, animals or detailed scenes. They occur when there is pathology in the occipitotemporal region causing either epileptic auras or field defects with hallucinations in the blind hemifield. Visual hallucinations that occur as the aura of epileptic seizures can involve a single hemifield or encompass the entire visual field. They are characteristically short-lived, lasting seconds or fractions of seconds. Hemianopic hallucinations are strictly unilateral, involving the hemianopic field, and are the projection of stored visual images onto the blind hemifield, which otherwise receives no physiological stimulation. Since they have a normal unaffected field for comparison, patients retain insight into their hallucinations. In Anton's syndrome of cortical blindness, however, pathology in both occipital lobes leads to complete loss of vision with hemianopic hallucinations in both hemifields, prompting patients to deny or underestimate the degree of visual loss.[36]

Visual cognition and agnosias

When patients fail to identify and recognize objects, it is usually because they have problems with visual perception.[37] When their basic visual functions are tested, they may have any combination of defects in their visual acuity, color vision, visual fields and eye movements. There is a small group of patients, however, whose lower visual perceptive functions remain intact, but are unable to identify or recognize objects visually. They can recognize objects by using other sensory modalities, for example by smell or touch, and do not have nominal aphasias, which would inhibit their ability to apply verbal labels to objects. Such patients have 'higher' cognitive impairments. They become confused when viewing objects with similar global (size, shape) or local (color, texture) features and cannot distinguish between them. Over the years, there have been papers on a number of well-studied patients with this clinical phenomenon, which has been termed visual object agnosia. Visual object agnosia in its pure form is a rare condition, and genuine visual agnosias are very difficult to diagnose clinically because they differ so subtly from visual perceptual disorders.[19,38]

The original attempt to classify visual agnosia was made by Lissauer in 1890, and since then several authors have refined the classification based on the specific hierarchical steps involved in object recognition. Different agnosias can be linked to variations between the cortical regions involved in the lesions of affected patients.[39] Commonly, multiple disseminated lesions are found bilaterally within the occipital lobes, sometimes extending into the left or both temporal lobes, disrupting the ventral stream. Etiologically, diffuse processes such as carbon monoxide poisoning and anoxia are frequent causes. The extent of visual agnosia is also variable between patients. Some exhibit agnosia for a discrete visual category such as objects, faces (prosopagnosia), letters (alexia) or places (topographical agnosia), while others experience problems in more than one category.[40,41]

Visual object agnosia

Patients have difficulty in selecting and integrating visual features that characterize a given object and distinguish it from other similar objects. Recognition is preserved in other sensory modalities, and the object can be identified when handled or its odour detected.[42]

In *apperceptive visual agnosias* there is a breakdown in high-level visual perception leading to an inability to generate a stable perceptual representation of an object. Such patients cannot name, copy or recognize visually presented objects, but can do so with auditory or tactile cues. Tests of basic visual perception, for example visual acuity, contrast sensitivity, line orientation discrimination or color identification, are performed correctly.[43,44]

Associative visual agnosia occurs when there is a breakdown in retrieving stored knowledge about the object which normally allows it to be recognized. Other high-level visual processes, such as copying figures or written material, matching photographs taken from unusual views, or block design, are correct.[45]

Prosopagnosia

Patients with prosopagnosia fail to recognize familiar faces, even those of family members in extreme cases, and have difficulty in learning new faces. Familiar people are correctly identified by their voices, clothes or gait.[46] Although it can occur in isolation, it is often observed in association with other functional visual deficits such as achromatopsia and visual agnosia. Most patients have an additional left visual field defect, which is either a hemianopia or an upper quadrantinopia. Although the most obvious disturbance in such patients is impaired facial recognition, they may also show an inability to distinguish between objects belonging to other object categories, such as buildings, animals or cars.[47] Prosopagnosia appears to be related to a lesion in the occipitotemporal region which damages or disconnects the inferior visual association cortex from the right temporal cortex.[48] The right temporal cortex becomes completely disconnected when the lesion is combined with disruption to interhemispheric transfer of visual information from the left visual cortex, by section of the callosal fibers.[24,49–51]

Alexia without agraphia

Patients cannot identify individual letters or construct meaningful words from written text, despite the fact that they have no difficulty in visualizing the words or writing from memory.[52]

Reports of patients with visual agnosias who have been followed up for prolonged periods, in excess of 40 years in one case, conclude that spontaneous recovery can take place but is rare and incomplete.

Motion perception

Only one patient with a well-documented disturbance of motion perception (akinotopsia) has been reported. The disorder was highly specific for motion, the patient having no difficulty in seeing colors, form or depth. Her problems included crossing roads, because the exact positions of moving cars were difficult for her to judge, or pouring drinks into a cup, because the fluid appeared to be frozen and she could not follow the rising meniscus, such that the cup overflowed. She had bilateral lesions affecting a region at the lateral occipitotemporal junction, which has been shown to be specifically activated during motion perception with PET scanning.[53–55]

The converse effect, the perception of motion of an object without detection of any other visual attribute of the moving object, was described by Riddoch.[56] This may occur in scotomatous areas of the visual field resulting from lesions of the posterior visual pathways, and is known as the Riddoch phenomenon. It may reflect intact function in subcortical areas.

References

1. Rizzo M. The role of the striate cortex: evidence from human lesion studies. In Peters L, Rockland KS (eds) *Cerebral Cortex* (New York: Plenum Press, 1994): 505–40.

2. Tootell RBH, Hadjikhani NK, Mendola JD et al. From retinopathy to recognition: fMRI in human visual cortex (Reviews). *Trends Cog Sci* (1998) **2(5):** 174–83.

3. Livingstone MS, Hubel DH. Psychophysical evidence for separate channels for the perception of form, color, movement, and depth. *J Neurosci* (1987) **7(11):** 3416–68.

4. Kennard C. Visual perceptual defects. *Bailliere's Clin Neuro* (1993) **2**.

5. Rizzo M, Barton JJS. Central disorders of visual function. In Miller NR, Newman NJ (eds) *Clinical Neuro-Ophthalmology* (Williams and Wilkins, 1998).

6. Zeki S, Watson JD, Lueck CJ et al. A direct demonstration of functional specialization in human

visual cortex. *J Neurosci* (1991) **11(3):** 641–9.

7. Goodale MA, Milner AD. Separate visual pathways for perception and action. *Trends Neurosci* (1992) **15(1):** 20–5.

8. Jeannerod M, Decety J, Michel F. Impairment of grasping movements following a bilateral posterior parietal lesion. *Neuropsychologia* (1994) **32(4):** 369–80.

9. Milner AD. Neuropsychological studies of perception and visuomotor control. *Philos Trans R Soc Lond B Biol Sci* (1998) **353(1373):** 1375–84.

10. Perenin MT, Vighetto A. Optic ataxia: a specific disruption in visuomotor mechanisms. I. Different aspects of the deficit in reaching for objects. *Brain* (1988) **111(Pt 3):** 643–74.

11. Ungerleider LG, Mishkin M. Two cortical visual systems. In Goodals MA, Mansfield RJW (eds) *Analysis of Visual Behaviour* (Cambridge MA: MIT Press, 1982): 549–86.

12. Holmes G. Disturbances of vision by cerebral lesions. *Br J Ophthalmol* (1918) **2:** 353–84.

13. Zeki S. *Inner Vision* (Oxford: Oxford University Press, 1999).

14. Cowey A, Stoerig P. The neurobiology of blindsight. *Trends Neurosci* (1991) **14(4):** 140–5.

15. Weiskrantz L. The Ferrier lecture, 1989. Outlooks for blindsight: explicit methodologies for implicit processes. *Proc R Soc Lond B Biol Sci* (1990) **239(1296):** 247–78.

16. Weiskrantz L, Barbur JL, Sahraie A. Parameters affecting conscious versus unconscious visual discrimination with damage to the visual cortex (V1). *Proc Natl Acad Sci USA* (1995) **92(13):** 6122–6.

17. Blythe IM, Kennard C, Ruddock KH. Residual vision in patients with retrogeniculate lesions of the visual pathways. *Brain* (1987) **110(Pt 4):** 887–905.

18. Pambakian AL, Kennard C. Can visual function be restored in patients with homonymous hemianopia? *Br J Ophthalmol* (1997) **81(4):** 324–8.

19. Damasio AR. Disorders of complex visual processing: agnosias, achromotopsia, Balint syndrome and related difficulties of orientation and construction. In Mesulum M, Davis M (eds) *Principles of Behavioural Neurology* (Philadelphia: FA Davis, 1985): 259–88.

20. Beauchamp MS, Haxby JV, Jennings JE, DeYoe EA. An fMRI version of the Farnsworth–Munsell 100-Hue test reveals multiple color-selective areas in human ventral occipitotemporal cortex. *Cereb Cortex* (1999) **9(3):** 257–63.

21. Lueck CJ, Zeki S, Friston KJ et al. The colour centre in the cerebral cortex of man. *Nature* (1989) **340(6232):** 386–9.

22. Rizzo M, Smith V, Pokorny J, Damasio AR. Color perception profiles in central achromatopsia. *Neurology* (1993) **43(5):** 995–1001.

23. Damasio A, Yamada T, Damasio H et al. Central achromatopsia: behavioral, anatomic, and physiologic aspects. *Neurology* (1980) **30(10):** 1064–71.

24. Meadows JC. The anatomical basis of prosopagnosia. *J Neurol Neurosurg Psychiatry* (1974) **37(5):** 489–501.

25. Plant GT. Disorders of colour vision. In Foster DH, Cronly-Dillon J (eds) *Inherited and Acquired Colour Vision Deficiencies: Fundamental Aspects and Clinical Studies. Vision and Visual Dysfunction* (Boca-Raton: CRC Press, 1991): 173–98.

26. Zeki S. A century of cerebral

achromatopsia. *Brain* (1990) **113(Pt 6):** 1721–77.

27. Zeki S. *A Vision of the Brain* (Oxford: Blackwell, 1993).

28. Meadows JC. Disturbed perception of colours associated with localized cerebral lesions. *Brain* (1974) **97(4):** 615–32.

29. Kolmel HW. Peduncular hallucinations. *J Neurol* (1991) **238(8):** 457–9.

30. Critchley M. Types of visual perserveration: 'Paliopsia' and 'illusory visual spread.' *Brain* (1951); **74:** 267–99.

31. Bender MB, Feldman M, Sobin AJ. Palinopsia. *Brain* (1968) **91(2):** 321–38.

32. Bender MB. Polyopia and monocular diplopia of cerebral origin. *Arch Neurol* (1945) **54:** 323–38.

33. Ffytche DH, Howard RJ, Brammer MJ et al. The anatomy of conscious vision: an fMRI study of visual hallucinations. *Nat Neurosci* (1998) **1(8):** 738–42.

34. Ffytche DH, Howard RJ. The perceptual consequences of visual loss: 'positive' pathologies of vision. *Brain* (1999) **122(Pt 7):** 1247–60.

35. Lance JW. Simple formed hallucinations confined to the area of a specific visual field defect. *Brain* (1976) **99(4):** 719–34.

36. Manford M, Andermann F. Complex visual hallucinations. Clinical and neurobiological insights. *Brain* (1998) **121(Pt 10):** 1819–40.

37. Farah MJ. *Visual Agnosia* (Cambridge MA: MIT Press, 1990).

38. Caramazza A. The interpretation of semantic category specific deficits: what do they reveal about the organisation of conceptual knowledge in the brain? *Neurocase* (1998) **4:** 265–72.

39. Humphreys GW, Riddoch MJ. The fractionation of visual agnosia. In Humphreys GW, Riddoch MJ

(eds) *Visual Object Processing: a Cognitive Neuropsychological Approach* (Hove: Lawrence Erlbaum, 1987): 281–306.

40. Riddoch MJ, Humphreys GW, Gannon T et al. Memories are made of this: the effects of time on stored visual knowledge in a case of visual agnosia. *Brain* (1999) **122**(Pt 3): 537–59.

41. Rumiati R, Humphreys GW, Riddoch MJ, Bateman A. A visual object agnosia without alexia or prosopagnosia. *Vis Cogn* (1994) **1:** 181–94.

42. Farah MJ. Distinguishing perceptual and semantic impairments affecting visual object recognition. *Vis Cogn* (1997) **4:** 199–206.

43. Ferreira CT, Ceccaldi M, Giusiano B, Poncet M. Separate visual pathways for perception of actions and objects: evidence from a case of apperceptive agnosia. *J Neurol Neurosurg Psychiatry* (1998) **65(3):** 382–5.

44. Warrington EK, James M. Visual apperceptive agnosia: a clinico-anatomical study of three cases. *Cortex* (1988) **24(1):** 13–32.

45. Carlesimo GA, Casadio P, Sabbadini M, Caltagirone C. Associative visual agnosia resulting from a disconnection between intact visual memory and semantic systems. *Cortex* (1998) **34(4):** 563–76.

46. Damasio AR, Damasio H, Van Hoesen GW. Prosopagnosia: anatomic basis and behavioral mechanisms. *Neurology* (1982) **32(4):** 331–41.

47. Buxbaum LJ, Glosser G, Coslett HB. Impaired face and word recognition without object agnosia. *Neuropsychologia* (1999) **37(1):** 41–50.

48. Perrett DI, Hietanen JK, Oram MW, Benson PJ. Organization and functions of cells responsive to faces in the temporal cortex.

Philos Trans R Soc Lond B Biol Sci (1992) **335(1273):** 23–30.

49. Bentin S, Deouell LY, Soroker N. Selective visual streaming in face recognition: evidence from developmental prosopagnosia. *Neuroreport* (1999) **10(4):** 823–7.

50. Eimer M, McCarthy RA. Prosopagnosia and structural encoding of faces: evidence from event-related potentials. *Neuroreport* (1999) **10(2):** 255–9.

51. Kanwisher N, McDermott J, Chun MM. The fusiform face area: a module in human extrastriate cortex specialized for face perception. *J Neurosci* (1997) **17(11):** 4302–11.

52. Warrington EK, Shallice T. Word-form dyslexia. *Brain* (1980) **103(1):** 99–112.

53. Rizzo M, Nawrot M, Zihl J. Motion and shape perception in cerebral akinetopsia. *Brain* (1995) **118(Pt 5):** 1105–27.

54. Zeki S. Cerebral akinetopsia (visual motion blindness). A review. *Brain* (1991); **114(Pt 2):** 811–24.

55. Zihl J, von Cramon D, Mai N, Schmid C. Disturbance of movement vision after bilateral posterior brain damage. Further evidence and follow up observations. *Brain* (1991) **114(Pt 5):** 2235–52.

56. Riddoch G. Dissociation of visual perception due to occipital injuries, with special reference to appreciation of movement. *Brain* (1917) **40:** 15–57.

7
Cognitive dysfunction in hydrocephalus

Joanna L Iddon

Summary

The neuropsychological studies carried out thus far suggest that intellectually preserved, non-demented patients with hydrocephalus, in general, demonstrate a specific pattern of impairment of critical 'executive' functions, unrelieved by shunting, in the presence of preserved performance on tasks with a smaller executive component. These findings are important, because such functions are essential for effective performance in a complex world and have implications for real-life functioning.

In addition, if idiopathic 'normal pressure' hydrocephalus (NPH) is not diagnosed early and remains untreated, the functional deficits appear to broaden to include a global pattern of both cortical gray and subcortical white matter change, so causing a severe and permanent change in all aspects of mental functioning. Importantly, in this subgroup, some cognitive improvement is observed following shunting in some cases. This pattern of progressive deterioration demonstrates the importance of differential diagnosis and appropriate treatment early on in NPH and lends support to the use of objective neuropsychological assessment as part of the clinical diagnosis.

Neuropsychological assessment and cognitive profiling in hydrocephalus appears to be starting to explain the anecdotally reported difficulties associated with individuals in this group, and is particularly interesting against the background of preserved social and intellectual functioning. In contrast, individuals with spina bifida (SB) with no associated hydrocephalus do not appear to demonstrate significant cognitive impairment, although issues of low self-esteem due to physical abnormalities are potentially confounding factors.

The logical next step in the clinical management of the cognitive dysfunction associated with subtypes of hydrocephalus is to try to develop pharmaceutical and behavioral management strategies.

Introduction

In this chapter I will discuss some of the known cognitive and behavioral sequelae in two specific subtypes of hydrocephalus; (1) NPH, acquired, most commonly, in later life; and (2) developmental hydrocephalus (DH), acquired pre- or perinatally. I will begin with a brief overview of the pathology and treatment of hydrocephalus in general.

Pathology and treatment of hydrocephalus

Hydrocephalus (Greek 'hydro' (water), 'cephalus' (head)) is an abnormal accumulation of cerebrospinal fluid (CSF) in the ventricles of the brain. CSF is produced in the ventricles and circulates freely in a healthy brain before being absorbed into the bloodstream. CSF crucially acts as a kind of 'flotation cushion' for the brain and spinal cord, protecting against injury. It also acts to nourish the brain, containing nutrients and proteins, and carries away waste products, thus regulating healthy, balanced brain function. This process is impaired in hydrocephalus, where there is an imbalance between the amount of CSF produced and the rate at which it is absorbed. As CSF builds up, the ventricles become enlarged and pressure inside the head increases. Sustained malfunction of the CSF system causes irreversible cell death.[1] Hydrocephalus is an incurable disorder but can be treated via the insertion of a surgical 'shunt'. This is effectively an advanced 'drainage' system, where a flexible piece of tube is inserted into the ventricular system of the brain, diverting the flow of CSF into another region of the body, most usually the abdominal cavity. Although a highly innovative treatment, a shunt is prone to blockage and malfunction, so ongoing management is essential.

Normal pressure hydrocephalus

Introduction

Adults

NPH is an acquired syndrome, usually occurring in adulthood, with an idiopathic cause or occurring secondary to other neurosurgical complications including head injury, stroke and hemorrhage. It was first characterized[2] as ventricular dilation accompanied by a progressive triad of a gait disturbance, 'dementia' and incontinence. It must be confirmed by the demonstration of a raised CSF outflow resistance. There is now a broad consensus in the literature[1,3] that the physical symptoms can largely be relieved by insertion of a CSF shunt, in up to 65–70% of patients with a known cause and in 30–50% of idiopathic cases. Incontinence is usually the latter symptom in progressed and untreated NPH.[4]

The precise nature of the mental changes and their response to shunt surgery has recently begun to be clarified.

Progression of NPH

One of the problems with the characterization of the 'dementia' syndrome in NPH is that it has often been viewed as a single clinical entity. This is partly because, usually, only basic measures such as the Mini-Mental State Examination (MMSE) are used to assess cognitive function. Although the MMSE is a useful initial examination for determining whether a patient falls into the dementing range, and for determining the severity of dementia, it is less useful for assessing 'higher' cognitive capacity. I will discuss two main groups in turn, since it is likely that NPH is progressive and proceeds from a relatively mild pattern of 'executive' dysfunction without 'classical' dementia (higher functioning) to a more marked global 'classic' dementia (lower functioning) ('classic' dementia is defined here by a score of less than 24 on the MMSE). It is of note that most studies do not differentiate these groups, and thus mixing of groups is probable. Interpretation of results from the papers, reviewed in this chapter, is against a background of the findings from Iddon et al.[4]

Higher-functioning patients with NPH

It is most likely to be the case that during the early stages of NPH there is a specific pattern of 'executive' mental impairment. Studies of cognitive function in patients with NPH have reported disproportionately poor performance, both pre- and post-shunt, on tests of frontal 'executive' function — that is, tests sensitive to damage in the frontal lobe or related frontosubcortical areas.[4,5–9] For example, Caltagirone et al[5] administered a mental deterioration battery including measures of word fluency, memory, reasoning, copying and attentional set-switching. This study showed that a group of NPH patients were significantly more impaired on the tests purported to assess frontal lobe involvement (word fluency and attentional switching) and thus concluded that alongside the symptoms of inertia and apathy, 'frontal' impairment is one of the most frequent and earliest signs of mental deterioration in this disorder, showing no improvement post-shunt. Gustafson and Hagberg,[6] Thomsen et al[8] and Stambrook et al[10] all reported a similar pattern, including impairment on tests assessing attention, concentration, planning and memory.

Recently, Iddon et al[4] confirmed that in the absence of classical dementia (Figure 7.1) patients were specifically impaired on tests of executive function such as attentional set-shifting (Figure 7.2), while remaining relatively unimpaired on tests of posterior cortical function. A battery of tests was specifically chosen to 'profile' the pattern of dysfunc-

High-functioning NPH and Alzheimer's patients

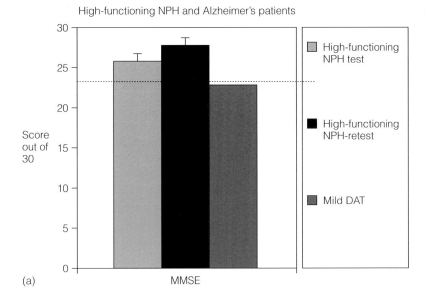

(a)

Low-functioning NPH patients

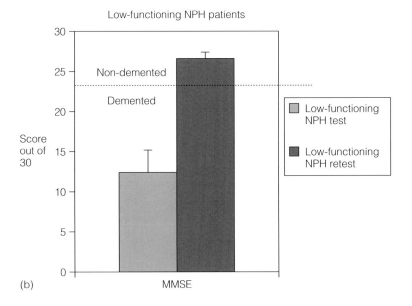

(b)

Figure 7.1

Pre- and post-shunt performance of high- and low-functioning patients with idiopathic NPH on the (a, b) MMSE and (c, d) KOLT. Patients with Alzheimer's disease are also compared with the high-functioning NPH patients on the MMSE (Iddon et al[4]). DAT: dementia of the Alzheimer type; KOLT: Kendrick Object Learning Test; MMSE: Mini-Mental State Examination; NPH: 'normal pressure' hydrocephalus.

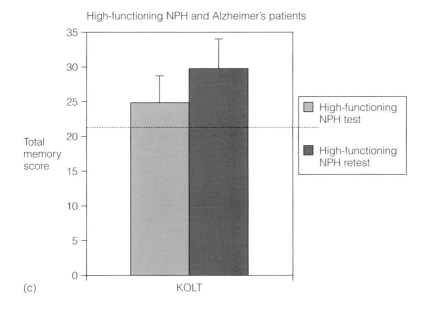

(c)

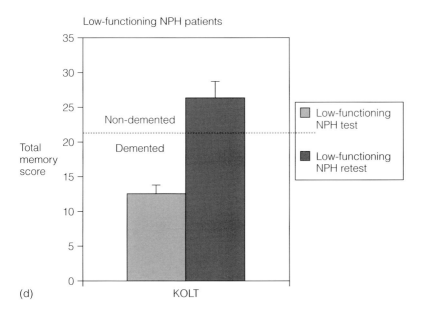

(d)

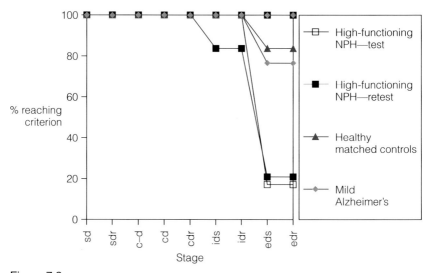

Figure 7.2

Performance of high-functioning NPH patients pre- and post-shunt, patients with
Alzheimer's disease and control subjects on the CANTAB Attentional Set Shifting Task
(Iddon et al[4]). NPH: 'normal pressure' hydrocephalus. sd: simple discrimination; sdr: simple
discrimination reversal; c-d: compound-discrimination; cd: compund discrimination; cdr:
compund discrimination reversal; ids: intra dimensional shift; idr: intra dimensional reversal;
eds: extra dimensional shift; edr: extra dimensional reversal.

tion mainly taken from the Cambridge Neuropsychological Test Automated Battery (CANTAB) (see Fray et al[11] for review).

The findings of these studies suggest a specific pattern of impairment
of critical executive functions, unrelieved by insertion of a shunt, important because such functions are essential for effective performance in a
complex world and have implications for real-life functions such as
decision-making and social cognition. Disinhibition, apathy, lability and
mania are also symptoms often observed in patients with NPH similar to
other neuropsychiatric disorders with 'subcortical'-type dysfunction.[12,13] It
appears that, if left untreated, these functional deficits broaden to a more
severe and global pattern of both cortical gray and subcortical white matter change, so causing a severe and permanent change in all aspects of
mental functioning.

Lower functioning patients with NPH

Iddon et al[4] assessed a group of 'classically' demented patients pre- and
post-shunt. Dementia was confirmed by a score of less than 24/30 on the
MMSE and less than 22 on the Kendrick Object Learning Test (KOLT)
(Figure 7.1). The remarkable finding was that, post-shunt, these patients

showed an impressive reversal of dementia on these basic tests (Figure 7.1). This was in keeping with subjective reports by the patients and their relatives about the significant improvements in activities of daily living, for example washing, dressing and cooking. This group remained impaired on more complex cognitive tasks. Other studies have reported significant improvements in general cognitive functioning in demented patients post-shunt surgery, particularly on memory tests,[10,14–16] although such studies have reported on a range of impairment levels, without differentiating, and often include mixed groups. (Mixed groups are primarily reported, for example, see Caltagirone et al,[5] who included 7 idiopathic cases, and 11 NPH secondary to subarachnoid hemorrhage, severe head trauma or an infectious central nervous system (CNS) disorder. Also, Stambrook et al[10] reported on 14 patients with hydrocephalus attributable to factors such as subarachnoid hemorrhage, craniotomy and others. Only eight cases were considered idiopathic. In contrast, Iddon et al[4] included an initial group of over 40 subjects but only included true idiopathic cases to confirm the 'subgroup' patterns of impairment. 'Well-defined' groups are most useful,[4] but cause complications in drawing definite conclusions in clinical studies due to resultant small numbers.)

Techniques used in the assessment of NPH

Historically, acute hydrocephalus has been associated with reduced frontal cerebral blood flow (CBF), possibly as the result of the stretching of the anterior cerebral arteries over the corpus callosum, for which there is some angiographic and doppler evidence. Ventricular enlargement may preferentially stretch the longest nerve fibers as they circumnavigate the ventricles; hence the gait and bladder disturbance. Projections of the cholinergic fibers from the nucleus basalis to the cortical neurons involved in memory might be stretched and could be involved in depressing CBF metabolism. It should be noted, though, that evidence for a preferential reduction in frontal cerebral blood flow and oxidative/glucose metabolism in NPH is contradictory. It is difficult to compare series, because of mixing of idiopathic with secondary cases and failure to base the diagnosis on robust techniques such as intracranial pressure (ICP) monitoring and CSF outflow resistance measurements. Many of the tomographic techniques used are semiquantitative. In brief, five groups have reported no evidence of frontal hypoperfusion,[17–21] while two groups described subcortical and inferior frontal/temporal hypoperfusion.[22,23] No consistent regional changes in cerebral oxygen or glucose consumption have been found by three separate groups using positron emission tomography (PET).[24–26]

Magnetic resonance imaging (MRI) techniques have been used to assess the effects of periventricular and deep white matter lesions on outcome after shunting.[27,28] Both studies concluded that, in general, the degree of improvement depended on the severity of damage to these different regions but that patients with severe white matter lesions may still benefit from shunting. Iddon et al[4] found that patterns of structural change on MRI corresponded well with the patterns of functional change in the majority of the patients. The use of MRI (to assess structural change) and neuropsychology (to assess functional change) is a powerful combination to assess brain damage and resultant dysfunction.

Early prediction and differential diagnosis of NPH

Often, subtle cognitive decline begins to take place long before physical changes become apparent in neurological disorders, so sensitive neuropsychological tests may be crucial, non-invasive aids to diagnosis. The pattern of cognitive impairment in the early stages of NPH is predominantly of 'executive' impairment, only later becoming more global. This contrasts markedly with the pattern observed in patients with questionable dementia/mild cognitive impairment and very mild Alzheimer's disease, who are more specifically impaired on tests sensitive to damage in posterior regions.[4,29] In terms of measurable pathological differences, Golomb et al[30] observed that hippocampal size strongly correlates with severity of dementia as determined by the MMSE score, revealing that there is a smaller degree of atrophy of the hippocampal formation in many patients with NPH compared with controls and patients with dementia of the Alzheimer type (DAT). This is also in keeping with the finding that there is no hippocampal atrophy in classic cases of NPH.[3] NPH and DAT are often confused because of their initial presentation with similar patterns of cortical ventricular change and complaints of deteriorating memory. Differential diagnosis is important because NPH is treatable, and trials of novel drug treatments for DAT require accurate diagnosis. A greater understanding of the neuropsychology of NPH might also aid in the 'fine tuning' of shunts and the development of novel techniques such as pharmaceutical cognitive enhancement and behavioral management strategies.

Developmental hydrocephalus

Cause and incidence

Developmental hydrocephalus can occur either pre- or perinatally in roughly 1 in every 500 children born, and is thought to be caused by a complex interaction of genetic and environmental factors. There are several different causes, including aqueductal stenosis, spina bifida, intraventricular hemorrhage, meningitis, head trauma and cysts. Bradbury[31] broadly categorized four main areas: (1) imbalance between production and drainage of CSF — usually due to a blockage of CSF pathways within the ventricles, subarachnoid space or arachnoid granulations, due to a tumor, malformations, subarachnoid fibrosis, meningitis, prematurity, Dandy–Walker syndrome, spina bifida, tuberous sclerosis; (2) developmental abnormalities — these are very rare disorders, such as Smith–Lemli–Opitz syndrome and Meckel syndrome; (3) destruction of brain tissue with associated cerebral atrophy and ventricular dilation — usually a result of pre- or perinatal brain damage in infants; and (4) mixed hydrocephalus — when there are several pathologies. Epilepsy is also common in children with hydrocephalus;[32] this can be another complicating disorder in management and research, and occurs in about 40% of cases. Another interesting anomaly is that 50% of patients with DH are left-handed, as compared to about 15% in the general population (Iddon et al, unpublished observations). It is unclear what the explanation might be for this.

Advances in the surgical treatment (shunt) of DH have reduced the risk of mental retardation and improved many aspects of physical functioning. But it is still the case that individuals with DH do not seem to develop properly in terms of cognitive, behavioral and emotional function. This can result in limited educational and occupational achievements as well as causing distress to the sufferers and relatives, who do not understand the problems that their children are experiencing — often, parents are blamed for poor handling. The majority of the studies of cognitive function have been carried out in children.

Cognitive dysfunction in children with hydrocephalus

One of the most frequently reported problems in children with hydrocephalus is distractibility, and it has been suggested that this may partially account for at least some of the cognitive and language problems that this patient group exhibits. For example, Horn et al[33] assessed primary school children with DH and controls on a non-verbal task during which irrelevant stimuli were present or absent. The two groups performed similarly when no irrelevant stimuli were present, but that when irrelevant stimuli were present, members of the DH group were much more distractible. This finding may suggest that those in the DH group were less able to filter out interference. Tew[34] showed in another observational study that 7-year-old hydrocephalic children had shorter attention spans and slightly more behavioral problems in school compared to normal children. This conclusion was based on subjective accounts by teachers rather than on quantifiable measures.

Other studies have investigated memory in hydrocephalic children. Cull and Wyke[35] assessed 10 children on a task requiring the learning of unrelated verbal material, and the subjects were found to be significantly impaired. Lumenta and Skotarczak[36] carried out a longitudinal study assessing cognitive function in hydrocephalic teenagers. Possibly the most comprehensive study to date, this was a post hoc analysis of the data of 233 children with DH who had undergone a shunt operation between 1964 and 1984. Psychological examination was carried out on 115 of patients, of whom, according to the authors, 62.8% showed unimpaired performance, while 29.8% showed problems with memory and concentration, poor intellectual performance and decreased performance in school. In another study in a group of 9–20-year-olds, Dorman et al[37] found that while children with DH could usually complete a number of different neuropsychological batteries (the Halstead Reitan and the Luria–Nebraska), they were still overall impaired on different tasks completed. This study did not distinguish between different age or intelligence subgroups within the sample, which may be an important factor.

DH is also associated with a pattern of language dysfunction described as the 'chatterbox syndrome',[38] also known as the 'Cocktail Party Syndrome',[39] as characterized by poor comprehension in the presence of preserved vocabulary and syntactical skills. Other groups have found contradictory evidence suggesting that vocabulary skills are not intact, but that this impairment may partially be accounted for by distractibility.[33] Several other groups have reported speech to have poor narrative content,[40,41] often associated with bizarre speech.[42] Thompson et al[43] neuropsychologically assessed pre-school infants with DH and found lower levels of performance on measures of verbal and non-verbal cognitive skills as compared to healthy children, a finding also reported by Fletcher et al.[44,45]

Intelligence may be an important factor to take into account in this group. Hagberg[46] found that lower IQ and neurological abnormalities were particularly associated with children with behavioral problems. More specifically, Taylor[40] reported good performance on verbal intelligence tasks and picture vocabulary but much poorer performance on tests of reasoning and comprehension. There have also been several reports of poor visuospatial and perceptual skills in young children with DH,[34,47] which Billard et al[48] suggested actually caused poor performance on IQ tests. In contrast, Ingram and Naughton[38] reported that intelligence was in the normal range in the majority of hydrocephalus patients. Another study[49] suggested that in a substantial number of cases, hydrocephalus does not cause overt intellectual disabilities or consequent handicaps in school or employment. Anecdotally, however, the more common reality is that many individuals suffering from these disorders, despite scoring in the 'normal' intelligence range on psychometric tests, are often paradoxically low achievers who find it difficult to cope in terms of living, and struggle to function independently. As has been pointed out,[49] normality on the Wechsler Adult Intelligence Scale (WAIS) does not necessarily mean normal intellect.

To summarize, cognitive impairment in children with hydrocephalus seems to be predominantly associated with poor attention (distractibility), memory (possibly associated with poor strategy), reasoning, monitoring and language skills. It is of note that such deficits are similar to those often exhibited in individuals with damage to the frontal lobe or related areas and may largely account for the regularly reported significant behavioral and emotional issues in children with DH.

Cognitive dysfunction in adults with DH

There is only one study to date in young adults with hydrocephalus.[50] In total, over 100 patients completed a neuropsychological test battery, including measures of visual and spatial recognition memory, spatial span, spatial working memory, attentional set-shifting (assessing cognitive flexibility, rule-learning and abstraction), visuospatial and verbal strategy, verbal recall, and verbal fluency. An emotional judgment task was also administered, shown previously to be impaired in individuals with autism.[51] Preliminary analysis shows that individuals with 'normal' intelligence show a specific pattern of frontal 'executive' dysfunction, in the presence of preserved intellect. As with the NPH patients previously described, this pattern of impairment suggests that individuals with hydrocephalus perform particularly poorly on tests requiring the integration of different cognitive processes, probably associated with attentional dysfunction, inflexibility of thought and a lack of ability to improve performance via the use of strategies, while remaining relatively well preserved on tests tapping executive skills less. It was of note that performance was also preserved on the emotional judgment task, which arguably measures emotional intelligence. These results suggest a core pattern of neural damage and resultant 'executive' cognitive impairment, in the presence of preserved emotional and traditional intelligence. MRI data are currently being collected in the same group of patients to set the functional data against a structural background.

Spina bifida

A complicating factor is the presence of SB, which is 80% concomitant with DH. Perhaps surprisingly, given the localization of damage (spinal rather than neural), some studies have suggested that SB (rather than DH) is the main cause of cognitive dysfunction.[34,52,53] It is of note (and concern) that these studies did not take into account the presence of DH. Other studies contrast with this approach, showing that SB children score closer to the 'normal' range on cognitive,[35] although performance is still below average.[54] Iddon et al (unpublished data) found that adults with SB without concomitant hydrocephalus had largely preserved cognitive function, lending support to the argument that DH is the primary cause of cognitive dysfunction, rather than SB.

It is of note that studying individuals with SB is quite difficult in practice, because of the low incidence of non-concomitant cases, so it is difficult to collect large samples. Also, the physical abnormalities associated with SB complicate the interpretation of cognitive findings, as disablement can cause low self-confidence and, in turn, low achievement. Several studies have highlighted these complicating factors when assessing behavior and self-confidence in relation to SB. For example, Landry[55] investigated goal-directed behavior in young children during videotaped play sessions. This study reported that the children with SB spent less time engaged in task-oriented behaviors and more time simply manipulating the toys, compared to non-disabled peers. Other studies have assessed perceived self-confidence and self-esteem in children with SB and concluded that such issues are particularly pertinent in young girls with SB, related to physical appearance.[56] Moreover, in other studies, pre-adolescent children showed feelings of anxiety and intellectual[57] and physical[58] inferiority in relation to non-disabled peers. In contrast, Campbell[59] and Spaulding and Morgan[60] reported no significant difference on measures of self-confidence and global worth in individuals with SB.

Schooling is also an important issue to take into account. Lord et al[61] carried out a study in California assessing the social and academic implications of mainstream and special schools in 31 adolescents with SB. They administered a vocabulary test and found that those children in specialist classes had poorer scores than those in mainstream schools. Simpson and Hemmer[49] also suggested that, despite the many advantages of special schools, such as protection, special teaching skills and medical treatment, these could be offset by isolation from normal life and a lack of competitive spirit and excellence.

A theory for the specific pattern of cognitive dysfunction

In any subtype of hydrocephalus it is likely that there is an underlying structural disorder or brain damage that leads to the seemingly specific behavioral and cognitive sequelae. The neural damage that takes place subcortically due to the build-up of CSF and consequent pressure is very likely to cause permanent damage to frontosubcortical connections. A speculative explanation is that damage occurs to corticosubcortical connections, through lesions of the fibers (white matter). This may be the result of changes in pressure in the 3rd and 4th ventricles that impair the functioning of frontosubcortical circuitry, although it is unclear in which area. A similarly speculative explanation has been suggested by Fishman.[62] In NPH, this damage is acquired and disrupts brain function. In DH, the developing brain is likely to be damaged early on, resulting in long-term and irreversible damage to developing circuits that appears not to be compensated for by the developing brain. Sobkowiak[63] reported that there is slow myelination in the congenital hydrocephalic brain as well as changes in the prefrontal cortex on electrophysiological measures, which may be caused by damage 'downstream'. The resultant cognitive dysfunction and slow social and emotional development may be a result of such abnormal neural development. Thus, to date, the (probably overly simplistic) theoretical neural explanation postulated here for the specific pattern of 'executive' impairment in hydrocephalus is that dysfunction in subcortical regions of the brain causes damage to frontosubcortical circuits, resulting in a specific pattern of cognitive dysfunction. It certainly seems logical that a build-up of fluid in the ventricles of the brain will result in damage and dysfunction such as that demonstrated in shunted hydrocephalus. If such pressure is sustained, severe impairment and white matter damage will occur, as demonstrated in the lower-functioning patients with NPH.

However, it is also possible that the insertion of a shunt may cause damage to periventricular white matter and thus cause secondary cognitive impairment. Weller and Shulman[64] suggested that it was possible for significant changes to occur in the white matter of hydrocephalic brains following shunt insertion. The ventricles may return to normal in response to shunting, but the expanded white matter remains thick and spongy. If this is the case, shunting may be related to permanent subcortical damage. A number of other studies have suggested that shunts may be detrimental to cognitive and mental function;[65-68] for example, Anderson and Plewis[68] showed in a large cohort of patients ($N = 96$) that patients with shunted hydrocephalus had lower mean scores on all tests compared with children without shunts, particularly on the non-verbal tasks. It is, however, of note that the findings in the NPH study[4] dispute this hypothesis, since the specific pattern of cognitive impairment was present both pre- and post-shunt. Thus, although a shunt dramatically improves life-expectancy, whether it is associated with mental dysfunction is still a matter of debate.

References

1. Pickard JD. Normal pressure hydrocephalus. *Clin Neurol* (1991) **1:** 151–64.

2. Hakin S, Adams RD. The special clinical problem of symptomatic hydrocephalus with normal cerebrospinal fluid pressure. Observations on cerebrospinal fluid hydrodynamics. *J Neurol Sci* (1965) **2:** 307–27.

3. Vanneste JA. Three decades of normal pressure hydrocephalus: are we wiser now? *J Neurol Neurosurg Psychiatry* (1994) **57(9):** 1021–5.

4. Iddon JL, Pickard JD, Cross JJL et al. Specific patterns of cognitive impairment in patients with idiopathic 'normal pressure' hydrocephalus and Alzheimer's disease: a pilot study. *J Neurol Neurosurg Psychiatry* (1999) **67(6):** 723–31.

5. Caltagirone C, Gainotti G, Masullo

C et al. Neurophysiological study of normal pressure hydrocephalus. *Acta Psychiatr Scand* (1982) **65(2):** 93–100.

6. Gustafson L, Hagberg B. Recovery in hydrocephalic dementia after shunt operation. *J Neurol Neurosurg Psychiatry* (1978) **41(10):** 940–7.

7. Berglund M, Gustafson L, Hagberg B. Amnestic-confabulatory syndrome in hydrocephalic dementia and Korsakoff's psychosis in alcoholism. *Am J Psychiatry* (1979) **150(9):** 1431–2.

8. Thomsen AM, Borgeson SE, Bruhn P, Gjerris F. Prognosis of dementia in normal pressure hydrocephalus after a shunt operation. *Ann Neurol* (1986) **20:** 304–10.

9. Torkelson RD, Leibrock LG, Gustavson JL, Sundell RR. Neurological and neuropsychological effects of cerebral spinal fluid shunting in children with assumed arrested ('normal pressure') hydrocephalus. *J Neurol Neurosurg Psychiatry* (1986) **48(8):** 799–806.

10. Stambrook M, Cardosa ER, Hawryluk GA et al. Neuropsychological changes following the neurosurgical treatment of normal pressure hydrocephalus. *Arch Clin Neuropsychol* (1988) **3:** 323–30.

11. Fray PJ, Robbins TW, Sahakian BJ. Neuropsychiatric applications of CANTAB. *Int J Geriatr Psychiatry* (1996) **11:** 329–36.

12. Mega MS, Cummings JL. Frontal-subcortical circuits and neuropsychiatric disorders. *J Neuropsychiatry* (1994) **6(4):** 358–70.

13. Whitehouse PJ. The concept of subcortical and cortical dementia: another look. *Ann Neurol* (1986) **19(1):** 1–6.

14. Malm J, Kristensen B, Karlsson T et al. A predictive value of cerebrospinal fluid dynamic tests in patients with the idiopathic adult hydrocephalus syndrome. *Arch Neurol* (1995) **52(8):** 783–9.

15. Chen IH, Huang CI, Liu HC, Chen KK. Effectiveness of shunting in patients with normal pressure hydrocephalus predicted by temporary, controlled resistance continuous lumbar drainage: a pilot study. *J Neurol Neurosurg Psychiatry* (1994) **57(11):** 1430–2.

16. Raftopoulos C, Deleval J, Chaskis C et al. Cognitive recovery in idiopathic normal pressure hydrocephalus: a prospective study. *Neurosurgery* (1994) **35(3):** 397–405.

17. Graff-Radford NR, Rezai K, Godersky JC et al. Regional cerebral blood flow in normal pressure hydrocephalus. *J Neurol Neurosurg Psychiatry* (1987) **50:** 1589–96.

18. Vorstrup S, Christensen J, Gjerris F et al. Cerebral blood flow in patients with normal pressure hydrocephalus before and after shunting. *J Neurosurg* (1987) **66(3):** 379–87.

19. Mamo HL, Meric PC, Ponsin JC et al. Cerebral blood flow in hydrocephalus. *Stroke* (1987) **18(6):** 1074–80.

20. Matsuda M, Nakasu S, Nakazawa T, Handa J. Cerebral hemodynamics in patients with normal pressure hydrocephalus. Correlation between cerebral circulation time and dementia. *Surg Neurol* (1990) **34:** 396–401.

21. Kimura M, Tanaka A, Yoshinaga S. Significance of periventricular hemodynamics in normal pressure hydrocephalus. *Neurosurgery* (1992) **30:** 701–4.

22. Waldemar G, Shmidt-Jes F, Delecluse F et al. High resolution SPECT with (^{99m}Tc)–*d,l*-HMPAO in normal pressure hydrocephalus

before and after shunt operation. *J Neurol Neurosurg Psychiatry* (1993) **56:** 655–64.

23. Kristenson B, Malm J, Fagerlund M et al. Regional cerebral blood flow, white matter abnormalities and cerebrospinal fluid hydrodynamics in patients with idiopathic adult hydrocephalus syndrome. *J Neurol Neurosurg Psychiatry* (1996) **60:** 282–8.

24. Brooks DJ. Beaney RP, Powell M. Studies of cerebral oxygen metabolism, blood flow, and blood volume, in patients with hydrocephalus before and after surgical decompression, using positron emission tomography. *Brain* (1986) **109:** 613–28.

25. Jagust WJ, Friedland RP, Budinger TF. Positron emission tomography with (^{18}F) fluorodeoxyglucose differentiates normal pressure hydrocephalus from Alzheimer's disease. *J Neurol Neurosurg Psychiatry* (1985) **48:** 1091–6.

26. Tedeschi E, Hasselbach SG, Waldemar G et al. Heterogeneous cerebral glucose metabolism in normal pressure hydrocephalus. *J Neurol Neurosurg Psychiatry* (1995) **59:** 608–15.

27. Krauss JK, Droste DW, Vach W et al. Cerebrospinal fluid shunting in idiopathic normal pressure hydrocephalus of the elderly: effects of periventricular and deep white matter lesions. *Neurosurgery* (1996) **39(2):** 292–9.

28. Pickard JD, Newton H, Greene A et al. A prospective study of idiopathic normal pressure hydrocephalus. *J Neurol Neurosurg Psychiatry* (1992) 55–518 (abstract).

29. Sahakian BJ, Morris RG, Evenden JL et al. A comparative study of visuospatial memory and learning in Alzheimer type dementia and Parkinson's disease. *Brain* (1988) **111:** 695–718.

30. Golomb J, de Leon MJ, George AE et al. Hippocampal atrophy correlates with severe cognitive impairment in elderly patients with suspected normal pressure hydrocephalus. *J Neurol Neurosurg Psychiatry* (1994) **57:** 590–3.

31. Bradbury MWB. Anatomy and physiology of cerebrospinal fluid. In Schurr PH, Polkey CE (eds) *Hydrocephalus* (Oxford: Oxford Medical Publications, Oxford University Press, 1993).

32. Blaauw G. Hydrocephalus and epilepsy. *Z Kinderchirurg* (1978) **25:** 341–5.

33. Horn DG, Lorch RF, Culatta B. Distractibility and vocabulary deficits in children with spina bifida and hydrocephalus. *Dev Med Child Neurol* (1985) **27(6):** 713–20.

34. Tew BJ, Laurence KM. The clinical and psychological characteristics of children with 'cocktail party' syndrome. *Z Kinderchirurg* (1979) **28:** 360–7.

35. Cull C, Wyke MA. Memory function of children with spina bifida and shunted hydrocephalus. *Dev Med Child Neurol* (1984) **26:** 177–83.

36. Lumenta CB, Skotarczak U. Long-term follow up of 233 patients with congenital hydrocephalus. *Child's Nervous System* (1995) **11(3):** 173–5.

37. Dorman C, Laatsch LK, Hurley AD. The applicability of neuropsychological test batteries for assessment of the congenitally brain disordered. *Int J Clin Neuropsychol* (1985) **7(2):** 111–17.

38. Ingram TTS, Naughton JA. Paediatric and psychological aspects of cerebral palsy associated with hydrocephalus. *Dev Med Child Neurol* (1962) **4:** 287–92.

39. Hagberg B, Sjorgen I. The chronic brain syndrome of infantile hydrocephalus. A follow-up study of 63

spontaneously arrested cases. *Am J Dis Children* (1966) **112(3):** 189–96.

40. Taylor EM. *Psychological Appraisal of Children with Cerebral Deficits* (Cambridge, MA: Harvard University Press, 1961).

41. Dennis M, Jacennik B, Barnes MA. The content of narrative discourse in children and adolescents after early-onset hydrocephalus and in normally developing age peers. *Brain Language* (1994) **46:** 129–65.

42. Swisher LP, Pinsker EJ. The language characteristics of hyperverbal hydrocephalic children. *Dev Med Child Neurol* **13:** 746–55.

43. Thompson NM, Chapieski L, Miner ME et al. Cognitive and motor abilities in preschool hydrocephalics. *J Clin Exp Neuropsychol* (1991) **13(2):** 245–58.

44. Fletcher JM, Francis DJ, Thompson NM et al. Verbal and nonverbal skill discrepancies in hydrocephalic children. *J Clin Exp Neuropsychol* (1992) **14:** 593–609.

45. Fletcher JM, Bohan TP, Brandt ME et al. Morphometric evaluation of the hydrocephalic brain: relationships with cognitive development. *Child's Nervous System* (1996) **12(4):** 192–9.

46. Hagberg B. The sequelae of spontaneously arrested infantile hydrocephalus. *Dev Med Child Neurol* (1962) **4:** 583–7.

47. Miller E, Sethi L. The effects of hydrocephalus perception. *Dev Med Child Neurol* (1971) **13(suppl 25):** 77–81.

48. Billard C, Santini JJ, Nargeot MC et al. Which future for children with hydrocephalus? Neurological, intellectual and visual outcome in 77 children with non-tumoral hydrocephalus. *Arch Fr Pediatrie* (1987) **44(10):** 849–54.

49. Simpson D, Hemmer R. Social aspects of hydrocephalus. In Schurr PH, Polkey CE (eds) *Hydrocephalus* (Oxford: Medical Publications, Oxford University Press).

50. Iddon JL, Morgan DJR, Sahakian BJ. Cognitive dysfunction in patients with congenital hydrocephalus and spina bifida: evidence for a dysexecutive syndrome? *Eur J Pediatr Surg* (1996) **6(Suppl I):** 41.

51. Baron-Cohen S, Jolliffe T, Mortimore C, Robertson M. Another advanced test of theory of mind: evidence from very high functioning adults with autism or asperger syndrome. *J Child Psychol Psychiatry* (1997) **38(7):** 813–22.

52. Snow JH, Prince M, Souheaver G et al. Neuropsychological patterns of adolescents and young adults with spina bifida. *Arch Clin Neuropsychol* (1994) **9(3):** 277–87.

53. Culatta B, Young C. Linguistic performance as a function of abstract task demands in children with spina bifida. *Dev Med Child Neurol* (1992) **34(5):** 434–40.

54. Tew B. 'The Cocktail Party Syndrome' in children with hydrocephalus and spina bifida. *Br J Disord Communication* (1975) **14:** 447–50.

55. Landry S. Goal-directed behaviour and perception of self-competence in children with spina bifida. *J Pediatr Psychol* (1993) **18(3):** 389–96.

56. Appleton PL, Minchom PE, Ellis NC et al. The self-concept of young people with spina bifida: a population-based study. *Dev Med Child Neurol* (1994) **36(3):** 198–215.

57. Ineichen R. Towards co-ordinated care of spina bifida children. *Social Work Today* (1973) **4:** 321–4.

58. Fletcher JM, Brookshire BL,

Landry SH et al. Behavioural adjustment of children with hydrocephalus: relationships with etiology, neurological and family status. *J Pediatr Psychol* (1995) **20(1):** 109–25.

59. Campbell S. Early prenatal diagnosis of neural tube defects by ultrasound. *Clin Obstet Gynecol* (1977) **20(2):** 351–9.

60. Spaulding BR, Morgan SB. Spina bifida and their parents: a population prone to family dysfunction. *J Pediatr Psychol* (1986) **11:** 359–74.

61. Lord J, Varzos N, Behrman B et al. Implications of mainstream classrooms for adolescents with spina bifida. *Dev Med Child Neurol* (1990) **32:** 20–9.

62. Fishman R. Normal pressure hydrocephalus and arthritis. *N Engl J Med* (1985) **312(19):** 1255–6.

63. Sobkowiak CA. Effect of hydrocephalus on neuronal migration and maturation. *Eur J Pediatr Surg* (1992) **2(Suppl 1):** 7–11.

64. Weller RO, Shulman K. Infantile hydrocephalus: clinical, histological and ultrastructural study of brain damage. *J Neurosurg* (1972) **36:** 255–6.

65. Spain B. Verbal and performance ability in pre-school children with spina bifida. *Dev Med Child Neurol* (1974) **16:** 773–80.

66. Anderson EM. Cognitive deficits in children with spina bifida and hydrocephalus: a review of the literature. *Br J Educat Psychol* (1973) **43:** 257–68.

67. Anderson EM, Spain B. *The Child with Spina Bifida* (London: Methuen, 1977).

68. Anderson EM, Plewis I. Impairment of a motor skill in children with spina bifida cystica and hydrocephalus: an exploratory study. *Br J Psychol* (1977) **68:** 61–70.

8
Dementia of the Alzheimer type

Shibley Rahman, Rachel Swainson and
Barbara J Sahakian

Summary

Introduction

Alois Alzheimer in 1907 described the cerebral cortex of a 55-year-old woman with a progressive dementia, noting the presence of abnormal nerve cells that contained neurofibrillary tangles and neuritic plaques. The prevalence of the disorder varies with age: about 1 in 1000 for the age range 40–65, rising to 1 in 50 for 65–70, 1 in 20 for 70–80, and 1 in 5 for those aged 80+.

Diagnostic criteria

The unequivocal diagnosis of dementia of the Alzheimer type (DAT) rests upon histopathological evidence at brain autopsy or biopsy. Clinical diagnosis is reliant upon a careful history. The report of the NINCDS-ADRDA Work Group on Alzheimer's Disease documents now well-established criteria for probable DAT. Other supportive tools include neuropsychological assessment, including the Mini-Mental State Examination (MMSE), and clinical rating scales such as the Clinician Interview Based Impression of Change (CIBIC). Furthermore, a range of possible investigative tools includes conventional neuropsychological tests, computer-based neuropsychological assessment, and structural and functional neuroimaging. Neuropsychology is crucial to diagnosis.

Neuropathology

The morphology of DAT includes cerebral atrophy, deposition of beta A4 amyloid (senile plaques and amyloid angiopathy), and neuritic changes (neuritic plaques, neurofibrillary tangles and neuropil threads). Four genes are associated with Alzheimer's disease. Three of these — the amyloid precursor protein (APP) gene on chromosome 21, the presenilin 1 gene on chromosome 14 and the presenilin 2 gene on chromosome 1 — are autosomal dominant genes associated with early-onset disease. Variation of another gene (*ApoE*) is also associated with Alzheimer's disease later in life. This gene has three forms: *ApoE2*, *ApoE3* and *ApoE4*. *ApoE2* seems to protect against Alzheimer's, while *ApoE4* seems to make it more likely. Furthermore, because of their chromosomal defect, people with Down's syndrome are also more likely to develop Alzheimer's disease.

Main neuropsychological findings

Clinically, the presenting problem in patients with DAT is often difficulty in new learning and memory, clinically usually forgetfulness of a minor degree, which may be difficult to distinguish from the effects of normal aging. The most profound impact is on episodic memory, usually with both verbal and non-verbal material affected. DAT also results in poor attention, with increased levels of distractibility and poor concentration, leading to difficulties in conversation, or following a news item on the television or in a newspaper article. There may be difficulty in performing everyday tasks, due to deficits in executive functioning. Assessment of neuropsychology is vital for early diagnosis, as well as differential diagnosis. We outline the rationale for two particular tests, paired associates learning and delayed matching to sample, that may be useful for this purpose, and their underlying scientific rationale. This is useful in the light of recent developments in therapies for DAT.

Introduction

Dementia of the Alzheimer type, or Alzheimer's disease, is the most common cause of dementia in the elderly, accounting for approximately 60–80% of cases. Alois Alzheimer in 1907 described the cerebral cortex of a 55-year-old woman with a progressive dementia, noting the presence of abnormal nerve cells that contained neurofibrillary tangles and neuritic plaques. This particular type of dementia is of considerable importance, as it is thought to affect approximately 5% of persons aged over 65 years, and 11% of the population between 80 and 85 years of age (24% older than 85). The Alzheimer's Disease Society estimated that, at the beginning of the year 2000, there were approximately 750 000 people with dementia living in the UK, of whom 400 000 had DAT.

A major objective of this chapter is to critically evaluate the evidence which may allow us to develop predictive tests for this disorder. The early diagnosis of DAT is crucial for effective care of both patients and carers, and specifically allows intervention using suitable drugs. Neuropsychology is a major component of the diagnosis of DAT, and we will therefore give an account of the main methods of neuropsychological assessment that are currently being adopted. We will also discuss what is currently known about the natural history of the neuropsychological deficits in DAT and consider the major domains of cognitive dysfunction that are represented in this disorder. There have been several recent developments in our understanding of the function of medial temporal lobe structures in memory, and in our knowledge of the staging of neuropathological deficits. A synthesis of both lines of evidence indicates that, while DAT is undoubtedly a distressing disorder, considerable progress has been made into which functional deficits occur and why. This offers substantial hope for the future.

Neuropathology

A key feature of DAT is that neurodegeneration is progressive, and this conclusion from neuropathological studies has been further corroborated from findings in vivo, using neuroimaging techniques such as positron emission tomography (PET).[1,2] The unequivocal diagnosis of DAT rests upon histopathological evidence at brain autopsy or biopsy (review: Jellinger and Bancher[3]). The morphology of DAT includes cerebral atrophy, deposition of beta A4 amyloid (senile plaques and amyloid angiopathy), and neuritic changes (neuritic plaques, neurofibrillary tangles and neuropil threads). In the earliest stages of disease, the pathology is known to affect medial temporal lobe structures, including the parahippocampal and entorhinal cortex (see the staging of hierarchical spreading of neuritic changes described by Braak and Braak[4]). This concurs with the initial cognitive deficits seen in patients with the formation of new memories. Important findings by Braak and Braak[4] indicate specifically that only the entorhinal region, a major port of entry for neocortical data in transit to limbic components of the medial temporal lobe, is affected in the mildest cases of DAT (reviews: Braak et al[5] and Gomez-Isla et al[6]). Encouragingly, there seems to be consistency in this finding across the literature.[7,8] The entorhinal region lies in a critical path in neural systems related to memory, receiving afferents from widespread association and limbic areas, projecting to the dentate gyrus of the hippocampal formation, receiving afferents from the hippocampus (HC) and sending efferents back to association neocortex.[9] Selective lamina within the entorhinal cortex may be selectively vulnerable,[6] contributing functionally to the compromise of memory-related neural systems.

Further review of the neurochemical literature regarding DAT reveals that neurons of the nucleus basalis of Meynert and cortical cholinergic axons are severely depleted in DAT.[10,11] A substantial literature indicates a consistent loss of basal forebrain cholinergic neurons in DAT, ranging from 30% to 90%. The loss of cortical cholinergic neurons is usually most severe (up to 85%) in inferotemporal, mid-temporal and entorhinal cortex and amygdala; less severe (40–70%) in prefrontal, parietal and hippocampal complex; and light (4–30%) in primary visual, motor and anterior cingulate cortex. This has proven of enormous interest for drugs which ameliorate the cholinergic deficit, for example the cholinesterase inhibitors.[12]

Diagnosis

The report of the NINCDS-ADRDA Work Group on Alzheimer's Disease documents now well-established criteria for probable DAT which have been found to produce good inter rater agreement in their application.[13] The criteria for the clinical diagnosis of probable DAT include: dementia established by clinical examination and documented by the MMSE, Blessed Dementia Scale, or a similar examination and confirmed by neuropsychological tests; deficits in two or more areas of cognition; progressive worsening of memory and other cognitive functions; no disturbance of consciousness; onset between ages 40 and 90, most often after age 65; and absence of systemic disorders or other brain diseases that in and of themselves could account for the progressive deficits in memory and cognition. The diagnosis is supported by: progressive deterioration of specific cognitive functions such as language (aphasia), motor skills (apraxia), and perception (agnosia); impaired activities of daily living and altered patterns of behavior; family history of similar disorders, particularly if confirmed neuropathologically; and laboratory results of normal lumbar puncture, normal pattern or non-specific changes in EEG, and evidence of cerebral atrophy on computerized tomography with progression documented by serial observation.

The diagnosis of dementia requires a careful clinical history with reliable informants.[14] This enables other causes of dementia to be excluded, and also enables identification of risk factors for DAT, for example head trauma, advanced age, Down's syndrome, or a history of dementia in first-degree relatives.[15] Despite considerable advances in both the genetic research and clinical management studies (review: Ganguli[16]), there is at present no reliable predictive test for most forms of DAT (review: Green et al[17]). To examine the extent of problems of the patients with DAT, a gamut of possible investigative tools includes conventional neuropsychological tests, computer-based neuropsychological assessment, and structural and functional neuroimaging. Neuropsychology contributes substantially to the diagnosis of dementia,[18] and, at an early stage, may precisely identify cognitive disorders, not necessarily accompanied by clinical complaints. Indeed, the NINCDS-ADRDA criteria are based on neuropsychological symptoms. The contribution of neuropsychology to the detection of DAT will be the focus of this chapter.

It is now known that, in the clinical diagnosis of DAT, magnetic resonance imaging (MRI) helps to improve the diagnostic accuracy, and, recently, new MRI-based techniques for performing volumetric measurement of cortical and subcortical structures have been developed. Many patients with minimal cognitive impairment already have brain changes accentuated within the hippocampal region, and around 70% of these patients may develop clinical dementia within a 4-year period;[19] longitudinal study has shown that hippocampal atrophy is a sensitive and specific predictor of future DAT for patients with minimal cognitive impairment. However, it is notable that a recent study demonstrated that the appearance of diffuse cerebral and medial temporal atrophy only occurred in patients with familial Alzheimer's disease once they were clinically affected.[20]

Recent years have provided new information about dementias using techniques such as functional MRI (fMRI). Functional neuroimaging techiques such as PET and single photon emission computed tomography (SPECT) have been used under resting conditions to measure abnormal patterns of regional cerebral blood flow and cerebral metabolic rate for glucose in patients with particular neuropsychological profiles, and to attempt to correlate the two.[21,22] Activation studies with PET permit the visualization of neural activity actively engaged in cognitive operations with good spatial resolution of the order of 1 cm, but relatively poor temporal resolution in comparison to information-processing tasks and event-related potentials. The finding of activation in cortical areas of patients with DAT requires qualified interpretation, as to whether there is a reallocation of cortical areas to perform a task or there is compensation for neuropathological changes which have occurred in the brain region relative to controls.[23]

The natural history of neuropsychological deficits

While some traditional teaching confusingly leaves one with the message that DAT is characterized by a global cognitive impairment, it is now being accepted that the initial deficit of the syndrome may be manifested as problems in memory and attention, which progress very gradually before impairments become apparent in other cognitive domains such as language, semantic memory and visuospatial function.[13,21,24]

In modern research in neuropsychology, a major advance has been the realization that many cognitive domains are not unified concepts, such as memory,[25] attention [26] and executive function, but instead may be divided into separate subsystems at both a functional and a neuroanatomical level. A careful consideration of the animal studies, human cognitive neuropsychology, neuropathology and neuroimaging has led, for example, to the identification of subtypes of memory, particularly in identification of the hippocampal complex as a crucial area in the encoding of new memories.[27] The main dichotomy is between declarative and non-declarative memory. Declarative memory includes memories for events (episodic) and facts (semantic), in which the memory content can be described or declared through verbalization and/or visualization, and depends on the integrity of the medial temporal lobe system (i.e. HC and related structures, including entorhinal, perirhinal and parahippocampal cortices).[28] In non-declarative memory, experience alters behavior non-consciously without providing any memory context: this includes skill-learning, priming, and non-associative memory (e.g. habituation, sensitization). In DAT, while episodic and semantic memory can be impaired, non-declarative memory remains relatively preserved.

Clinically, the presenting problem in patients with DAT is often difficulty in new learning and memory,[29] clinically usually forgetfulness of a minor degree, which may be difficult to distinguish from the effects of normal aging. The most profound impact is on episodic memory, usually with both verbal and non-verbal material affected. The anterograde amnesia results from both a failure to encode new information and rapid forgetting of new material. The crucial role of the entorhinal and perirhinal cortices in successful completion of visual recognition memory tasks has been highlighted in work using rats[30,31] and monkeys,[32,33] and it is therefore perhaps not surprising that episodic memory deficits may represent one of the earliest deficits in patients with DAT. It is important to note that, even within the domain of episodic memory, there may be heterogeneity in performance. Although the majority of DAT patients show the classic anterograde amnesia, some DAT patients show relatively specific evidence of short-term memory deficits in either or both the verbal and visual modalities. Retrograde memory loss has a temporally graded pattern, with sparing of more distant memories. Working memory as judged by digit span is generally normal early on in the disease.

A number of recent studies claim that attentional impairments represent the first non-mnemonic deficits in DAT. Attention, like memory, is not a unitary construct: aspects of vigilance and sustained as well as covert and overt visuospatial attention are affected in early, mild DAT. In contrast, attentional set-shifting is relatively spared in the mild stages of DAT, but deficits appear with increasing disease severity. Patients in the very early stages of DAT may show a reduced control in the spatial focus of attention, which contributes to deficits in spatial memory, reading, spelling, confrontation naming and letter cancellation. Language is typically normal on informal assessment. However, mild anomia on formal naming tests and poor generation of exemplars on category fluency may be found. Visuospatial functioning is good on simple bedside assessment, but deficits may become apparent on formal assessment, manifested as an inability to copy diagrams. In contrast with patients with frontal dementias, patients with DAT generally have well-preserved personality and do not show marked behavioral disturbance in the mild stages of the disease.

Later in the disease, impaired memory and attention results in marked temporal disorientation. Impairment in working memory is found. Distractibility and executive dysfunction occur which may reflect disconnection of corticocortical tracts. Breakdown of semantic memory leads to word-finding difficulties, diminished vocabulary, semantic paraphasic errors in spontaneous conversation, poor naming ability, reduced generation of exemplars on category fluency testing, and a loss of general knowledge. Marked visuospatial deficits are usually apparent, manifested as an inability of patients to find their way around when driving, or to judge distances. Although there is considered to be incomplete agreement about the actual order of decline in the various domains because of heterogeneity across the different samples which have been studied and the difficulty of comparing all the functions together using equally sensitive methods, it appears that, in general, the course of deterioration across various cognitive domains in DAT is consistent with a posterior-to-anterior spread of pathology in the cerebral cortex.

The major domains of cognitive performance

Studies comparing the current cognitive performance of diagnosed DAT patients with that of healthy control subjects have highlighted differences between these populations in a number of areas of cognition — principally memory (episodic and semantic), attention and executive function. These will be considered in turn.

Memory and new learning

Effects on anterograde episodic memory, or the ability to acquire new memories of events, are most noticeable to the early DAT patient and their family in everyday life,[29] for instance forgetting conversations, appointments, or information from a recently watched TV program. The key role played by hippocampal and related temporal lobe structures, e.g. entorhinal cortex and subiculum, in episodic memory is now firmly established (reviews: Squire[27] and Murray[34]; see also Murray[35]) and doubtless underlies the particular vulnerability of these functions in early DAT. Episodic memory deficits are probed via a number of traditional psychological tests, often requiring recall of verbal lists or information (e.g. the California Verbal Learning Test (CVLT)[36]) and logical memory from the Wecshler Memory Scale (WMS).[37] The deficits are present in a variety of conditions, e.g. recognition as well as free or cued recall, and visual as well as verbal modalities.

There is some controversy over the exact nature of the episodic memory deficit, for example whether it stems from a primary impairment of storage with an increased rate of forgetting,[38] impairments in retrieval potentially related to strategic or executive deficits, or poor registration or learning of information,[39] possibly resulting partly from attentional disruption (see below).

The impairment of knowledge-based, or semantic, memory later in the course of DAT probably reflects the spread of pathology from medial temporal lobe structures to the temporal neocortex proper.[24] There is forgetting of over-learned material such as people's names and infrequently used items. Testing with confrontation naming and generative naming (verbal fluency) tasks suggests that impairments are primarily due to breakdown in the structure of semantic knowledge (degradation of stored representations), which is augmented by poor retrieval strategies.[40] Semantic memory deficits can augment those in episodic memory, leading to even greater impairments on cued recall tasks where control subjects, but not DAT patients, are able to make use of semantic cues to improve recall.[41]

Attention

Patients and their carers report that DAT brings increased levels of distractibility and poor concentration, leading to difficulties in conversation, or following a news item on the television or in a newspaper article. Although some aspects of attention appear to be spared in early DAT — e.g. immediate memory (digit span[42]), simultaneous matching-to-sample and attentional set-shifting,[43,44] — there seems to be no question that other aspects of attention, including focused attention and vigilance,[45] are susceptible to disruption in DAT. Selective attention — evaluated clinically using the visual cancellation task and the digit cancellation task — does not appear to be impaired in patients with mild DAT.[46] The finding that patients with mild DAT are unimpaired on intra- and extradimensional shifting[44] concurs with this finding. Interestingly, Sahakian et al[43] reported a double dissociation of memory and attentional deficits when comparing patients with Parkinson's disease (PD) and DAT. On the tasks used in this study, a subgroup of mild DAT patients were found to have memory deficits but no problems with attentional set-shifting, whereas the opposite is true for PD, reflecting perhaps that the memory deficits in DAT represent temporal lobe dysfunction, whereas the cognitive deficits in PD are related to frontostriatal dysfunction.

The improvement in attentional function seen after certain cholinergic therapeutic interventions such as nicotine or cholinesterase inhibitor administration[47,48,49] strongly suggests that it is the loss of acetylcholine throughout the cortex, subsequent to destruction of the forebrain nucleus basalis of Meynert, which is responsible for the poor attentional function. An alternative proposal is that the pathology within the cortex affects the transmission of information between cortical regions. Studies in experimental animals, such as those by Robbins and colleagues, using analogous tasks to those used in patients with DAT also suggest a key role for the cholinergic system arising from the nBM.[50]

Executive function

Observation of patients with DAT can reveal that they have difficulty in performing everyday tasks, because of deficits in executive functioning. Executive function, or control processes which optimize efficiency of subordinate psychological processes in certain (e.g. novel or involving a degree of conflict) situations,[51] can be somewhat difficult to define and may include a number of distinct factors. It is also notoriously difficult to measure accurately when the subordinate processes themselves are disrupted, as they often are in DAT. Nevertheless, it seems that impairments in some aspects of executive function may contribute to the profile of impaired memory in DAT[52] for example by impairing the search for appropriate items during phonemic fluency tasks.[53] The ability to perform in 'dual-task' situations is a classic example of a situation in which a superordinate or supervisory control process could be implemented to improve performance. It seems that DAT patients find it particularly difficult to perform dual tasks adequately and that this is not an effect simply of difficulty on overall processing capacity.[54]

Methods of neuropsychological assessment

The degree of functional cognitive dysfunction in DAT is best evaluated with neuropsychological assessment. It is particularly vital in the measured outcome of drug trials that provide measurement of cognitive impairment across several stages of disease, have alternative forms to avoid practice effects, and have high inter rater and retest reliability.

The MMSE is easy to administer, measures relevant areas of cognition, is available in multiple languages, and has available longitudinal data.[55] It shows good test–retest and inter rater reliability, is relatively easy to administer, and can follow decline in patients going into the later stages of dementia. Its major disadvantages are that it does not cover all domains of cognitive functioning, is insufficiently sensitive for the early detection of dementia, and is relatively insensitive to change. It may also be subject to considerable bias from sociodemographic variability in subjects.

The Alzheimer Disease Assessment Scale (ADAS) is another attempt to measure specifically gross cognitive deficits considered to be characteristic of patients with DAT, and measures the severity of dysfunction in both cognitive and non-cognitive domains.[56] The cognitive part (ADAS-cog) has 11 items and a maximum score of 70, and measures memory, language and praxis. A score of 70 means that the patient is profoundly demented, and a score of 0 means that the patient made no errors at all. It therefore provides a broad coverage of cognitive functioning and is frequently used as an outcome measure. The non-cognitive part of the scale consists of 10 items, and includes measures of mood state and behavioral changes (ADAS-*non cog*). However, members of the International Working Group on the Harmonization of Dementia Drug Guidelines were recently critical of the ADAS-*cog*, stating that 'a generally acknowledged limitation of the ADAS-*cog* is that it lacks a subtest for attention/concentration'.

The Clinical Global Impression of Change (CGIC) and the CIBC are scales which measure improvement or worsening in condition since the last assessment. The CGIC is completed by the attending physician, supposed to be blind to the results of neuropsychological testing, and without input from relatives or caregivers. An important criticism is that, at present, a number of CGIC scales have not been validated, but are nevertheless being employed in clinical trials. Performance on memory testing appears to influence the ratings more than other features of dementia. The main themes considered in the CIBIC are functional independence, social appropriateness and mental clarity.

Most recently, computerized neuropsychological testing batteries have been receiving much attention from investigators in the field of dementia. Conventional neuropsychological tests are popular because of their ease of administration and the existence of normative data. These tests are available in standardized versions, and therefore allow performance to be compared across studies as well as with the performance of other cognitive domains such as semantic memory and visuospatial functions. Many conventional neuropsychological tests tend to suffer from ceiling effects in normal volunteers, a lack of specificity, and poor temporal resolution. Many of the tests load quite heavily on functions of working memory, episodic memory and low-level visuospatial abilities. Recent technological advances have been exploited for the development instead of computerized neuropsychological assessments which are reproducible and accurately timed. These tests therefore have high temporal resolution and may allow comparison of results across studies and linking of deficits to the anatomy of pathology.

The Cambridge Neuropsychological Test Automated Battery (CANTAB) is an example of these batteries, and has extensive normative data.[57,58] The existence of extensive normative data from a large (*N* about 800) sample of normal community-dwelling elderly volunteers, which also takes into account the premorbid functioning of the patients, makes the use of such batteries extremely useful. Finally, the existence of graded difficulty levels within each test reduces the common problem of floor and ceiling effects. The theoretical rationale of the tests is based upon two main themes: (1) adapting tests from animal neuropsychological paradigms that have proved successful in elucidating the neural substrates of certain types of cognitive function; and (2) undertaking a componential analysis of the processes underlying particular forms of cognitive function. The CANTAB battery is therefore of use also in psychopharmacological studies. The tests are comprehensive in terms of the range of cognitive functions that they assess, including the domains of attention, visual learning and memory, working memory and planning. One of the advantages of CANTAB is that various tests have been validated on neurosurgical cases with well-defined cortical excisions, and additional neural validation has been provided by a growing set of neuroimaging data.

The need for neuropsychological assessment

Neuropsychological assessment in patients with DAT has a number of aims, including: (1) early diagnosis; and (2) differential diagnosis. Each of these clinical applications inevitably requires different combinations of neuropsychological tests.

Early diagnosis, for example within the context of a memory clinic, is clearly important, enabling the development of a clear plan for care, rationalization of drug treatment, and the commencement of appropriate treatment when it is of most value.[59] As the elderly population of the developed world increases and the number of people with dementia also grows, there is continual interest in the problems that people with dementia face. There is now considerable optimism in the treatment of the presenile dementias, particularly as any drug that could delay the onset of symptoms should have a serious impact upon the number of people affected before natural death occurs. With this optimism has come the growing realization that therapeutic strategies in dementia should have very specific aims — to delay the progress of the disorder that is causing a progressive decline, to treat a range of emergent cognitive deficits, to ameliorate associated behavioral and affective disturbances, thereby reducing the consequences of functional disability and improving quality of life, and to address fully the needs of the caregiver. While work is ongoing to define those factors in already-diagnosed DAT patients who will derive most benefit from treatment with the new acetylcholinesterase (AChE) inhibitors, there is also a strong need to predict which individuals, as yet undiagnosed with DAT, will go on to develop the disease proper. Intervention at this early stage could allow progress of the disease to be arrested, or at least slowed, such that the patient's level of functioning remained at an acceptable level. Unfortunately, until recently, the development of the early detection of DAT has been somewhat hindered by the lack of elderly normative data.

The differential diagnosis includes delirium and depression, which both need to be excluded. If cognitive changes develop over a very short period of time, the diagnosis is likely to be delirium, not dementia. Delirium is an acute state of fluctuating awareness that develops over hours or days and is caused by medical conditions such as liver or kidney failure, urinary tract infection or hypoglycemia, and is usually reversible.

Examination during a lucid interval may show a relative preservation of intellectual faculties. Dementia can also be extremely difficult to differentiate from depression in the elderly. There is remission in depression, whereas dementia is progressive; also, patients with depression are often slow to answer in mental status testing. Psychomotor retardation and insomnia with early-morning waking are commonly present in depression. Depressed, elderly patients exhibit a generalized profile of deficits, with impairments in tests shown to be sensitive to temporal or prefrontal cortical dysfunction. The depressed may also exhibit an abnormal response to negative feedback which may contribute to different forms of cognitive dysfunctioning.[29] DAT may also be confused with focal degenerative disorders which indicate a more restricted form of progressive neurodegeneration limited to a particular part of the cerebral cortex, as may be the case for semantic dementia and frontal variant, frontotemporal degeneration.

Which tests will be most useful in predicting DAT?

No neuropsychological test is likely to be a true predictor of disease; rather, a test may be sensitive enough to detect impairments produced by the small degree of damage incurred at the earliest stages of disease, months or years before a clinical diagnosis of DAT would be reached. It is possible that it may also detect this damage before changes would be detectable using structural or functional imaging techniques, but such a direct comparison has yet to be carried out. The neuroanatomical staging findings of Braak and Braak[4] show us that those areas which are susceptible to the earliest damage remain among the worst affected throughout the course of the disease; thus, the tests for which patients in the mild stages of probable DAT are most impaired may well turn out to be the most sensitive tests in predicting DAT.

Concepts behind the development of accurate predictive neuropsychological tests

Patients with purely amnesic symptoms, although not fulfilling clinical criteria for a diagnosis of probable DAT, show a high rate of conversion to DAT and therefore may be seen as being in the prodromal stages of the disease;[60] however, impaired memory is a feature of other conditions, such as depression[61] and other dementias, as well as of normal aging, so it is essential that the amnesia of preclinical DAT can be characterized specifically in order to be useful in early diagnosis. Because memory function is now well accepted to be composed of a number of facets which are to some degree separable (e.g. episodic, semantic, procedural memory), it is reasonable to assume that the significant damage within the entorhinal and hippocampal regions which characterizes this preclinical phase of DAT[4] may be detectable with suitably directed neuropsychological tests. The deficits in anterograde episodic memory (memory for new events) which is evident in the earliest stages of DAT in fact probably reflects damage to the hippocampal formation,[62,63] and it is likely that a predictive test for DAT would assess this type of memory.

However, caution must be exercised for a number of reasons when developing and using such a test.

Heterogeneity of neuropathology and symptoms in DAT

It is not necessarily the case that the pattern of neuropathology is consistent across individuals.[52,64] Patients may present with a progressive parietal lobe syndrome[65] or a progressive aphasia.[66] The study of single cases can therefore be very useful in understanding the range of cognitive deficits in DAT. Such heterogeneity poses a problem for the utility of a single task in predicting DAT. If such a test relies for its usefulness on tapping the functions of the area(s) of the brain which receive the earliest damage in DAT, it would be unlikely to detect the onset of the disease in a patient whose initial damage was restricted to another area, say, the parietal lobe.[67]

Benefits of repeat testing

Because of the wide range of cognitive ability within the healthy population, an impaired score from a neuropsychological test at any single point in time would be unlikely to constitute unequivocal evidence of DAT, particularly with high-performing individuals whose dementia brought their scores down to the average level. Conversely, patients with a low-functioning baseline may be falsely considered as showing deterioration without reference to appropriate normative data. Unlike verbal IQ, which can be predicted with some degree of accuracy using tests such as the National Adult Reading Test (NART),[68] there is no available test for premorbid memory function. Consideration of the history of the patient is therefore important; for example, indicators of a high level of premorbid cognitive function may include patients who were well educated, well read and successful in a job, whereas a low level could include poor scholastic performance. This difficulty may be relatively simply overcome by employing repeat testing over a number of months and using the decline in score as the predictive measure. This is particularly appropriate, of course, in the study of dementias for which *progressive* decline in cognitive abilities is a core feature. Such an approach is proving to be valuable in both the neuropsychological and structural imaging realms,[20] and should also aid in the differential diagnosis of dementia from conditions which produce non-progressive cognitive complaints, such as depression.

The need for specificity as well as sensitivity

Although brain function is accepted to be to some degree modularized, such that particular areas have responsibilities for implementing particular cognitive functions, there is also a high degree of intercommunication between these modules, and neuroimaging studies show us that a large proportion of the brain is active during any given task. It is, therefore, a more useful approach to consider the distributed neuronal network necessary to perform a task. A way of increasing the specificity of a predictive task is to also administer a task which would be expected to show a lack of impairment in DAT. Neuropsychological tasks have been identified which are relatively more sensitive to frontotemporal lobar degeneration (FTLD), Huntington's disease (HD) and PD than to mild DAT. For example, it is useful to note that patients with mild frontal variant of FTLD (fvFTLD), as well as showing marked behavioral changes which are traditionally considered to be hallmarks of the condition, may demonstrate cognitive deficits akin to those of patients with defined neurosurgical lesions affecting the ventromedial or orbital prefrontal cortex in reversal learning and decision-making.[69] Interestingly, a preliminary analysis indicates that patients with mild DAT do not show these reversal deficits.[70] A full overview of the nature of cognition in this disorder, and other 'frontostriatal' pathologies such as PD and HD, may be found in Rahman et al.[70]

Extrapolating from clinical studies to use of tests with patient populations

Measures of accuracy for tests used to discriminate between patient populations must always be interpreted with caution, as they depend critically on the nature of the populations against which accuracy of the test is assessed (see Figure 8.1 for definitions of sensitivity and specificity).

Evidence for the use of certain tests in early neuropsychological detection

A number of studies have taken the approach of simply comparing matched groups of patients diagnosed with DAT and healthy control subjects and assessing the accuracy of neuropsychological measures in appropriately distinguishing these populations. Such studies are a useful first step in finding predictive markers of DAT. In this context, high sensitivity is found in episodic recall such as the logical memory stories of the

Sensitivity = Number of patients failing test
 Total patient cases

i.e. How many patients will a particular test assign correctly?

Specificity = Number of non-patients* failing test
 Total non-patient cases

i.e. How many non-patients will a particular test assign correctly?

*This may include other patient groups, as well as healthy controls for a more stringent measure of specificity

Figure 8.1

Definitions of 'sensitivity' and 'specificity'.

WMS, especially when tasks also involve semantic cueing.[71,72] Solomon et al[73] found that combining scores from four neuropsychological tests (cued recall, category fluency, orientation and clock-drawing) produced a model with 100% accuracy for differentiating probable DAT from healthy controls. However, the *selectivity* of tasks to DAT was not stringently assessed with this type of study design, because there is much more overlap of symptoms with those of depression and other forms of dementia than with normal aging, and, indeed, distinguishing DAT from such conditions is a more relevant problem in clinical practice.[74] Varma et al[75] showed that the NINCDS-ADRDA criteria which are used to make a clinical diagnosis of probable DAT are only 23% specific for DAT when assessed retrospectively (after neuropathological confirmation at postmortem) against cases of FTLD. Neuropsychological measures were shown to be more useful in differentiating the following two disorders — orientation and praxis (relatively specific for DAT) and problem-solving (relatively specific for FTLD). The attentional set-shifting task from the CANTAB battery may prove to be useful in differentiating FTLD and DAT, as described above.

Unfortunately, relatively little work has been done on accurately differentiating DAT and elderly depression by neuropsychological measures. This is a particularly troublesome differentiation to make, as depression may be part of the symptomatology of dementia — many recently diagnosed DAT patients subsequently develop depressive symptoms[76] possibly due to pathology within some of the same structures as are damaged in DAT,[77] and the symptomatology of depression appears to change as DAT becomes established.[78] Distinguishing the two conditions, where possible, will be necessary in order to optimize their treatment, and this may be best done by characterizing fine-grained neuropsychological profiles of the disorders.[79] Ongoing studies are currently underway which will attempt to further characterize and differentiate these disorders.[80]

The best way to be sure that tests give accurate *predictive* measures is to use them longitudinally (repeated testing over time) with a currently non-demented population and, following diagnosis by clinical or pathological criteria, retrospectively evaluate task performance against outcome (i.e. how many patients who performed below a certain cut-off went on to receive the diagnosis). A test intended for use in screening for DAT among the general population should ideally be assessed in an epidemiological study, where recruitment is carried out in a non-selective way and a large group of subjects is followed up over time in order to give a realistic picture of the actual incidence rates in the general population. Such studies have shown that poor recall and learning are associated with a later diagnosis of DAT and, in addition that recognition, naming and 'control' ('executive') aspects of tasks may be predictive for DAT.[81,82]

Epidemiological studies are necessarily very extensive and expensive in terms of both the numbers of subjects needing to be recruited and the time needed to follow them up, owing to the relatively low conversion rate to DAT in the general population. There are also problems with drop-out of subjects, leading to analytical considerations. Much smaller, shorter-duration studies are feasible when subjects are those at high risk of conversion to DAT. Fox et al[20] followed patients with a 50% genetic risk of developing familial DAT (FAD), first testing them when they were clinically non-demented and when both they and close family members felt that they had suffered no cognitive decline. Scores at this stage on tests of performance IQ and verbal recognition memory were significantly poorer among the eight patients who went on to fulfill the criteria for probable DAT within 5 years than among those who remained well. However, the accuracy (sensitivity and specificity) of these measures in distinguishing the healthy and demented groups was not reported.

The most appropriate patients for intervention therapies in the near future are probably those who have already begun to show some symptoms of DAT but are as yet in the very early stages. These cases cannot fulfill criteria for probable DAT and may referred to as having isolated memory loss,[83] 'questionable dementia'[84] or 'mild cognitive impairment'.[71] The rates of conversion to DAT are higher among such subjects than in the general population (e.g. 12% per year compared with 1–2% per year in the study by Petersen et al[71]). Tierney et al[85] showed that a combination of scores from the Rey Auditory Verbal Learning Test and the Mental Control subtest of the WMS predicted which patients would develop probable DAT within 2 years with a sensitivity of 76% and a specificity of 94%.

The quest to develop more accurate predictive measures continues. As described previously, computerized tests may provide the reliability of administration (standardized feedback timings of presentation, etc.) necessary for a measure which could be used to aid diagnosis. Two CANTAB (CeNeS Ltd) tests — paired associates learning (PAL) and delayed matching to sample (DMTS) — may be of use in this respect. DMTS is a classic test of episodic memory, and is used in a large amount of research. In this task, each item (an abstract colored pattern) must be stored over a short time and then selected from among distractor items. The CANTAB version of this task has been shown to be differentially sensitive to different types of neural damage in humans. The DMTS procedure has previously been found to be sensitive to the mnemonic impairments in patients with temporal lobe lesions or bilateral amygdalo-hippocampectomies.[86] Even more specifically, the DMTS test is a test of visual recognition memory, which evidence from studies in non-human primates suggests is dependent on the rhinal cortex,[34] known to be affected early in DAT. While mild DAT patients show delay-dependent deficits, the impairments of patients with PD, or patients with neurosurgical temporal lobe excisions and amygdalohippocampectomy, appear not to be related to the length of delay; frontal lobe excisions do not significantly impair performance.[43,87] Interestingly, particularly in relation to the hypothesis that cholinergic abnormalities contribute to cognitive deficits in DAT, the muscarinic receptor antagonist scopolamine significantly impairs accuracy of performance on the DMTS task in a dose- and delay-dependent manner.[88]

The second task (PAL) utilizes the finding that some forms of associative learning may be especially sensitive to DAT. We have demonstrated striking deficits on the CANTAB (CeNeS Ltd; www.cenes.com) PAL episodic memory task even in mild DAT. Previous neuropsychological findings[87] and current findings from similar associative learning tasks suggest that the visuospatial PAL test may be sensitive to damage to regions including the parahippocampal gyrus and entorhinal cortex. In this task, subjects have to learn the location of a number of patterns, with levels increasing in difficulty from 1 to 8 patterns, and up to 10 chances given at each level until all patterns are placed correctly (otherwise the task terminates). Ability to perform this task is impaired by frontal as well as temporal lobe excisions,[87] probably because it may be performed using 'conditional' rules (e.g. when shown pattern A, touch box 1); the more difficult stages of the task are also sensitive to PD.[43] In contrast, 'implicit' learning (where memories are not available to conscious report) appears to be relatively unaffected in DAT. This further distinguishes DAT from 'subcortical dementias' such as PD and HD, which can impair implicit learning, probably due to striatal lesions.[89,90]

These tests have been shown to discriminate well between probable DAT and control patients, and also to signal the onset of DAT among patients with questionable dementia (QD).[84,91] In the latter study, a group of 21 QD subjects, along with groups of probable DAT and healthy control subjects, was assessed at 6-monthly intervals using these tasks. Errors made on the PAL task did not discriminate QD patients from controls at time of entry to the study, but significant group differences were apparent after 12 months. Moreover, the *decline* in performance (increase in errors) over 12 months appeared to split the QD cases into roughly equal subgroups, whose scores either declined or remained stable. The authors hypothesized that the subgroup whose scores declined may be incipient DAT cases, and in fact all of these patients have now received a clinical diagnosis (Figure 8.2).

These questions are being addressed in an ongoing study by our group[80] using the same tasks as those used by Fowler et al but along with a large number of other computerized and traditional non-computerized tests and incorporating repeat testing of elderly depressed as well as mild DAT, QD and elderly control groups. Analyses from this study[80] indicate that the PAL task discriminates very well between mild probable DAT and depression. This is a good indication that this test may also be useful in predicting which QD patients (who have memory impair-

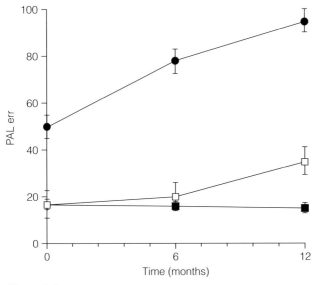

Figure 8.2

The total errors to criterion (PAL err) on the CANTAB paired associates learning task. Errors to criterion denotes how many errors were made before the completion of the test, so that a larger score indicates greater difficulty with the task. An adjusted score is used for participants *not* completing the test: participants who do not reach a set are allocated the error score of the lowest-performing individual attempting that set. [Key: Filled circles = patients with dementia of the Alzheimer type; open squares = patients with questionable dementia; filled squares = normal control volunteers.] (Redrawn from Fowler et al[91]).

ments but reach the diagnosis criteria for neither DAT nor depression) will develop DAT within a 2-year period. The crucial part of this study — retrospective evaluation of initial neuropsychological performance following diagnosis of probable DAT in a proportion of the sample — has yet to reach the analysis stage, but this will hopefully help to clear up some of the outstanding issues listed above, as well as crucially extending the assessment of these computerized studies in differentiating DAT from depression in the elderly.

Neural substrates underlying episodic memory deficits in DAT

We have demonstrated that two computerized tasks sensitive to mnemonic function — CANTAB PAL and DMTS — are useful in identifying deficits in DAT. It is instructive to consider the possible reasons for this in the light of the current literature delineating the brain systems of memory function.

Since the early reports that medial temporal lobe damage leads to serious problems in anterograde memory function, notably with patient HM, who received a bilateral temporal lobectomy and suffered a severe impairment in acquiring new memories,[92] a huge amount of effort has been devoted to animal studies to elucidate the functional effects of lesions of structures within the medial temporal lobe, with the aim of identifying the cause of the memory impairments in humans. Until recently, work from a number of laboratories had led to the idea that the medial temporal lobe was responsible for forming new declarative memories. The evidence in fact suggested that a number of temporal lobe structures, including the HC proper, amygdala and surrounding 'perihippocampal' cortex, acted together to encode and consolidate declarative memory, such that the greater the area of tissue damage, the more severe the memory loss (the effect of 'mass action'). One of the tasks most frequently used in such studies is the delayed non-matching to sample test (DNMTS), the matching analog of which has been shown to be so sensitive to DAT in humans. However, recent evidence suggests that the traditional aspirative lesion was removing more than the areas intended for lesion in these experiments, and that the HC and amygdala may in fact be less important in episodic memory function than had been thought.[34,35] Although some authors still argue for an essential role of HC in DNMTS,[93] the rhinal cortex — including perirhinal and entorhinal cortices — has now assumed prominence as subserving the type of visual episodic recognition memory necessary for DMTS or DNMTS performance,[34,94] a view now being corroborated by imaging evidence with healthy human volunteers.[95] This new evidence may help to explain the high degree of sensitivity of the DMTS task in DAT, as it is the transentorhinal and entorhinal cortices that suffer the most damage early on in

DAT, and continue to be among the worst affected areas throughout the course of the disease.[4,6] The integration of evidence from human and animal studies is obviously helpful in allocating dissociable functions to the various regions of the medial temporal lobe system. Nevertheless, there are likely to be a number of significant differences between human and other animals in terms of which particular brain areas participate in which cognitive functions, and indeed there may be no strict anatomical or connective homology between all of the areas mentioned.

One important difference, for example, is that while DNMTS is used to test the memory of monkeys, who spontaneously choose the novel item in an array, DMTS is used with humans, whose natural tendency appears to be to match stimuli. Thus, when the alternative task is used in either group, a factor of inhibition of the natural response is probably recruited, substantially altering the nature of the task, recruiting additional brain areas such as prefrontal cortex, and rendering it liable to impairments from rather different lesions.[95] Another difficulty has been identified with regard to the nature of semantic memory function. Bussey and Murray[96] have recently nominated the perirhinal cortex as being crucial for knowledge about objects rather than particular visual features, thus being 'semantic' in nature. In humans, it is an established finding that the anterior lateral temporal neocortex is the area of primary importance in the semantic deficits of patients with semantic dementia and in DAT.[24,97,98] It may be that task differences account for a degree of this discrepancy, particularly with regard to whether novel, or familiar, stimuli are employed. DNMTS in the animal studies essentially demands the animal to make a familiarity judgment when shown a number of stimuli, one of which is familiar because it has been seen in an identical format previously, whereas the material used with semantic dementia patients typically tests recollection of items which were familiar prior to testing (such as commonly used words in a word-list recognition task). It turns out that when such considerations are taken into account, there may be room for much agreement between the apparently contradictory evidence,[96] and an important lesson to be learned from these studies is that, at the very least, a great deal of care must be taken in extrapolating findings from monkeys to humans. Simons et al[99] and Graham et al[100] have contributed much to the discussion of the relationship between episodic and semantic memory, and have recently suggested that sensory and perceptual information and semantic memory work in concert to support new learning. It is an intriguing empirical question how patients with the temporal cortical damage sustained in semantic dementia would perform on the DMTS task, which is so sensitive to DAT.

The PAL task is very different in a number of respects from the DMTS task. First, its requirement to remember the location of a visual stimulus does not just tax the type of 'visual' memory used in DMTS, that of remembering the visual features of a particular object. The position of this object within a spatial array comprises information about the context of the object, particularly its spatial context, and as such may involve the 'dorsal' visual processing stream as well as the 'ventral' stream which is involved with the analysis of the object itself.[101] This implicates brain areas which receive information from at least two physically distant areas of association cortex and therefore may be subserved by hierarchically 'higher' levels of the visual memory system than are necessary for tasks which depend on purely visual information. This may implicate the rhinal cortex which is active in cross-modal association memory between visual and tactual information,[102] in keeping with the polymodal nature of its extrinsic neuronal connectivity. Further evidence comes from the imaging study of Owen et al,[103] which showed that the entorhinal cortex was activated particularly in the retrieval of stimulus–location as compared with a location memory control condition. In relation to this, PAL may load upon aspects of 'object-in-scene' memory, which appears to depend more upon hippocampal than perirhinal function.[94] A further factor for consideration is that, unlike D(N)MTS tasks, it is not a familiarity judgment which is required in PAL. Rather, a cue is given which constitutes one part of a learned stimulus–location association, and the subject is required to retrieve the missing piece of information. This requirement may be seen as being rather strategic in nature, thus being aided by the prefrontal circuitry, which has been implicated in memory retrieval.[104] It is clear that there exist exciting avenues for research in explaining precisely the subtle functional deficits exhibited by patients in the mildest stages of DAT, that, in the light of structural and functional neuroimaging evidence, can throw light upon the neural substrates of episodic and semantic memory.

From diagnosis to treatment

Further exciting developments in research into DAT have built upon the now well-established 'cholinergic hypothesis of geriatric dysfunction'.[105,106] This hypothesis generated much interest in the functions of central cholinergic systems and the neuropathological substrates underlying DAT. The synaptic loss, neuronal atrophy and degeneration of cholinergic nuclei in the basal forebrain may be associated with reduced cholinergic activity in the hippocampus and a cortical loss of choline acetyltransferase, an enzyme that produces acetylcholine in the neurons (review: Perry[11]). Central cholinergic pathways have been found to have an important role in attentional function, as well as the processing and storage of information and memory. Perry et al[10] had previously demonstrated that the degree of cholinergic abnormality correlated with mental state scores obtained from patients with DAT shortly before their death. Furthermore, systemic administration of the muscarinic acetylcholine receptor antagonist scopolamine to normal volunteers was found to reproduce many of the deficits in attention, visuospatial functions and language seen in DAT.[105] Importantly, cholinergic deficiency has been linked to a number of behavioral manifestations of DAT.[107] Certainly, the cholinergic deficit hypothesis continues to fuel the studies of mechanisms of actions of systemically administered cholinergic drugs in patients with DAT.

Conclusion

Dementia of the Alzheimer type is the most common form of dementia. An understanding of the nature of the cognitive deficits in this important disorder is vital for its early detection, and can only properly be obtained within the context of known neuropathological changes which occur early in the disease. Cognitive deficits may be found early in the disease, primarily within the domains of memory, attention and executive function. However, it is becoming increasingly clear that tests which load upon visual recognition learning and memory and which have been previously extremely well validated may have a prominent role in identifying DAT. Diagnosis has traditionally been difficult, given the possibility of delirium, depression or focal neurological diseases being responsible for the symptoms presented in the clinic. Correct identification of DAT through the application of recently developed neuropsychological tests clearly has promise for the practical management of patients and carers. This is obviously crucial for assessing the efficacy of any intervention, whether aimed at symptoms, neuroprotection, or both.

Acknowledgements

The work was completed with the MRC Link Grant to Barbara J Sahakian, Professor John R Hodges, Professor Trevor W Robbins and Dr James Semple, and within the MRC Co-operative Group in Brain, Behaviour and Neuropsychiatry. Shibley Rahman is funded by a MRC Research Studentship and the University of Cambridge School of Clinical Medicine. Rachel Swainson is funded by the MRC Link Grant to Barbara J Sahakian, Professor John R Hodges, Professor Trevor W Robbins, and Dr James Semple.

References

1. Haxby JV, Grady CL, Koss E et al. Longitudinal study of cerebral metabolic asymmetries and associated neuropsychological patterns in early dementia of the Alzheimer type. *Arch Neurol* (1990) **47(7):** 753–60.

2. Smith D, Jobst KA, Edmonds Z et al. Neuroimaging and early Alzheimer's disease. *Lancet* (1996) **348(9030):** 829–30.

3. Jellinger KA, Bancher C. Neuropathology of Alzheimer's disease: a critical update. *J Neural Transm Suppl* (1998) **54:** 77–95.

4. Braak H, Braak E. Neuropathological staging of Alzheimer-related changes. *Acta Neuropathol (Berl)* (1991) **82(4):** 239–59.

5. Braak H, Griffing K, Braak E. Neuroanatomy of Alzheimer's disease. *Alzheimer's Res* (1997) **3:** 235–47.

6. Gomez-Isla T, Price JL, McKeel DW et al. Profound loss of layer II entorhinal cortex neurons in very mild Alzheimer's disease. *J Neurosci* (1996) **16(14):** 4491–500.

7. Hyman BT, Van Hoesen GW, Kromer LJ, Damasio AR. Perforant pathway changes and the memory impairment of Alzheimer's disease. *Ann Neurol* (1986) **20(4):** 472–81.

8. Arnold SE, Hyman BT, Van Hoesen GW, Damasio AR. Some cytoarchitectural abnormalities of the entorhinal cortex in schizophrenia. *Arch Gen Psychiatry* (1991) **48(7):** 625–32.

9. Rosene DL, Van Hoesen GW. Hippocampal efferents reach widespread areas of cerebral cortex and amygdala in the rhesus monkey. *Science* (1977) **198(4314):** 315–17.

10. Perry EK, Tomlinson BE, Blessed G et al. Correlation of cholinergic abnormalities with senile plaques and mental test scores in senile dementia. *Br Med J* (1978) **2:** 1457–9.

11. Perry EK. The cholinergic hypothesis — ten years on. *Br Med Bull* (1986) **42:** 63–9.

12. Rahman S, Gregory CA, Sahakian BJ. Drug interventions in dementia. In Hodges JR (ed.) *Early Onset Dementia* (Oxford: Oxford University Press, 2000).

13. McKhann G, Drachman D, Folstein M et al. Clinical diagnosis of Alzheimer's disease: report of the NINCDS-ADRDA Work Group under the auspices of Department of Health and Human Services Task Force on Alzheimer's Disease. *Neurology* (1984) **34(7):** 939–44.

14. Gauthier S, Panisset M. Current diagnostic methods and outcome variables for clinical investigation of Alzheimer's disease. *J Neural Transm Suppl* (1998) **53:** 251–4.

15. Cummings JL, Benson DF. *Dementia: a Clinical Approach* (Boston: Butterworths, 1992).

16. Ganguli M. The use of screening instruments for the detection of dementia. *Neuroepidemiology* (1997) **16(6):** 271–80.

17. Green RC, Clarke VC, Thompson NJ et al. Early detection of Alzheimer disease: methods, markers and misgivings. *Alzheimer Dis Assoc Disord* (1997) **11(Suppl 5):** S1–5.

18. Pasquier F. Early diagnosis of dementia: neuropsychology. *J Neurol* (1999) **246(1):** 6–15.

19. De Leon MJ, Convit A, De Santi S, et al. Contribution of structural neuroimaging to the early diag-

nosis of Alzheimer's disease. *Int Psychogeriatr* (1997) **9(Suppl 1):** 183–90.

20. Fox NC, Warrington EK, Seiffer AL et al. Presymptomatic cognitive deficits in individuals at risk of familial Alzheimer's disease. A longitudinal prospective study. *Brain* (1998) **121(9):** 1631–9.

21. Grady CL, Haxby JV, Horwitz B et al. Longitudinal study of the early neuropsychological and cerebral metabolic changes in dementia of the Alzheimer type. *J Clin Exp Neuropsychol* (1988) **10(5):** 576–96.

22. Parasuraman R, Greenwood PM, Haxby JV, Grady CL. Visuospatial attention in dementia of the Alzheimer type. *Brain* (1992) **115(Pt 3):** 711–33.

23. Becker JT, Minthun MA, Aleva K et al. Alterations in functional neuroanatomical connectivity in Alzheimer's disease. Positron emission tomography of auditory verbal short-term memory. *Ann NY Acad Sci* (1996) **17(777):** 239–42.

24. Hodges JR, Graham N, Patterson K. Charting the progression in semantic dementia: implications for the organisation of semantic memory. *Memory* (1995) **3(3–4):** 463–95.

25. Tulving E. Episodic and semantic memory. In Tulving E, Donaldson W (eds) *The Organisation of Memory* (New York and London: Academic Press, 1972).

26. Posner MI, Petersen SE. The attention system of the human brain. *Annu Rev Neurosci* (1990) **13:** 25–42.

27. Squire LR. Memory and the hippocampus: a synthesis from findings with rats, monkeys and humans. *Psychol Rev* (1992) **99(2):** 195–231. [Published erratum appears in *Psychol Rev* (1992) **99(3):** 582.]

28. Zola-Morgan S, Squire LR, Alvarez-Royo P, Clower RP. Independence of memory functions and emotional behavior: separate contributions of the hippocampal formation and the amygdala. *Hippocampus* (1991) **1(2):** 207–20.

29. Robbins TW, Elliott R, Sahakian BJ. Neuropsychology — dementia and affective disorders. *Br Med Bull* (1996) **52(3):** 627–43.

30. Mumby DG, Pinel JPJ. Rhinal cortex lesions and object recognition in rats. *Behav Neurosci* (1994) **20:** 18.

31. Zhu XO, Brown MW, Aggleton JP. Neuronal signalling of information important to visual recognition memory in rat rhinal and neighbouring cortices. *Eur J Neurosci* (1995) **7(4):** 753–65.

32. Gaffan D, Murray EA. Monkeys (Macaca fascicularis) with rhinal cortex ablations succeed in object discrimination learning despite 24-hr intertrial intervals and fail at matching to sample despite double sample presentations. *Behav Neurosci* (1992) **106(1):** 30–8.

33. Muenier M, Bachavelier J, Mishkin M, Murray EA. Effects on visual recognition of combined and separate ablations of the entorhinal and perirhinal cortex in rhesus monkeys. *J Neurosci* (1993) **13:** 5418–32.

34. Murray EA. What have ablation studies told us about the neural substrates of stimulus memory? *Semin Neurosci* (1996) **5:** 10–20.

35. Murray E. Memory for objects in nonhuman primates. In Gazzaniga M (ed.) *The New Cognitive Neurosciences.* (Cambridge, MA: MIT Press, 2000): 753–63.

36. Delis D, Kramer J, Kaplan E, Ober B. *California Verbal Learning Test: Research Edition* (New

York, NY: Psychological Corporation, 1987).

37. Wechsler D. *Wechsler Memory Scale — Revised* (San Antonio, CA: Psychological Corporation, 1987).

38. Hart R, Kwentus J, Taylor J, Harkins S. Rate of forgetting in dementia and depression. *J Consult Clin Psychol* (1987) **55(1):** 101–5.

39. Greene J, Baddeley A, Hodges JR. Analysis of the episodic memory deficit in early Alzheimer's disease. Evidence from the doors and people test. *Neuropsychologia* (1996) **34(6):** 537–51.

40. Chertkow H, Bub D. Semantic memory loss in dementia of Alzheimer's type. What do various measures measure? *Brain* (1990) **113(2):** 397–417.

41. Masur D, Sliwinski M, Lipton R et al. Neuropsychological prediction of dementia and the absence of dementia in healthy elderly persons. *Neurology* (1994) **44:** 1427–32.

42. Small B, Fratiglioni L, Almkvist O et al. Cognitive predictors of incident Alzheimer's disease: a prospective longitudinal study. *Neuropsychology* (1997) **11(3):** 413–20.

43. Sahakian BJ, Morris RG, Evenden JL et al. A comparative study of visuospatial memory and learning in Alzheimer-type dementia and Parkinson's disease. *Brain* (1988) **111:** 695–718.

44. Sahakian BJ, Downes JJ, Eagger S et al. Sparing of attentional relative to mnemonic function in a subgroup of patients with dementia of the Alzheimer type. *Neuropsychologia* (1990) **28:** 1197–213.

45. Sahakian B, Coull J. Nicotine and tetrahydroaminoacridine:

evidence for improved attention in patients with dementia of the Alzheimer type. *Drug Dev Res* (1994) **31:** 80–8.

46. Vitaliano PP, Russo J, Breen AR et al. Functional decline in the early stages of Alzheimer's disease. *Psychol Aging* (1986) **1(1):** 41–6.

47. Sahakian B, Jones G, Levy R et al. The effects of nicotine on attention, information-processing and short-term memory in patients with dementia of the Alzheimer type. *Br J Psychiatry* (1989) **154:** 797–800.

48. Sahakian BJ, Coull JT. Tetrahydroaminoacridine (THA) in Alzheimer's disease: an assessment of attentional and mnemonic function using CANTAB. *Acta Neurol Scand Suppl* (1993) **149:** 29–35.

49. Jones GM, Sahakian BJ, Levy R et al. Effects of acute subcutaneous nicotine on attention, information processing and short-term memory. *Psychopharmacology (Berl)* (1992) **108(4):** 485–94.

50. Robbins TW, McAlonan G, Muir JL, Everitt BJ. Cognitive enhancers in theory and practice: studies of the cholinergic hypothesis of cognitive deficits in Alzheimer's disease. *Behav Brain Res* (1997) **83(1–2):** 15–23.

51. Norman D, Shallice T. Attention to action. Willed and automatic control of behaviour. In Davidson R, Schwartz G, Shapiro D (eds) *Consciousness and Self Regulation*, Vol. 4 (New York: Plenum Press, 1986): 1–18.

52. Becker J. Working memory and secondary memory deficits in Alzheimer's disease. *J Clin Exp Neuropsychol* (1988) **10(6):** 739–53.

53. Zec R. Neuropsychological functioning in Alzheimer's disease. In

Parks R, Zec R, Wilson R (eds) *Neuropsychology of Alzheimer's Disease and Other Dementias* (Oxford: Oxford University Press, 1993).

54. Baddeley A, Della Sala S, Spinnler H. The two-component hypothesis of memory deficit in Alzheimer's disease. *J Clin Exp Neuropsychol* (1991) **13(2):** 372–80.

55. Folstein, MF, Folstein, SE, McHugh, PR: 'Mini-mental state'. A practical method for rating the cognitive state of patients for the clinician. *J Psychiat Res* (1975) **12:** 189–98, 1975.

56. Rosen WG, Mohs RC, Davis KL. A new rating scale for Alzheimer's disease. *Am J Psychiatry* (1984) **141(11):** 1356–64.

57. Robbins TW, James M, Owen AM et al. Cambridge Neuropsychological Test Automated Battery (CANTAB): a factor analytic study of a large sample of normal elderly volunteers. *Dementia* (1994) **5(5):** 266–81.

58. Robbins TW, James M, Owen AM et al. A study of performance on tests from the CANTAB battery sensitive to frontal lobe dysfunction in a large sample of normal volunteers: implications for theories of executive functioning and cognitive aging. Cambridge Neuropsychological Test Automated Battery. *J Int Neuropsychol Soc* (1998) **4(5):** 474–90.

59. Bayer AJ, Pathy MS, Twining C. The memory clinic. A new approach to the detection of early dementia. *Drugs* (1987) **33(Suppl 2):** 84–9.

60. Hodges JR. The amnestic prodrome of Alzheimer's disease. *Brain* (1998) **121(9):** 1601–2.

61. Rosenstein L. Differential diagnosis of the major progressive dementias and depression in middle and late adulthood: a summary of the literature of the early 1990s. *Neuropsychol Rev* (1998) **8(3):** 109–66.

62. Hyman B, Van Hoesen G, Damasio A, Barnes C. Alzheimer's disease: cell-specific pathology isolates the hippocampal formation. *Science* (1984) **225:** 1168–70.

63. Deweer B, Lehircy S, Pillon B et al. Memory disorders in probable Alzheimer's disease: the role of hippocampal atrophy as shown with MRI. *J Neurol Neurosurg Psychiatry* (1995) **58:** 590–7.

64. Baddeley A, Bressi S, Della Sala S et al. The decline of working memory in Alzheimer's disease. *Brain* (1991) **114:** 2521–42.

65. Crystal HA, Horoupian DS, Katzman R, Jotkowitz S. Biopsy-proven Alzheimer disease presenting as a right parietal lobe syndrome. *Ann Neurol* (1982) **12:** 186–8.

66. Kirshner HS, Webb WG, Kelly MP, Wells CE. Language disturbance. An initial symptom of cortical degenerations and dementia. *Arch Neurol* (1984) **41:** 491–6.

67. Mackensie Ross S, Graham N, Stuart-Green L et al. Progressive biparietal atrophy: an atypical presentation of Alzheimer's disease. *J Neurol Neurosurg Psychiatry* (1996) **61:** 388–95.

68. Nelson HE. National Adult Reading Test (NART) Test Manual (Windsor: NFER-Nelson, 1982).

69. Rahman S, Sahakian BJ, Hodges JR et al. Specific cognitive deficits in mild frontal variant frontotemporal dementia. *Brain* (1999) **122(8):** 1469–93.

70. Rahman S, Robbins TW, Sahakian BJ. Comparative cognitive neuropsychological studies of frontal lobe function:

implications for therapeutic strategies in frontal variant frontotemporal dementia. *Dement Geriatr Cogn Disord* (1999) **10(suppl 1):** 15–28.

71. Petersen R, Smith G, Waring S et al. Mild cognitive impairment — Clinical characterisation and outcome. *Arch Neurol* (1999) **56:** 303–8. [Published erratum appears in *Arch Neurol* (1999) **56(6):** 760.]

72. Zakzanis KK. Quantitative evidence for neuroanatomic and neuropsychological markers in dementia of the Alzheimer's type. *J Clin Exp Neuropsychology* (1998) **20(2):** 259–69.

73. Solomon P, Hirschoff A, Kelly B et al. A 7-minute neurocognitive screening battery highly sensitive to Alzheimer's disease. *Arch Neurol* (1998) **55:** 349–55.

74. Knopman DS. The initial recognition and diagnosis of dementia. *Am J Med* (1998) **104(4A):** 2S–12S.

75. Varma AR, Snowden JS, Lloyd JJ et al. Evaluation of the NINCDS-ADRDA criteria in the differentiation of Alzheimer's disease and frontotemporal dementia. *J Neurol Neurosurg Psychiatry* (1999) **66(2):** 184–8.

76. Chen P, Gaguli M, Mulsant B, DeKosky S. The temporal relationship between depressive symptoms and dementia. *Arch Gen Psychiatry* (1999) **56:** 261–6.

77. Fioravanti M. The quest for distinction between old-age depression and dementia. *Arch Gerontol Geriatr* (1998) **suppl 6:** 201–6.

78. Ritchie K, Gilham C, Ledesert B et al. Depressive illness, depressive symptomatology and regional cerebral blood flow in elderly people with subclinical cognitive involvement. *Age Ageing* (1999) **28:** 385–91.

79. O'Carroll R, Curran S, Ross M et al. The differentiation of major depression from dementia of the Alzheimer type using within-subject neuropsychological discrepancy analysis. *Br J Clin Psychology* (1994) **33:** 23–32.

80. Swainson R, Galton CJ, Hodges JR et al. Early detection and differential diagnosis of Alzheimer's disease and depression. *Dementia and Geriatric Cognitive Disorders* (in press).

81. Jacobs D, Sano M, Dooneief G et al. Neuropsychological detection and characterization of preclinical Alzheimer's disease. *Neurology* (1995) **46:** 957–62.

82. Fabrigoule C, Rouch I, Taberly A et al. Cognitive process in preclinical phase of dementia. Brain (1998) **121:** 135–41.

83. Bowen J, Teri L, Kuknull W et al. Progression to dementia in patients with isolated memory loss. *Lancet* (1997) **349(9054):** 763–5.

84. Fowler K, Saling M, Conway E et al. Computerized delayed matching to sample and paired associate performance in the early detection of dementia. *Appl Neuropsychol* (1995) **2:** 72–8.

85. Tierney M, Szalai J, Snow W et al. Prediction of probable Alzheimer's disease in memory-impaired patients: a prospective longitudinal study. *Neurology* (1996) **46:** 661–5.

86. Owen AM, Sahakian BJ, Semple J et al. Visuo-spatial short-term recognition memory and learning after temporal lobe excisions, frontal lobe excisions or amygdalo-hippocampectomy in man. *Neuropsychologia* (1995) **33(1):** 1–24.

87. Owen AM, Morris RG, Sahakian

BJ et al. Double dissociations of memory and executive functions in working memory tasks following frontal lobe excisions, temporal lobe excisions or amygdalo-hippocampectomy in man. *Brain* (1996) **119:** 1597–615.

88. Robbins TW, Semple J, Kumar R et al. Effects of scopolamine on delayed-matching-to-sample and paired associates tests of visual memory and learning in human subjects: comparison with diazepam and implications for dementia. *Psychopharmacology* (1997) **134:** 95–106.

89. Butters N, Heindel W, Salmon D. Dissociation of implicit memory in dementia: neurological implications. *Bull Psychonomic Soc* (1990) **28(4):** 359–66.

90. Knowlton BJ, Mangels JA, Squire LR. A neostriatal habit learning system in humans. *Science* (1996) **273:** 1399–402.

91. Fowler K, Saling M, Conway E et al. Computerized neuropsychological tests in the early detection of dementia: prospective findings. *J Int Neuropsychol Soc* (1997) **3:** 139–46.

92. Scoville WB, Milner B. Loss of recent memory after bilateral hippocampal lesions. *J Neurol Neurosurg Psychiatry* (1957) **20:** 11–21.

93. Zola S, Squire L, Teng E et al. Impaired recognition memory in monkeys after damage limited to the hippocampal region. *J Neurosci* (2000) **20(1):** 451–63.

94. Gaffan D. Episodic and semantic memory and the role of the not-hippocampus. *Trends Cogn Sci* (1997) **1(7):** 246–8.

95. Elliott R, Dolan RJ. Differential neural responses during performance of matching and non-matching to sample tasks at two

delay intervals. *J Neurosci* (1999) **19:** 5066–73.

96. Bussey T, Murray E. Reply to: 'What does semantic dementia reveal about the functional role of the perirhinal cortex?' *Trends Cogn Sci* (1999) **3(7):** 249–50.

97. Graham KS, Hodges JR. Differentiating the role of the hippocampal complex and the neocortex in long-term memory storage: evidence from the study of semantic dementia and Alzheimer's disease. *Neuropsychology* (1997) **11(1):** 77–89.

98. Mummery CJ, Patterson K, Price CJ et al. A voxel-based morphometry study of semantic dementia: relationship between temporal lobe atrophy and semantic memory. *Ann Neurol* (2000) **47(1):** 36–45.

99. Simons JS, Graham KS, Hodges JR. What does semantic dementia reveal about the functional role of the perirhinal cortex? *Trends Cogn Sci* (1997) **3(7):** 248–9.

100. Graham KS, Simons JS, Pratt KH et al. Insights from semantic dementia on the relationship between episodic and semantic memory. *Neuropsychologia* (2000) **38:** 313–24.

101. Ungerleider LG, Mishkin M. Two cortical visual systems. In Ingle DJ, Goodale MA, Mansfield RJW (eds) *Analysis of Visual Behaviour* 549–89 (Cambridge, MA: MIT, 1982).

102. Goulet S, Murray EA. Effects of lesions of either the amygdala or anterior rhinal cortex on cross-modal association in humans? *Soc Neurosci Abstr* (1995) **21:** 1446.

103. Owen A, Milner B, Petrides M, Evans A. A specific role for the right parahippocampal gyrus in the retrieval of object-location: a positron emission tomography

study. *J Cogn Neurosci* (1996) **8(6):** 588–602.

104. Tulving E, Kapur S, Markowitsch H et al. Hemispheric coding/retrieval asymmetry in episodic memory: positron emission tomography findings. *Proc Natl Acad Sci USA* (1994) **91:** 2012–25.

105. Drachman DA, Sahakian BJ. The effects of cholinergic agents on human learning and memory. In Barbeau A, Growden JH, Wurt-man RJ (eds) *Nutrition and the Brain*, Vol. 5 (New York: Raven Press, 1979): 351–66.

106. Bartus RT, Dean RL, Beer B, Lippa AS. The cholinergic hypothesis of geriatric memory dysfunction. *Science* (1982) **217:** 408–14.

107. Cummings JL, Kaufer D. Neuropsychiatric aspects of Alzheimer's disease: the cholinergic hypothesis revisited. *Neurology* (1996) **47(4):** 876–83.

9
Huntington's disease

Andrew D Lawrence

Summary

A brief history of Huntington's disease

Huntington's disease (HD) is named after the American physician George Sumner Huntington (1850–1916) who provided an early description of the disease in 1872. In fact, there are a number of possible descriptions of the disorder in the literature preceding Huntington's paper. The first definite record of HD was in a letter by Charles Oscar Waters, published in 1842. It is highly likely, however, that HD has been with us for quite some time. Indeed, a vivid portrait of what looks very much like HD may be found in Pieter Brueghel's drawing of the St John's dance, a mixed pagan–Christian ritual serving as a defense against 'St John's disease', which dates back to the fourteenth century and the time of the Black Death.

Huntington had initially observed the disease in his father's medical practice in Easthampton, Long Island, New York, although his grandfather had earlier noted the disorder. Huntington's paper has been described as 'one of the most remarkable in the history of medicine'. It was presented to the Meigs and Mason Academy of Medicine at Middleport, Ohio on 15 February 1872 and published that year in *The Medical and Surgical Reporter*. All the cardinal features of HD, as recognized today, are described in this brief paper: adult onset, progressive course, choreic movements, intellectual impairment, psychiatric disturbance, and hereditary nature.

Diagnostic criteria

Huntington's disease is an autosomal, dominantly inherited disorder characterized phenotypically by involuntary movements (chorea), impaired voluntary movements, dystonia, marked loss of body weight, cognitive impairment, and emotional disturbances (including irritability and apathy). The gene HD, which is mutated in HD patients, has been mapped to chromosome 4p16.3. The mutation is an expanded polyglutamine repeat,

(CAG)$_n$, within exon 1 of the gene. In the normal population, the number of CAG repeats ranges from 6 to 35, whereas in HD the repeat length ranges from ~40 to 121. Age of onset of HD is inversely correlated with CAG-repeat length. Huntingtin, the product of the HD gene, is a 350-kDa protein of unknown function.

The diagnostic criteria for HD include: (1) a family history of typical Huntington chorea; (2) progressive motor disability with chorea or rigidity of no other cause; and (3) psychiatric disturbance with gradual dementia of no other cause. The disease is universal, affecting all races, and has the highest prevalence in Europe and North America, with 4–8 per 100 000 affected in Europe.

Neuropathology

Despite the finding that the gene encoding huntingtin is expressed ubiquitously, selective cell loss and fibrillary astrocytosis is observed in the brains of HD victims. The most striking changes are found within the striatum, with GABA-containing medium-spiny striatal projection neurons bearing the brunt of the pathology. Although the striatum suffers greatest damage, other neural structures are affected by HD. Subcortically, the substantia nigra, globus pallidus, subthalamic nucleus, amygdala, thalamus and hypothalamus are all affected, to varying degrees. The brainstem neurotransmitter systems appear to be relatively spared. Cortically, cerebellar, occipital, parietal, temporal (including hippocampus), primary motor, cingulate and prefrontal cortices have all been reported to show neuronal loss in HD.

Neuropsychiatric side-effects of treatment

Pharmacological treatment in HD is limited to reduction of chorea and psychiatric disturbances, often at the cost of further impairing voluntary movement, and, consequently, total functional capacity. Fetal striatal transplantation may be a feasible, safe and effective treatment for HD. Preliminary data suggest no worsening of cognitive function following bilateral striatal (caudate and putamen) grafts in a small group of advanced, non-demented HD patients.

Main neuropsychological findings

The cognitive impairment in HD encompasses a number of domains, most especially memory and 'executive' or control functions. In the domain of memory, episodic memory is impaired, especially in tests of free recall as compared to recognition. Semantic memory is relatively unaffected. Certain aspects of non-declarative memory are also impaired, including response learning and certain motor skills, especially those relying on predictive sequencing, while perceptual skills are relatively unimpaired.

Perhaps the major cognitive impairment in HD is a 'dysexecutive syndrome'. Particularly affected are executive aspects of memory (e.g. use of strategies, planning, working memory) and executive attention (e.g. behavioral regulation, 'set' processes). It is as yet unclear if the cognitive deficit in HD is the result of a unitary information-processing deficit, which cuts across a variety of cognitive domains.

Less vulnerable to HD are primary sensory and perceptual abilities (with the possible exception of face processing), and most aspects of language.

Introduction

Huntington's disease is an autosomal dominant neurodegenerative disease with midlife onset characterized by motor, cognitive and affective symptoms. The genetic mutation in HD, an unstable, expanded trinucleotide repeat (CAG_n) in the gene that encodes the protein huntingtin, leads to very characteristic neuropathological changes via mechanisms that are currently unknown.] The most striking changes are found within the striatum, with GABA-containing medium-spiny striatal projection neurons bearing the brunt of the pathology. There is a dorsal-to-ventral, anterior-to-posterior and medial-to-lateral progression of cell death, with the dorsomedial striatum affected earliest and relative sparing of the ventral striatum. Although the striatum suffers greatest damage, other neural structures are affected by HD. Subcortically, the substantia nigra, globus pallidus, subthalamic nucleus, amygdala, thalamus and hypothalamus are all affected, to varying degrees. The brainstem neurotransmitter systems appear to be relatively spared.[1] Cortically, cerebellar, occipital, parietal, temporal, primary motor, cingulate and prefrontal cortices have all been reported to show neuronal loss in HD.[1] Nevertheless, the striatum bears the brunt of neural damage in HD.

Systems-level architecture of the basal ganglia

The basal ganglia consist of the neostriatum (caudate and putamen), ventral striatum, globus pallidus, substantia nigra and subthalamic nucleus. Each of these nuclei has distinct functional subdivisions that include 'motor', 'oculomotor', 'associative', and 'limbic' territories.[2,3] The functional subdivisions are differentiated on the basis of their respective physiological properties and their interconnections with cortical and thalamic territories of the same functionalities. As a consequence of this organization, the basal ganglia can be viewed as components among a family of re-entrant loops that are organized in parallel, each taking its origin from a particular set of cortical fields, passing through the functionally corresponding portions of the basal ganglia and returning to parts of those same cortical fields by way of specific basal ganglia-recipient zones in the thalamus (Figure 9.1).[4] One of the remarkable features of

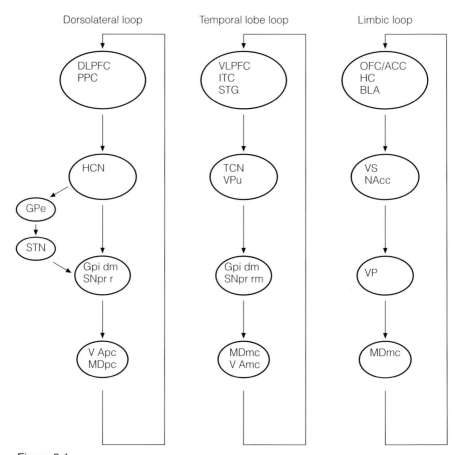

Figure 9.1

The schematic organization of corticostriatal anatomical circuits. Three of the parallel, segregated loops are shown. DLPFC, dorsolateral prefrontal cortex; PPC, posterior parietal cortex; VLPFC, ventrolateral prefrontal cortex; ITC, inferior temporal cortex; STG, superior temporal gyrus; OFC, orbitofrontal cortex; ACC, anterior cingulate; HC, hippocampus; BLA, basolateral amygdala; HCN, head of caudate nucleus; TCN, tail of caudate nucleus; VPu, ventral putamen; VS, ventral striatum; NAcc, nucleus accumbens; Gpi, internal segment of the globus pallidus; SNpr, substantia nigra, pars reticulata; VP, ventral pallidum; VA, ventral anterior thalamus; MD mediodorsal thalamus; Gpe, external segment of globus pallidus; STN, subthalamic nucleus; dm, dorsomedial; r, rostral; rm, rostromedial; pc, parvocellularis; mc, magnocellularis. For the sake of clarity, only one 'indirect loop' via Gpe and STN is shown.

basal ganglia circuitry is that functionally discrete 'channels' of informa-tion processing are maintained throughout the various corticobasal ganglia–thalamocortical pathways, in the face of layer-to-layer connectiv-ity that is highly convergent.[4] In addition to the 'motor' and 'oculomotor' loops (not shown), three circuits, the 'dorsolateral prefrontal', the 'limbic' and the 'temporal association cortex' circuits, may have particular rele-vance for understanding the nature of the cognitive deficit in HD. In the 'dorsolateral' loop, the dorsolateral prefrontal and parietal cortices project to the head and body of the caudate nucleus, which has connections through parts of the globus pallidus and substantia nigra to the ventral anterior group of thalamic nuclei and thus to the dorsolateral prefrontal cortex. In the 'limbic' loop, 'limbic' and related structures such as the amygdala, orbitofronal cortex and hippocampus project to the ventral striatum, which has projections through the ventral pallidum to the mediodorsal nucleus of the thalamus and thus to prefrontal and cingulate cortices. Finally, in the 'temporal lobe' loop, the inferior temporal cortex and the ventrolateral (inferior convexity) prefrontal cortex project to pos-terior and ventral parts of the striatum and the tail of the caudate, and, via thalamic relays, back to the ventrolateral prefrontal cortex. Part of the globus pallidus, probably the part influenced by the temporal lobe, pro-jects back, via thalamus, to area TE[5] (Figure 9.1).

It is clear from the anatomy of basal ganglia circuitry that the basal ganglia are ideally placed to influence neural processing in prefrontal and temporal lobe regions, particularly. Given that these areas have prin-cipally been recognized to be associated with 'executive functions' (see below) and memory, we will concentrate our focus on these two areas of cognitive function in HD.

The cognitive pathology of HD

Memory

An important development in the neuropsychological study of memory has been the realization that 'memory' can be usefully subdivided into a collection of component subsystems. These separate subsystems have been divided on a number of grounds, including evolutionary history, operating characteristics and anatomy.[6] The most influential distinction made is that between declarative and procedural memory.[7] Declarative memory was defined as stored knowledge concerning facts or events that have been experienced and can be represented symbolically, whereas procedural memory referred to information acquired when learn-ing a skill that is demonstrated by performance rather by than recalling facts or experiences. Anatomically, procedural memory and declarative memory were dissociated following damage to the medial temporal lobe

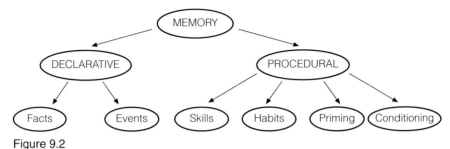

Figure 9.2

Squire's proposed taxonomy of memory and associated neural structures. (Adapted from Squire.[8]).

and diencephalon, as occurs in clinical amnesia. The original declarative–procedural distinction was revised by Squire and colleagues[8] following findings that amnesic patients displayed priming effects dependent on the retention of declarative memories. Squire now makes a distinction between declarative and non-declarative memory systems. Non-declarative memory includes a somewhat disparate collection of non-conscious memories, of which procedural memory is but one. Under the broad category of non-declarative memories, Squire includes phenomena such as priming, classical conditioning, non-associative learning, as well as skills and 'habits' — all of which are spared in the amnesic syndrome.[8] These current distinctions are shown diagrammatically in Figure 9.2.

In terms of operating characteristics, one property that has been used to dissociate these two systems is the awareness that subjects have for what is learned. According to Squire, declarative memory 'affords the capacity for conscious recollections about facts and events', whereas non-declarative memory 'does not appear to require awareness of any memory content'.[8] However, there are some problems with this notion. First, awareness is a subjective notion, and second, there is an inherent circularity in its application to the study of non-human animals. Further, we must note that Squire uses the terms 'declarative' and 'non-declarative' not as originally defined, but as synonyms for the terms 'explicit' and 'implicit' memory.[9] The term explicit refers to the conscious intention to learn or remember. In contrast, whenever something is learned that influences subsequent performance without conscious intention to recall the relevant memories, the behavior is said to be an instance of 'implicit memory'.

The distinction between explicit and implicit memory cuts across the distinction between declarative and procedural memory as originally defined.[10] Pavlovian conditioning in animals is clearly an example of implicit memory, as animals make no conscious effort to learn in conditioning experiments. However, modern theories of classical conditioning[11] postulate declarative memory as the basis for conditioning, if declarative memory is defined as memory for facts and experiences. The memories underlying classical conditioning are 'symbolic' in the sense that they 'represent' the CS (conditioned stimulus), US (unconditioned stimulus) and CS–US relation. Therefore, for Squire's taxonomy of memory to be valid, declarative memory must be defined as explicit memory, i.e. the capacity for *intentional* learning and recall.

Declarative memory

Declarative memory can be further subdivided into episodic and semantic memory according to the type of information that is stored.[12] Episodic memories are memories for personally experienced episodes in one's life that are dependent upon temporal and/or spatial cues for their retrieval. Most traditional verbal learning tasks used in cognitive psychology involve retrieval from episodic memory. In contrast, semantic memories are memories for facts about things-in-the-world and ideas, and are completely independent of contextual cues for their retrieval.

Short-term versus long-term memories and the concept of 'working memory'

A distinction has been traditionally made in the psychological literature between short-term and long-term memory. Short-term episodic memory is viewed as a limited-capacity storage system in which information rapidly degrades unless continuously rehearsed, whereas long-term memory is considered to be a more stable, permanent store. In more recent years, it has become apparent that, as is the case with long-term memory, short-term memory as a unitary construct is not useful.[13] In Baddeley's 'working memory' model, a limited-capacity 'central executive' (CE) holds control over two 'slave' systems: the 'articulatory loop' (AL), involved in the short-term storage of verbal information, and the 'visuospatial sketchpad' (VSSP), responsible for setting up and maintaining visuospatial images. The AL can further be divided into a phonological store, which holds speech-based information, and an articulatory control process, which recycles a limited amount of speech-based information.[13] The functions of the CE are far from fully mapped out, but bear resemblance to those functions of the brain called 'executive' or 'control' processes, and will be taken up further in the section on such processes (see below). The two 'slave' systems bear the most resemblance to earlier concepts of short-term episodic memory, and experiments that can be interpreted within the framework of these two subsystems will be the concern of this subsection.

The digit span task loads heavily on the AL. Digit span has consistently been found to be impaired in all but the earliest stages of HD,[14,15] although it is not clear to what extent dysarthria contributes to this impairment. HD patients also show abnormally rapid forgetting on the Brown–Peterson paradigm, in which distractor activity intervenes between presentation and recall.[14]

Spatial span tasks rely heavily on the functions of the VSSP. Orsini et al[16] and Lange et al[17] have reported reduced spatial spans in patients with advanced HD. Spatial span is also reduced in early HD, but there are some doubts about the contribution of motor problems to these deficits.[18] Mental imagery tasks also tap the functions of the VSSP. HD patients have been shown to be impaired on tasks requiring mental rotation/image manipulation.[14,15,19,20] Another task that would appear to rely heavily on the VSSP is the classic delayed-response (DR) task and variants such as delayed alternation (DA), in which a 'representation' of a stimulus must be held 'on-line' for a short period of time. Impairments on these tasks have been reported in patients following lesions to the dorsolateral prefrontal cortex.[21] Oscar-Berman et al[22] found impaired DA, but not DR, deficits in HD patients. However, these results are somewhat complicated, as both DR and DA performance involve high levels of inhibitory control, and these findings will be taken up further in the section on executive functions. In a recent study, Lange et al[17] found impairment in advanced HD patients on a task of spatial recognition memory, which bears some resemblance to the classic DR task. Deficits on this task, and on an equivalent pattern recognition memory task, also occur in early HD.[18,23]

Long-term episodic memory deficits have been exemplified by poor performance on tests of verbal learning and recall/recognition, such as list-learning and paired associates learning tasks. HD patients are impaired in learning paired associates[14,24] and in recalling short stories.[25] Granholm and Butters[26] found that HD patients were able to properly encode to-be-remembered items, suggesting that HD patients' memory impairment (at least for verbal stimuli) is not related to an encoding deficit.

A very important feature of the memory deficit in HD is that, at least early in the disease, verbal recognition memory tends to be spared relative to recall.[15,27,28] Further, HD patients' recall can be improved by the provision of retrieval cues and contextual/categorizing cues during stimulus presentation[15,27] This has led to the suggestion that the HD impairment is primarily a retrieval problem; this retrieval problem may be due to impairment in setting up plans for the systematic search of memory[14] and/or ineffective use of clustering strategies in encoding/retrieval.[29] The retrieval deficit hypothesis is supported by the findings of a 'flat' curve when HD patients are required to recall premorbidly acquired knowledge about faces, events and geography.[14,15,19]

However, it should be noted that HD patients do not always benefit from the aid to encoding/retrieval supplied by the provision of categorical cues and can show verbal recognition memory deficits.[30] This recognition impairment appears to be due primarily to an increase in false-positive errors.[30] It is still the case, however, that the magnitude of the free recall impairment exceeds that shown on recognition tasks.

It is also important to note that the relative sparing of recognition memory may only be the case for verbal stimuli. HD patients, even relatively early in the disease, can show profound face recognition impairments.[14,31,32] They also show deficits in tasks requiring them to memorize complex patterns and scenes.[14,15,17,18] We have recently shown non-delay-dependent deficits on a trial-unique version of the classic test of stimulus recognition memory, delayed matching-to-sample in HD patients,[23] suggesting that the visual recognition 'memory' impairment in HD might be due to factors other than a genuine memory impairment.

Semantic memory

The available evidence suggests that HD patients have relatively preserved semantic memories. HD patients are impaired on both letter and category fluency tests to a similar extent,[15,33] suggesting that their impairment reflects a more general retrieval deficit than any semantic memory impairment.[34] Indeed, the use of a cueing procedure improves the performance on semantic fluency tests in HD, but not in Alzheimer patients.[15] Further, the performance on semantic fluency tests correlates with performance on confrontation naming tasks in Alzheimer, but not HD, patients. Indeed, HD patients tend to make perceptual rather than semantic errors in confrontation naming.[15] More recently, performance on verbal fluency tasks has been examined using statistical techniques that allow investigators to examine the organization of semantic 'space' based on the clustering patterns that subjects produce. Chan et al[35] report an intact semantic 'space' in HD, but not Alzheimer, patients, in line with the above results. In addition, HD patients show a normal release from proactive interference effect, suggesting that patients can adequately encode information in a semantic manner and thus benefit from a shift in semantic categories.[36]

Non-declarative memory
Motor skills

A number of studies have reported that HD patients are impaired in their ability to learn the motor skills underlying performance of pursuit tracking tasks. On the rotor-pursuit task, HD patients show very little learning, even when matched with controls for initial performance levels.[37,38]

Recent evidence suggests that the basal ganglia may only be critical for the acquisition of skilled motor behavior involving the predictive sequencing of motor acts. HD patients are impaired on the serial reaction time task.[39,40] Further, HD patients fail to improve their performance on tasks requiring them to trace a route through a computerized maze. This deficit manifests itself in the HD patients' inability to improve their performance with predictable relative to unpredictable routes.[40] In contrast, HD patients are able to learn motor tasks that do not require the sequencing of movements, for example when they have to learn a mapping between perceptual cues and the appropriate motor response[38,40] and are not impaired on a computerized version of rotary pursuit in which they must keep a crosshair cursor on top of a moving circular target when the target moves randomly, but are impaired when the target moves in a predictable sequence.[41]

Very recently, Smith et al[42] have found that HD subjects' corrective responses to externally generated force pulses are greatly disturbed, indicating that HD subjects display aberrant responses to both external and self-generated errors. Smith et al[42] suggest that a dysfunction in error correction may characterize the motor control deficit in HD.

Perceptual Skills

In their original investigation of skill-learning in HD, Martone et al[43] reported that HD patients showed deficits in mirror-reading. The deficit consisted of a lengthening of the time taken to read horizontally inverted text. Over 3 days of training, HD subjects' performance did improve, but far less than that of controls. However, a difficulty with the finding of impaired mirror-reading in HD is the fact that HD patients exhibit aberrant eye movements. Indeed, baseline reading speeds of HD patients in the study of Martone et al[43] were significantly slower than those of controls. In contrast to such possibly impaired mirror-reading, Gabrieli et al[38] have found intact mirror-tracing in HD. Squire and colleagues have also reported intact artificial grammar-learning, a form of perceptual learning, in HD.[44]

Cognitive skills

One task that has been claimed to be a useful measure of cognitive skill-learning is the Tower of Hanoi (TOH). Butters et al[45] assessed the ability of amnesic patients and HD patients to learn a five-disk version of the TOH which required a minimum of 31 moves for solution. Amnesic patients were impaired, showing significantly less improvement in performance with practice than controls. A similar level of impairment was shown by advanced HD patients, while a group of early HD patients did not differ from controls. Saint-Cyr et al[25] examined HD patients' ability to learn three- and four-disk problems of a modified version of the TOH referred to as the 'Tower of Toronto' (TOT). A complex pattern of results was obtained: amnesic patients showed normal learning, despite profound declarative memory impairments. A group of advanced HD patients were impaired on both the declarative memory tests and the TOT. A group in the early stages of the illness exhibited a variable pattern of task performance; one subset had impaired declarative memory but normal learning of the TOT, and another subset had precisely the opposite pattern of results. The authors sought to explain this pattern in terms of neurological heterogeneity within the HD group. More recently, Yágüez et al[20] reported impaired performance on the 'Tower of Düsseldorf', another variant of the TOH.

However, 'Tower' problems are probably of little value in examining skill-learning, as they are not 'process pure', requiring a certain amount of forward planning ability and inhibitory control, and amnesic patients may fail to learn such puzzles depending on the degree of frontal lobe damage they have sustained.[46]

Habits

Habit learning refers to the formation of stimulus–response associations in which an arbitrary stimulus has to be linked to an arbitrary motor response through reinforcement.[47] In humans, this learning is characterized by two key features: lack of awareness of the algorithm learned, and a slow rate of acquisition. In experimental animals, habit-learning involves learning, in a slow, incremental fashion to associate stimulus cues and specific responses in order to obtain reinforcement, e.g. in visual-discrimination learning tasks. Such learning is impaired following striatal lesions.[48]

Some evidence for a deficit in visual-discrimination learning in HD comes from the work of Oscar-Berman and colleagues using tests of individual-pair (IP) and concurrent-pair (CP) discrimination learning. Oscar-Berman et al[49] compared the performance of amnesic and HD patients on a series of IP and CP visual discriminations. Both amnesic and HD patients were impaired in their ability to learn IP and CP discriminations. However, unlike HD patients, the amnesics' performance on the CP discriminations improved over time, and their performance on IP problems was better than for CP discriminations. In contrast, HD patients were unable to improve their performance over time with the CP discriminations, and their IP performance was no better than their CP performance. Oscar-Berman et al[49] concluded that this pattern of impairment was the result of increased sensitivity to interference in the amnesics, whereas the HD patients had an impairment in associative learning mechanisms. We have recently examined learning of a two-pair CP discrimination, and this is intact in early-stage HD patients.[50]

Perhaps the most compelling argument to date for a 'habit system' in humans comes from the work of Squire and colleagues. In their study,[44] subjects were given a series of probabilistic discriminations, presented as a 'weather forecasting' task. Subjects have to predict the weather based on the images on four cue cards, with there being a probabilistic association between a particular weather outcome and a particular cue card. The task can be considered a habit-learning task, as the probabilistic nature of the cue–outcome associations requires that learning occur across many trials. Thus, information about a single trial is not as reliable as information accrued across many trials, and hence learning is incremental in nature. Amnesic patients exhibited normal learning of the task despite profoundly impaired declarative knowledge for the nature of the cues and the task-training. In contrast, patients with HD failed to learn the probabilistic discrimination task, although they also showed impaired memory for the nature of the cues and task-training.[44] We have also shown impaired learning in HD patients of a probabilistic discrimination learning task.[50]

Priming
Priming refers to the increased ability to identify/detect a stimulus as a result of its recent presentation. Priming effects have been demonstrated for novel materials having no pre-existing representations, suggesting that priming is based on the sensory-perceptual traces created by stimulus presentation. Across a number of studies, HD patients have been found to reliably exhibit intact lexical, semantic and perceptual priming effects.[15,37] However, HD patients exhibit impaired adaptation-level effects, e.g. weight-biasing and prism adaptation, possibly due to a deficit in motor programming.[37]

Conditioning
Woodruff-Pak and Papka[51] examined eyeblink classical conditioning in HD. There were no differences in production of conditioned responses (CRs) between HD patients and control subjects, but the timing of the CR was abnormal in HD. The authors suggested that the striatum might play a role in optimizing the timing of the CR.

Executive/control functions in HD

The term 'executive function' encompasses several aspects of cognitive function and generally refers to those mechanisms by which individuals adapt to novelty and control (thus optimizing) performance.[52] The principal theoretical framework we have for understanding the operation of executive functions is the supervisory system model of Norman and Shallice.[53] The theory follows the basic tenets of all theories of executive functions, that is the separation between routine and non-routine behaviors.[54] In this model, four components of cognitive processing are postulated: (1) modules, (2) schemata, (3) contention scheduling, and (4) the supervisory attentional system (SAS). Components 1, 2 and 3 are related to routine behavior. Basic cognitive processes are carried out in modules, which are controlled by schemata, routine programs for the control of overlearned behaviors. Hierarchies of schemata allow the co-ordination of complex, but routine, activities. Contention scheduling is the term used by Norman and Shallice to describe the (lateral inhibitory) mechanisms that control competition between schemata. Schemata are activated by particular triggers, which can be perceptions or the outputs of other schemata. The fourth unit is the 'executive' component of behavior, the SAS. This system acts to deal with non-routine behaviors and functions primarily under conditions of task/situational novelty when there are no known or only weakly related schemata available for task solution and thus error-correction mechanisms are maximally challenged; in demanding circumstances where planning and goal-monitoring mechanisms are maximally challenged; when decision-making/conflict resolution is required; and when inappropriate schemata must be inhibited. In its original manifestation,[53] the SAS was presumed to act by modulating contention scheduling. More recent revisions of the model[55] posit that the SAS works by constructing and implementing temporary new schemata (which may be existing but weakly activated schemata or adaptations of pre-existing schemata), which can take the place of the schemata triggered by contention scheduling alone, and which in turn are capable of controlling lower-level schemas so as to provide a procedure for achieving goals. In either case, the SAS can be said to function by top-down activation, inhibition or modification of schemata.[55,56] There is currently some debate as to whether the SAS is fractionable or represents the workings of a single, limited-capacity 'resource'.[52]

The prefrontal cortex is that region of the brain classically associated with executive processes. Indeed, the terms 'executive function' and 'frontal function' have often been used synonymously. However, it is important to note that there is not necessarily equivalence between 'executive functions' and 'frontal functions'. It is proving useful to consider 'circuit models' of executive functions in relation to the anatomical diversity of the frontal cortex and its connections with other cortical and subcortical regions, just as detailed knowledge of the anatomy of the medial temporal lobe and midline diencephalic systems is proving useful in the study of the amnesic syndrome. The combination of cognitive and anatomical data represents a powerful technique for the study of executive functions.

The notion that HD represents some form of 'dysexecutive syndrome' has some ecological validity, given the findings that many early-stage HD patients describe difficulties with planning, organizing and scheduling their day-to-day activities.[15] Somewhat surprisingly, then, the existing literature on executive functioning in HD is relatively sparse. The findings to date can be considered under the headings 'executive aspects of memory' and 'executive attention'.

Executive aspects of memory

There appears to be remarkable 'family resemblance' between those memory tasks sensitive to HD and those sensitive to damage to the frontal lobes. Thus, like frontal lobe patients,[57] HD patients are impaired on tasks of free recall relative to recognition,[15] and when they do show recognition memory impairment it appears to be like that of frontal lobe patients, i.e. an increase in false-positive errors, suggesting that some rule for making/verifying decisions when uncertain, rather than memory per se, is impaired.[30] Like frontal lobe patients, HD patients show flat remembering curves for remote memories, impaired memory for source, impaired delayed-response performance, impaired conditional associative learning,[58,59] and impaired frequency judgments,[60] although unlike frontal lobe patients, HD patients appear to show intact 'feelings of knowing'.[19] It has been suggested that all of these tasks require executive processes such as the setting up of plans for retrieval, monitoring and verifying of output, creation of new schemata, and inhibition of irrelevant responses.[55] However, there are some problems with declaring that HD patients' memory problems are a result of executive dysfunction. For example, HD patients are impaired on tasks such as span tasks, which seem to require relatively little in the way of executive control. Some authors have suggested that this is because even the simplest span tasks require considerable monitoring.[61] However, this approach is clearly unsatisfactory. In these studies, executive dysfunction is inferred on a post hoc basis rather than operationalized experimentally and measured directly. We cannot use these findings as unequivocal evidence for impaired executive control of memory.

Is there more direct evidence for an executive memory deficit in HD? Baddeley[61] has equated the CE component of working memory with the SAS of Shallice, and researchers have developed tasks considered to tap the functions of this limited-capacity 'control mechanism'. One such task is the so-called 'working memory span' (WMS) task.[62] This task involves remembering and then recalling the terminal words in a series of sentences. The subject's WMS is the maximum number of sentences that can be processed while retaining the final word. Gabrieli[63] found impaired WMS in HD patients and claimed that this represented an impairment in 'strategic working memory', as performance on the WMS task correlated highly with verbal fluency performance and performance on a self-ordered pointing task, which involves a great deal of monitoring. It is unclear, however, exactly what aspect of the 'CE' the WMS task is supposed to be tapping, and correlational evidence seems to be of little help in this regard. Indeed, the WMS task appears to relate more to theories of working memory that emphasize the role of 'active maintenance mechanisms' in control, rather than Baddeley's model, which postulates separate control (CE) and active storage mechanisms in working memory.[64]

Undoubtedly the best operationalized task of such putatively distinct executive aspects of working memory is the spatial working memory test used by Owen and colleagues.[65] This task is analogous to the 'radial maze', which measures working memory as defined in the animal-learning literature,[66] and in which rats are required to 'self-order' a series of choices in order to forage for food optimally. In addition to active maintenance, this task is considered to require the use of separate executive functions to optimize task performance by organizing and monitoring responses in order not to make redundant searches. In the computerized modification for humans as used by Owen et al,[65] subjects are required to search through an array of boxes for hidden 'tokens', hidden one at a time. Once a token is found and placed in a 'store' another token is hidden behind a different box, and no box is used twice to hide a token. Two types of error are possible: (1) between-search errors (BSEs) represent a return to a box used to hide a token on a previous trial; and (2) within-search errors (WSEs) represent a return to a box already shown not to hide a token within a particular trial. Importantly, successful performance in control subjects entails the use of a search strategy which involves retracing the route previously employed by the subject in searching through the array, 'editing' each search so as to avoid previously reinforced locations.[65] This strategy can be indexed, is uncontaminated by overall memory level, but correlates highly with performance. In frontal lobe patients, BSEs and WSEs are increased, the BSEs as a result of impaired use of such a strategy, while in other patient groups with more posterior damage, BSE scores are impaired but not strategy scores. Thus, mnemonic and executive aspects of performance can be dissociated.[65]

On this self-ordered spatial working memory task, early-stage HD patients made significantly more BSEs than controls, but were only mildly impaired in their use of an effective search strategy.[18,23] Patients with more advanced HD exhibit profound impairments on this task, with a very high degree of perseverative responding, which includes repetition of responses within the same search (WSE).[17] Thus, the self-ordered spatial working memory deficit in HD shows a discernible progression in which mechanisms that exert a control over responding show a graded breakdown. Monitoring of responses with respect to previous self-ordered searches is disrupted prior to the monitoring of responses within the same sequence. Rich et al[24] have reported similar deficits in self-ordered searching in HD.

The ability to set up plans and monitor their action is clearly an example of executive control of memory 'resources'.[67] Impaired planning has been inferred from impairments in picture arrangement and clock-drawing,[68] but, as with working memory, 'planning' in these examples is poorly operationalized. We have examined the performance of HD patients on the Tower of London (TOL), the classic test of planning, sensitive to frontal lobe lesions.[56] Across all problems, early-stage HD patients are only impaired on the most stringent index of planning, the number of 'perfect' solutions, and only make more excess moves than controls on the most difficult, five-move problems.[18]

Patients with early HD were also impaired in terms of their initial and subsequent thinking times, after correction for motor slowing. These results are consistent with previous findings of bradyphrenia in HD.[14] In advanced HD patients, there is a far more pronounced deficit, with impairments even at the level of the simplest two- and three-move problems. Thus, again, there is a discernible progression in HD, from the high-level selection of the appropriate responses in order to complete quite complicated plan-solution paths, to the more basic level of selection of responses in routine, easy solutions, consistent with hierarchical neural network models of planning.[69]

Executive attention and the concept of 'set'

The concept of 'set' has for a long time been associated with basal ganglia function.[70] In general terms, 'sets' are 'tendencies', 'dispositions', or a 'readiness', and their effect on cognition is one of 'guidance', 'facilitation', or 'selection'.[71] The most widely used definition of set is that of Buchwald et al.[70] 'Set is defined as a relatively persisting predisposition to behave in a particular way on the occurrence of a given stimulus'. Buchwald et al[70] distinguish between response set and cognitive set. Response set refers to the relatively short-term biasing effects that enable the smooth initiation and execution of a series of movements. A normal cognitive set was defined as the ability to discriminate a situational context and make an appropriate response to a given signal. Robbins and Brown,[72] in similar fashion to Buchwald et al,[70] define 'response set' as the 'prior assignment of probability of selection from the repertoire of available responses', and present data from rats to suggest that the striatum is a critical structure for 'response set'. Cognitive set is a 'set to respond according to abstract aspects of input, that is not tied to a particular motor response'.[72]

There is some evidence for impaired response set in HD. Jahanshahi et al[73] employed a simple (SRT) and a choice (CRT) task to study HD patients, and found that, unlike controls, who were able to respond faster in the SRT as compared to the CRT task, there was no SRT/CRT difference in the HD patients. Thus, HD patients were not engaged in the response set necessary to confer a speed advantage to SRT as compared to CRT. Further, HD patients are not able to use a response set for selecting the appropriate response in a task requiring sequential button presses;[74] and Georgiou et al[75] found an impairment in shifting attention from expected to unexpected locations on a vibrotactile CRT task. HD patients also make inappropriate response selections on differential reinforcement for low rates of responding schedules,[22] show exaggerated stimulus–response incompatibility effects,[76] and show inappropriate response selections on a variety of target detection tasks.[77] This has been suggested to be because of a fundamental problem in inhibiting unwanted responses,[76] and Swerdlow et al[78] have suggested that HD patients have problems even in inhibiting basic reflexes, such as inhibition of the startle reflex. Tasks which rely upon the involuntary shifting of attention, in contrast, are unaffected by HD.[79,80]

In terms of cognitive set, there are conflicting findings. The classic set test in clinical neuropsychology is the Wisconsin Card Sorting Test

(WCST). In this concept-learning task, subjects must learn by experimenter-provided feedback to sort a deck of cards, initially by one of the perceptual dimensions of shape, color or number, and then to shift their selection to one of the other two dimensions and then the remaining dimension, and then to repeat their series of choices. This task involves the acquisition, maintenance and shifting of cognitive set.

Josiassen et al[81] examined the performance of early-stage HD patients on the WCST. They suggested that HD patients were impaired only in shifting, and not in forming or maintaining attentional set, as they made more 'perseverative' than 'non-perseverative' errors. However, the WCST is not a 'process-pure' task,[56] and can be solved using a number of different strategies.[82] Furthermore, the measure of perseverative errors used by Josiassen and colleagues can catch errors made for a number of different reasons. Indeed, using other concept-formation tasks, Oscar-Berman et al[83] and Hanes et al[84] suggested that HD patients perform poorly on such tasks for a variety of reasons.

Other authors have suggested that HD patients have problems in shifting cognitive set, as they show impaired performance on the Trail Making Task and the Stroop interference task.[15] However, HD patients have difficulties on parts of the task that do not necessitate shifting set, that is, they are slower on trails A and have difficulties on the non-interference stages of the Stroop,[85] so it is difficult to conclude from these studies that HD patients have a particular problem in shifting set.

In order to study cognitive set in a purer form than in traditional concept-learning tasks, and to facilitate comparisons between humans and monkeys, Roberts et al[86] 'deconstructed' the WCST into its constituent elements. These researchers reasoned that the WCST involves a series of extradimensional shifts (EDS), as construed in animal-learning theory. In an EDS, attention to compound stimuli is transferred from one perceptual dimension to another (e.g. from color to shape) on the basis of changing reinforcement. In the task devised by Roberts et al,[86] subjects must learn a series of visual discriminations that culminate in an EDS. Control tests for EDS performance include the ability to alter specific stimulus–reward associations (reversal learning) and the ability to maintain cognitive set and thus successfully shift performance to novel exemplars of the same dimension (intradimensional shift). Frontal lobe patients have specific deficits at the EDS stage of the task,[87] whereas Parkinson's disease patients have difficulty throughout the task,[88] suggesting that frontal lobe patients have a specific deficit in overcoming a bias to respond to a previously reinforced dimension, whereas PD patients have more basic learning deficits.

In our study of early-stage HD, the most striking deficit seen was in performance on the discrimination/shift-learning task. Patients were impaired specifically at the EDS stage, with fewer than 20% of patients able to reach the criterion of six consecutive correct responses within 50 trials.[18] This deficit appears to be one of perseveration.[50] Deficits in shift-learning might represent a 'core' cognitive deficit in HD, because of their presence in early-stage patients. In a study of a group of preclinical HD mutation carriers, we have demonstrated specific deficits at the EDS stage of the discrimination/shift-learning task, prior to the onset of overt clinical movement disorder, and in the absence of performance deficits on tasks such as the TOL.[89]

The increase in perseverative responding at the EDS stage in early-stage HD is not observed in the reversal-learning phases of this task. However, in advanced HD, we have shown that patients exhibit dramatic increases in the reversal phase of the task, preventing them from reaching the EDS stage. These deficits are truly perseverative, because the patients continue to select the formerly reinforced stimulus to a significant degree.[17] Analogous reversal-learning deficits in HD were first observed by Oscar-Berman et al.[90]

The results from the above studies suggest that perseverative behavior is a cardinal feature of HD, and that its expression varies according to the course of the disease. Connectionist simulations[91] have shown that shift and reversal learning are computationally distinct, and lesion studies have shown that deficits in shift and reversal learning are anatomically doubly dissociable. Lesions to the lateral prefrontal cortex impair shift, but not reversal learning, while lesions of ventral prefrontal cortex impair reversal, but not shift-learning.[92] These regions of the prefrontal cortex probably project to dorsal and ventral portions of the striatum, respectively,[93] and so the reversal- and shift-learning results are consistent with the known spread of pathology in HD, with those functions associated with dorsal striatum being impaired prior to those associated with more ventral regions of the striatum.[1]

Related findings have recently been made in the domain of language. Ullman et al[94] had patients produce past tenses of regular and novel words which are thought to require the use of an '–ed' suffixation 'rule' (e.g. looked, plugged), and irregular verbs (e.g. dug) which are thought to be retrieved from memory. Ullman and colleagues found overactive or excess –ed suffixation rule use in HD patients, who showed a pronounced over-regularization rate (e.g. producing 'digged' as the past tense of 'dig'), and showed numerous instances of the superfluous and perseverative addition of the '–ed' suffix, as if a 'suffixing rule' was overactive or disinhibited.

Relation of neuropathology to cognitive disorder: is cognitive dysfunction in HD due to cortical or striatal pathology?

Several lines of evidence suggest that the cognitive dysfunction in HD may result from degeneration of the striatum, rather than the cortex. Measures of caudate atrophy on computerized tomography (CT) and magnetic resonance imaging (MRI) correlate strongly with many cognitive measures, including Trail Making, Stroop, source memory, and Tower of Düsseldorf (TOD) performance.[15,20,95]

More direct evidence comes from functional, rather than structural, brain imaging, using positron emission tomography (PET) and single photon emission computerized tomography (SPECT) measures of regional cerebral blood flow (rCBF) and glucose metabolism. Resting measures of caudate metabolism have been shown to correlate with verbal memory, picture arrangement and WCST performance.[96,97] Furthermore, a SPECT activation study has shown that HD patients can activate frontal cortex normally when performing the WCST.[98] Not all studies, however, have found that cortical abnormalities contribute minimally to cognitive impairment. For example, Harris et al[99] found that MRI measures of global cortical atrophy bore a stronger relation to cognitive test performance than measures of striatal atrophy, and Hasselbalch et al[97] found that recognition memory, language and perceptual impairments were related to cortical, rather than striatal, blood flow as measured by SPECT. Clearly, then, not all of the cognitive impairment in HD can be related to 'striatal' pathology. It is tempting to speculate that the core features of the cognitive impairment in early-stage HD are related to striatal pathology, but the more global dementia of advanced HD may be related to cortical pathology.

In our own studies,[100] we have examined the relationship between PET measures of striatal neuronal loss and cognitive function in clinical HD subjects and presymptomatic HD mutation carriers. Striatal medium-spiny neurons express dopamine receptors. Dopamine receptor-binding potentials measured with PET thus provide a direct marker of basal ganglia pathology. We have shown a significant relationship between impaired executive functions and dopamine receptor-binding potentials, (Figure 9.3), suggesting that executive dysfunction in HD is indeed related to striatal neuronal loss. Brandt et al[107] also found a relationship between caudate dopamine D2 receptor binding and performance on the Trail Making and Symbol-Digit Coding tests. Furthermore, a recent correlational analysis of cognitive performance in HD patients with MRI-assessed cortical, striatal and thalamic volumes and PET measures of dopamine neurotransmission (dopamine transporter, D1 and D2 receptors) has shown quite clear relationships between both frontal cortex volumes and indices of striatal function with most of the cognitive tests employed.[102] This study helps to make the point that, from a functional perspective, the basal ganglia should not be viewed in isolation. It makes better sense to attempt to ascribe behavioral functions to entire circuits of interconnected neural structures than to individual structures themselves. The basal ganglia should be viewed as components of circuits organized in parallel and remaining largely segregated from one another.[4]

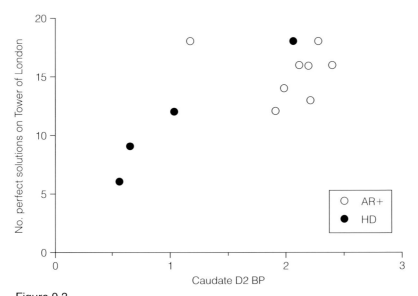

Figure 9.3

Relationship between caudate dopamine D2 receptor-binding potential (BP = B_{max}/K_D), measured using [¹¹C]raclopride PET, and planning performance (number of perfect solutions on a 'one-touch' version of the Tower of London task) in a group of clinical HD patients (HD) and presymptomatic HD mutation carriers (AR+). Rs (Spearman rank correlation coefficient) = 0.61, $P < 0.05$.[100]

Can the cognitive deficits in HD be related to a unitary, core-processing deficit? The cognitive pathology of HD in relation to models of information processing in the basal ganglia

From the results described, it is clear that HD is associated with cognitive deficits that can potentially be attributed to disruption of information processing mediated by different corticostriatal circuits (Figure 9.1). Thus, deficits in executive function might be associated with the 'dorsolateral' circuit; reversal learning might be associated with the 'temporal lobe' and/or the 'limbic' circuit; certain of the memory and visual impairments suggest an involvement of the 'temporal lobe' circuit; and the affective disturbance in HD might be associated with damage to the 'limbic' circuit. While the range of cognitive deficits in HD might be related to a diverse range of information-processing operations carried out by the striatum, it is possible that the principal forms of deficit outlined above for HD could be explained by a *unitary* cognitive processing deficit.

In recent times, several computational models of information processing in corticostriatal circuitry have been proposed.[103,104] There is a common computational theme running throughout such models, based on the unique neural architecture of these regions. The recurrent corticostriatal circuit architecture, in which virtually the entire cortex projects to the striatum, which then projects onto the smaller pallidum, before returning via the thalamus to specific cortical regions (Figure 9.1), suggests that some form of selection/modification/stabilization process may be occurring within this circuitry. Indeed, most researchers emphasize that the striatum plays a role in context-dependent response selection[105–107] or, more generally, the action selection problem.[108,109] Context-relevant information processing would allow the striatum to instruct cortical areas as to which sensory inputs or patterns of motor output are behaviorally significant in a given context. That is, the striatum, possibly under the influence of dopaminergic 'teaching signals',[110] might be performing some form of pattern classification computation, modifying coarsely coded cortical representations of memories, sensory features or motor intentions into stable representations which are context-appropriate.[106] We have produced a conceptual model which elaborates these ideas, and which suggests that many of the cognitive deficits seen in HD can be related to the breakdown of such an information-processing mechanism.[107]

Conclusions

In this chapter, I hope to have illustrated how the study of information-processing deficits in HD can be integrated with other approaches, including anatomy, neuroimaging, and computational modeling, thus leading to a richer framework in which to study the clinical cognitive neuroscience of HD and related disorders. It is hoped that such a unified approach will lead to advances not only in our understanding of information processing in basal ganglia circuitry, but also to therapeutic benefits for patients with basal ganglia disorders.

Acknowledgments

I would like to thank the Medical Research Council of Great Britain for financial support. This work is based upon research carried out by the author for the degree of Doctor of Philosophy at Darwin College, University of Cambridge. I would like to thank my thesis supervisors, Professor Trevor W Robbins and Dr Barbara J Sahakian, for their guidance and support.

References

1. Vonsattel JPG, DiFiglia M. Huntington disease. *J Neuropath Exp Neurol* (1998) **57:** 369–84.

2. Nakano K, Kayahara T, Ushiro H, Kuwabara H. The basal ganglia-thalamo-cortical connections with special reference to output neuronal distributions in macaque monkeys. In Ohye C, Kimura M, McKenzie JS (eds) *The Basal Ganglia V* (New York: Plenum Press, 1996): 19–26.

3. Smith Y, Shink E, Sidibé M. Neuronal circuitry and synaptic connectivity of the basal ganglia. *Neurosurg Clin North Am* (1998) **9:** 203–22.

4. Alexander GE. Anatomy of the basal ganglia and related motor structures. In Watts RL, Koller WC (eds) *Movement Disorders: Neurologic Principles and Practice* (New York: McGraw-Hill, 1997): 73–85.

5. Middleton FA, Strick PL. The temporal lobe is a target of output from the basal ganglia. *Proc Natl Acad Sci USA* (1996) **93:** 8683–7.

6. Schacter DL, Tulving E (eds) *Memory Systems 1994* (Cambridge, MA: MIT Press, 1994).

7. Winograd T. Frame representation and the declarative-procedural controversy. In Bobrow DG, Collins A (eds) *Representation and Understanding: Studies in Cognitive Science* (New York: Academic Press, 1975): 185–210.

8. Squire LR. Declarative and non-declarative memory: multiple brain systems supporting learning and memory. In Schacter DL, Tulving E (eds) *Memory Systems 1994*, (Cambridge, MA: MIT Press, 1994): 203–8.

9. Schacter DL, Chiu CYP, Ochsner KN. Implicit memory: a selective review. *Annu Rev Neurosci* (1993) **16:** 183–205.

10. Gillett E. Learning theory and intrapsychic conflict. *Int J Psychoanal* (1996) **77:** 689–707.

11. Dickinson A. *Contemporary Animal Learning Theory* (Cambridge: Cambridge University Press, 1980).

12. Tulving E. *Elements of Episodic Memory* (Oxford: Oxford University Press, 1983).

13. Baddeley A. *Working Memory* (Oxford: Clarendon Press, 1986).

14. Butters N. The clinical aspects of memory disorders: contributions from experimental studies of amnesia and dementia. *J Clin Exp Neuropsychol* (1984) **6:** 17–36.

15. Brandt J, Butters N. Neuropsychological characteristics of Huntington's disease. In Grant I, Adams KM (eds) *Neuropsychological Assessment of Neuropsychiatric Disorders* (New York: Oxford University Press, 1996): 312–41.

16. Orsini A, Fragassi NA, Chiacchio L et al. Verbal and spatial memory span in patients with extrapyramidal diseases. *Percept Motor Skills* (1987) **65:** 555–8.

17. Lange KW, Sahakian BJ, Quinn NP et al. Comparison of executive and visuospatial memory function in Huntington's disease and dementia of Alzheimer type matched for degree of dementia. *J Neurol Neurosurg Psychiatry* (1995) **58:** 598–606.

18. Lawrence AD, Sahakian BJ, Hodges JR et al. Executive and mnemonic functions in early Huntington's disease. *Brain* (1996) **119:** 1633–45.

19. Brandt J. Cognitive impairments

in Huntington's disease: insights into the neuropsychology of the striatum. In Boller F, Grafman J (eds) *Handbook of Neuropsychology*, Vol. 5 (Amsterdam: Elsevier, 1991): 241–64.

20. Yágüez L, Canavan AGM, Lange HW, Hömberg V. Motor learning by imagery is differentially affected in Parkinson's and Huntington's diseases. *Behav Brain Res* (1999) **102:** 115–27.

21. D'Esposito M, Postle BR. The dependence of span and delayed-response performance on prefrontal cortex. *Neuropsychologia* (1999) **37:** 1303–15.

22. Oscar-Berman M, Zola-Morgan SM, Öberg RGE, Bonner RT. Comparative neuropsychology and Korsakoff's syndrome. III. Delayed response, delayed alternation and DRL performance. *Neuropsychologia* (1982) **20:** 187–202.

23. Lawrence AD, Watkins LHA, Sahakian BJ et al. Visual object and visuo-spatial cognition in Huntington's disease: implications for information processing in cortico-striatal circuits. *Brain* (2000) **123:** 1349–64.

24. Rich JB, Bylsma FW, Brandt J. Self-ordered pointing performance in Huntington's disease patients. *Neuropsychiatr Neuropsychol Behav Neurol* (1996) **9:** 99–106.

25. Saint-Cyr JA, Taylor AE, Lang AE. Procedural learning and neostriatal dysfunction in man. *Brain* (1988) **111:** 941–59.

26. Granholm E, Butters N. Associative encoding and retrieval in Alzheimer's and Huntington's disease. *Brain Cogn* (1988) **7:** 335–47.

27. Butters N, Salmon DP, Granholm E et al. Neuropsychological differentiation of amnesic and dementing states. In Stahl SM, Iversen SD, Goodman EC (eds) *Cognitive Neurochemistry* (Oxford: Oxford University Press, 1987): 3–20.

28. Pillon B, Deweer A, Michon C et al. Are explicit memory disorders of progressive supranuclear palsy related to damage to striato-frontal circuits? Comparison with Alzheimer's and Huntington's disease. *Neurology* (1994) **44:** 1264–70.

29. Rich JB, Troyer AK, Bylsma FW, Brandt J. Longitudinal analysis of phonemic clustering and switching during word-list generation in Huntington's disease. *Neuropsychology* (1999) **13:** 525–31.

30. Brandt J, Corwin J, Krafft L. Is verbal recognition memory really different in Huntington's and Alzheimer's disease? *J Clin Exp Neuropsychol* (1992) **14:** 773–84.

31. Jacobs DH, Shuren J, Heilman K. Impaired perception of facial identity and facial affect in Huntington's disease. *Neurology* (1995): **45:** 1217–18.

32. Sprengelmeyer R, Young AW, Calder AJ et al. Loss of disgust: perception of faces and emotions in Huntington's disease. *Brain* (1996) **119:** 1647–65.

33. Rosser A, Hodges JR. Initial letter and semantic category fluency in Alzheimer's disease, Huntington's disease, and progressive supranuclear palsy [see comments]. *J Neurology Neurosurg Psychiatry* (1994) **57:** 1389–94. Comment in: *J Neurology Neurosurg Psychiatry* (1995) **58:** 520–1.

34. Rohrer D, Salmon DP, Wixted JT, Paulsen JS. The disparate effects of Alzheimer's disease and Huntington's disease on semantic memory. *Neuropsychology* (1999) **13:** 381–8.

35. Chan AS, Butters N, Salmon DP et al. Comparison of the semantic networks in patients with dementia and amnesia. *Neuropsychology* (1995) **9:** 177–86.

36. Wilson RS, Como PG, Garron DC et al. Memory failure in Huntington's disease. *J Clin Exp Neuropsychol* (1987) **9:** 147–54.

37. Heindel WC, Salmon DP, Butters N. Cognitive approaches to the memory disorders of demented patients. In Sutker PB, Adams HE (eds) *Comprehensive Handbook of Psychopathology* (New York: Plenum Press, 1993): 735–61.

38. Gabrieli JDE, Stebbins GT, Singh J et al. Intact mirror-tracing and impaired rotary-pursuit skill learning in patients with Huntington's disease: evidence for dissociable memory systems in skill learning. *Neuropsychology* (1997) **11:** 272–81.

39. Knopman D, Nissen MJ. Procedural learning is impaired in Huntington's disease; evidence from the serial reaction time task. *Neuropsychol* (1991) **29:** 245–54.

40. Willingham DB, Koroshetz WJ. Evidence for dissociable motor skills in Huntington's disease patients. *Psychobiology* (1993) **21:** 173–82.

41. Willingham DB, Koroshetz WJ, Peterson EW. Motor skills have diverse neural bases: spared and impaired skill acquisition in Huntington's disease. *Neuropsychology* (1996) **10:** 315–21.

42. Smith MA, Brandt J, Shadmehr R. Motor disorder in Huntington's disease begins as a dysfunction in error feedback control. *Nature* (2000) **403:** 544–9.

43. Martone M, Butters N, Payne M et al. Dissociations between skill learning and verbal recognition in amnesia and dementia. *Arch Neurol* (1984) **41:** 965–70.

44. Knowlton BJ, Squire LR, Paulsen JS et al. Dissociations within nondeclarative memory in Huntington's disease. *Neuropsychology* (1996) **10:** 538–48.

45. Butters N, Wolfe J, Martone M et al. Memory disorders associated with Huntington's disease: verbal recall, verbal recognition, and procedural memory. *Neuropsychologia* (1985) **23:** 729–43.

46. Joyce EM, Robbins TW. Frontal lobe function in Korsakoff and non-Korsakoff alcoholics: planning and spatial working memory. *Neuropsychologia* (1991) **29:** 709–23.

47. Mishkin M, Malamut B, Bachevalier J. Memories and habits: two neural systems. In Lynch G, McGaugh JL, Weinberger NM (eds) *Neurobiology of Learning and Memory* (New York: Guildford Press, 1984): 65–77.

48. Reading PJ, Dunnett SB, Robbins TW. Dissociable roles of the ventral, medial and lateral striatum on the acquisition and performance of a complex visual stimulus–response habit. *Behav Brain Res* (1991) **45:** 147–61.

49. Oscar-Berman M, Zola-Morgan SM. Comparative neuropsychology and Korsakoff's syndrome. II — two-choice visual discrimination learning. *Neuropsychologia* (1980) **18:** 513–25.

50. Lawrence AD, Sahakian BJ, Rogers RD et al. Discrimination, reversal, and shift learning in Huntington's disease: mechanisms of impaired response selection. *Neuropsychologia* (1999) **37:** 1359–74.

51. Woodruff-Pak DS, Papka M. Huntington's disease and eyeblink classical conditioning: normal learning but abnormal timing. *J Int Neuropsychol Soc* (1996) **2:** 323–34.

52. Burgess PW. Theory and

methodology in executive function research. In Rabitt P (ed.) *Methodology of Frontal and Executive Functions* (Hove: Erlbaum, 1998): 81–116.

53. Norman DA, Shallice T. Attention to action: willed and automatic control of behaviour. In Schwartz GE, Shapiro D (eds) *Consciousness and Self-Regulation* (New York: Plenum Press, 1986): 1–18.

54. Grafman J. Similarities and distinctions among current models of prefrontal cortical functions. *Ann NY Acad Sci* (1995) **769:** 337–68.

55. Stuss DT, Shallice T, Alexander MP, Picton TW. A multidisciplinary approach to anterior attentional functions. *Ann NY Acad Sci* (1995) **769:** 191–211.

56. Shallice T. *From Neuropsychology to Mental Structure* (Cambridge: Cambridge University Press, 1988).

57. Shimamura AP. Memory and the prefrontal cortex. *Ann NY Acad Sci* (1995) **769:** 151–9.

58. Sprengelmeyer R, Canavan AGM, Lange HW, Hömberg V. Associative learning in degenerative neostriatal disorders: contrasts in explicit and implicit remembering between Parkinson's and Huntington's diseases. *Mov Disord* (1995) **10:** 51–65.

59. Tucker J, Harding AE, Jahanshahi M et al. Associative learning in patients with cerebellar ataxia. *Behav Neurosci* (1996) **110:** 1229–34.

60. Strauss ME, Weingartner H, Thompson K. Remembering words and how often they occurred in memory-impaired patients. *Memory Cogn* (1985) **13:** 507–10.

61. Baddely A. Exploring the central executive. *Q J Exp Psychol* (1996) **49A:** 5–28.

62. Daneman M, Carpenter PA. Individual differences in working memory and reading. *J Verb Learn Verb Behav* (1980) **19:** 450–66.

63. Gabrieli J. Contribution of the basal ganglia to skill learning and working memory in humans. In Houk JC, Davis JL, Beiser DG (eds) *Models of Information Processing in the Basal Ganglia* (Cambridge, MA: MIT Press, 1995): 277–94.

64. O'Reilly RC, Braver TS, Cohen JD. A biologically-based computational model of working memory. In Miyake A, Shah P (eds) *Models of Working Memory: Mechanisms of Active Maintenance and Executive Control* (New York: Cambridge University Press, 1999): 375–412.

65. Owen AM, Morris RG, Sahakian BJ et al. Double dissociations of memory and executive functions in working memory tasks following frontal lobe excisions, temporal lobe excisions or amygdalo-hippocampectomy in man. *Brain* (1991) **119:** 1597–615.

66. Maki WS. Some problems for a theory of working memory. In Roitblat HL, Bever TG, Terrace HS (eds) *Animal Cognition* (Hillsdale, NJ: Lawrence Erlbaum Associates, 1984): 117–33.

67. Miller GA, Galanter E, Pribram KH. *Plans and the Structure of Behavior* (New York: Holt, Rinehart and Winston, 1960).

68. Rouleau I, Salmon DP, Butters N et al. Quantitative and qualitative analyses of clock drawing in Alzheimer's and Huntington's disease. *Brain Cogn* (1992) **18:** 70–87.

69. Dehaene S, Changeux JP. A hierarchical neuronal network for planning behaviour. *Proc Natl Acad Sci USA* (1997) **94:** 13293–8.

70. Buchwald NA, Hull CD, Levine MS, Villablanca J. The basal ganglia and the regulation of response and cognitive sets. In Brazier MAB (ed.) *Growth and Development of the Brain* (New York: Raven Press, 1975): 171–89.

71. Gibson JJ. A critical review of the concept of set in contemporary experimental psychology. *Psychol Bull* (1941) **38:** 781–817.

72. Robbins TW, Brown VJ. The role of the striatum in the mental chronometry of action: a theoretical review. *Rev Neurosci* (1990) **2:** 181–213.

73. Jahanshahi M, Brown RG, Marsden CD. A comparative study of simple and choice reaction time in Parkinson's, Huntington's and cerebellar disease. *J Neurol Neurosurg Psychiatry* (1993) **56:** 1169–77.

74. Georgiou N, Bradshaw JL, Philips JG et al. Reliance on advance information and movement sequencing in Huntington's disease. *Mov Disord* (1995) **10:** 472–81.

75. Georgiou N, Bradshaw JL, Phillips JG, Chiu E. The effect of Huntington's disease and Gilles de la Tourette's syndrome on the ability to hold and shift attention. *Neuropsychologia* (1996) **34:** 843–51.

76. Georgiou N, Bradshaw JL, Phillips JG et al. The Simon effect and attention deficits in Gilles de la Tourette's syndrome and Huntington's disease. *Brain* (1995) **118:** 1305–18.

77. Sprengelmeyer R, Lange HW, Hömberg V. The pattern of attentional deficits in Huntington's disease. *Brain* (1995) **118:** 145–52.

78. Swerdlow NR, Paulsen J, Braff DL et al. Impaired prepulse inhibition of acoustic and tactile startle response in patients with HD. *J Neurol Neurosurg Psychiatry* (1995) **58:** 192–200.

79. Filoteo VJ, Delis DC, Roman MJ et al. Visual attention and perception in patients with Huntington's disease. *J Clin Exp Neuropsychol* (1995) **17:** 654–67.

80. Tsai TT, Lasker A, Zee DS. Visual attention in Huntington's disease: the effect of cueing on saccade latencies and manual reaction times. *Neuropsychologia* (1995) **33:** 1617–26.

81. Josiassen RC, Curry LM, Mancall EL. Development of neuropsychological deficits in Huntington's disease. *Arch Neurol* (1983) **40:** 791–6.

82. Dehaene S, Changeux JP. The Wisconsin card sorting test: theoretical analysis and simulation of a reasoning task in a model neuronal network. *Cereb Cortex* (1991) **1:** 62–79.

83. Oscar-Berman M, Sax DS, Opoliner L. Effects of memory aids on hypothesis behaviour and focusing in patients with Huntington's chorea. *Adv Neurol* (1973) **1:** 717–28.

84. Hanes KR, Andrewes DG, Pantelis C. Cognitive flexibility and complex integration in Parkinson's disease, Huntington's disease, and schizophrenia. *J Int Neuropsychol Soc* (1995) **1:** 545–53.

85. Watkins LHA, Rogers RD, Lawrence AD et al. Impaired planning but intact decision making in early Huntington's disease: implications for specific frontostriatal pathology. *Neuropsychologia* (2000) **38:** 1112–25.

86. Roberts AC, Robbins TW, Everitt BJ. The effects of intra-dimensional and extra-dimensional shifts on visual discrimination learning in humans and non-human primates. *Q J Exp Psychol* (1988) **40B:** 321–41.

87. Owen AM, Roberts AC, Polkey CE et al. Extra-dimensional versus intra-dimensional set shifting performance following frontal lobe excision, temporal lobe excision or amygdalo-hippocampectomy in man. *Neuropsychologia* (1989) **29:** 993–1006.

88. Downes JJ, Roberts AC, Sahakian BJ et al. Impaired extra-dimensional shift performance in medicated and unmedicated Parkinson's disease: evidence for a specific attentional dysfunction. *Neuropsychologia* (1989) **27:** 1329–44.

89. Lawrence AD, Hodges JR, Rosser AE et al. Evidence for specific cognitive deficits in pre-clinical Huntington's disease. *Brain* (1998) **121:** 1329–41.

90. Oscar-Berman M, Zola-Morgan SM. Comparative neuropsychology and Korsakoff's syndrome. I — spatial and visual reversal learning. *Neuropsychologia* (1980) **18:** 499–512.

91. Krushke J. Dimensional relevance shifts in category learning. *Connection Sci* (1996) **8:** 225–47.

92. Dias R, Robbins TW, Roberts AC. Dissociation in prefrontal cortex of affective and attentional shifts. *Nature* (1996) **380:** 69–72.

93. Arikuni T, Kubota K. The organisation of prefrontocaudate projections and their laminar origin in the macaque monkey: a retrograde study using HRP gel. *J Comp Neurol* (1986) **244:** 429–51.

94. Ullman MT, Corkin S, Coppola M et al. A neural dissociation within language: evidence that the mental dictionary is part of declarative memory, and that grammatical rules are processed by the procedural system. *J Cogn Neurosci* (1997) **9:** 266–76.

95. Brandt J, Bylsma FW, Aylward EH et al. Impaired source memory in Huntington's disease and its relation to basal ganglia atrophy. *J Clin Exp Neuropsychol* (1996) **17:** 868–77.

96. Berent S, Giordani B, Lehtinen S et al. Positron emission tomographic scan investigations of Huntington's disease: cerebral metabolic correlates of cognitive function. *Ann Neurol* (1988) **23:** 541–6.

97. Hasselbalch SG, Öberg G, Sorensen SA et al. Reduced regional cerebral blood flow in Huntington's disease studied by SPECT. *J Neurol Neurosurg Psychiatr* (1992) **55:** 1018–23.

98. Goldberg TE, Berman KF, Moore E, Weinberger DR. rCBF and cognitive function in Huntington's disease and schizophrenia: a comparison of patients matched for performance on a prefrontal-type task. *Arch Neurol* (1990) **47:** 418–22.

99. Harris GJ, Aylward EH, Peyser CE et al. Single photon emission computed tomographic blood flow and magnetic resonance volume imaging of basal ganglia in Huntington's disease. *Arch Neurol* (1996) **53:** 316–24.

100. Lawrence AD, Weeks RA, Brooks DJ et al. The relationship between striatal dopamine receptor binding and cognitive performance in Huntington's disease. *Brain* (1998) **121:** 1343–55.

101. Brandt J, Folstein SE, Wong DF et al. D2 receptors in Huntington's disease: positron emission tomography findings and clinical correlates. *J Neuropsychiatr Clin Neurosci* (1990) **2:** 20–7.

102. Bäckman L, Robins-Wahlin TB, Lundin A et al. Cognitive deficits in Huntington's disease are predicted by dopaminergic PET

markers and brain volumes. *Brain* (1997) **120:** 2207–17.

103. Houk JC, Davis JL, Beiser DG. *Models of Information Processing in the Basal Ganglia* (Cambridge, MA: MIT Press, 1995).

104. Wickens J. Basal ganglia: structure and computations. *Network: Comput Neural Syst* (1997) **8:** R77–109.

105. Rolls ET. Neurophysiology and cognitive functions of the striatum. *Rev Neurol (Paris)* (1994) **150:** 648–60.

106. Beiser DG, Hua SE, Houk JC. Network models of the basal ganglia. *Curr Opin Neurobiol* (1997) **7:** 185–90.

107. Lawrence AD, Sahakian BJ, Robbins TW. Cognitive functions and corticostriatal circuits: insights from Huntington's disease. *Trends Cogn Sci* (1998) **2:** 379–88.

108. Hikosaka O. Basal ganglia — possible role in motor co-ordination and learning. *Curr Opin Neurobiol* (1991) **1:** 638–43.

109. Redgrave P, Prescott TJ, Gurney K. The basal ganglia: a vertebrate solution to the selection problem? *Neuroscience* (1999) **89:** 1009–23.

110. Schultz W. Reward responses of dopamine neurons: a biological reinforcement signal. In Gerstner W, Germond A, Hasler M, Nocoud J-D (eds) *Lecture Notes in Computer Science 1327* (Berlin: Springer, 1997): 3–12.

10
Parkinson's disease

John E Harrison, Isabel Stow, and Adrian M Owen

Introduction

Neuropsychology is a slightly ghoulish discipline, dependent upon nature's caprice to provide experimental material with which to work. Neuropsychologists seeking to make links between brain and cognition rarely (i.e. only in surgical cases) have control of where and how large a lesion will be made. Most brain injury is a fairly messy affair, usually the result of disease, traumatic injury or cerebrovascular accident. These unpredictable and heterogeneous causes of brain lesions mean that instances of two or more identical lesions will be vanishingly rare. One reason for neuropsychologists' apparent preoccupation with single cases is simply a paucity of good study materials.

In this wild and unpredictable landscape it is small wonder that so many investigators should have settled upon the disorder of Parkinson's disease (PD) as the focus of their study. At first look, the disease appears to offer an excellent model of basal ganglia dysfunction, as the best evidence supports the view that PD is caused by damage to the pars compacta of the substantia nigra. It seems that not only is the disorder homogeneous with regard to its signs and symptoms, but also that the focused pathology is responsible for the cardinal signs of tremor, rigidity, bradykinesia and postural instability. Add in the fact that a ready supply of study subjects is available from any neurologists' outpatient clinic, and one ostensibly has an excellent model with which to investigate basal ganglia function. On paper, then, it seems that the neuropsychological study of any patient group diagnosed as having PD provides the opportunity to establish both the changes in cognition caused by the disorder and to determine the role of the basal ganglia in normal subjects. Given the apparently discrete lesion found in PD and the apparent homogeneity of signs and symptoms in the disorder, it is a surprise to discover that opinion regarding the nature of cognitive dysfunction in PD ranges from a very specific subset of 'frontostriatal' symptoms to a widespread and general deterioration of intellectual function. The cognitive dysfunction literature for PD runs to literally hundreds of publications, and a review of all these topics is unachievable in so short a chapter. Broadly speaking, however, the deficits that have been most commonly described across four decades of research fall into three major categories: (1) memory impairments;[1–7] (2) visuospatial impairment;[8–10] and (3) impairments of 'executive functions', including concept formation and attentional set-shifting ability,[6,7,11–17] planning,[6,18–21] and working memory.[6,19,20,22–27]

Against this background, it is perhaps not surprising that no clear consensus has been reached as to whether any or all of these deficits can be understood in terms of the disruption of a common underlying mechanism.

In this chapter, we will attempt to illustrate some of the difficulties attached to understanding the cognitive changes reported in PD patients by focusing on just two specific domains within which deficits have been reliably reported:

1. verbal fluency, both phonological and semantic;
2. performance on rule-learning and attentional set-shifting tasks.

Our main criterion for selection is familiarity with the reported literature, usually through having reported studies of our own. However, the areas we have selected will amply illustrate the marked variation in cognitive skills that is evident in the performance of PD patients. We will review PD performance in these specified areas of cognition, where possible using meta-analytic techniques to report both the findings of specific studies and a summary of their findings. The graphical method we shall use consists of 'tree plots', a representation commonly used in meta-analysis. We have found these plots to be an efficient method of showing difference scores, statistical significance, power to detect effects and evidence of publication bias. We conclude by reviewing the patient selection criteria adopted by authors as a way of determining the true cognitive sequelae of PD. An explanation of tree plots is provided in the legend to Figure 10.1. Given our acknowledgment that variability in cognitive dysfunction is the norm in PD, summarizing the facts about a particular cognitive domain is something of a challenge. However, the effect of pooling studies is to strengthen any 'real' effect through the increased power afforded by having a larger sample. The meta-analyses will include studies with different inclusion and exclusion criteria (an issue discussed below), but the sheer weight of numbers should compensate for any particularly unusual results caused by this, and Figure 10.1 provides a graphical illustration of notable inconsistencies. Thus the result summaries we provide are best viewed as being 'more true than they are not'.

In the first part of the chapter, we will provide an introduction to the identified and proposed reasons for the marked heterogeneity that has been reported in the cognitive performance of PD patients, providing some account of why such differences might exist between subjects. If one samples from the population of PD patients with no regard to factors such as depression, dementia, comorbid disease, and drug-induced cognitive deficits, and then compares with a matched normal group, poorer performance is often a characteristic of the PD group. It would seem, therefore, that the most effective way of determining cognitive change caused by PD would be to use subjects carefully screened for factors such as depression and dementia mentioned above. However, this raises two issues, one practical and the other theoretical. First, screening patients for all the factors mentioned above leaves small sample sizes that may then not be big enough to demonstrate a 'real' effect, and also do not reflect the disease population as a whole. Second, and more important, this procedure may remove patients of 'legitimate' interest, metaphorically 'throwing the baby out with the bathwater', as some coexisting conditions such as depression and dementia may in fact be part of the disease process itself and therefore worthy of investigation.

Established and proposed sources of cognitive variability in PD

Comorbid disease

Not knowing the cause, or causes, of PD precludes grouping patients by etiology. The absence of a diagnostic test for PD means that patients are diagnosed based on the presence of the signs and symptoms of the disorder. A positive response to anti-parkinsonian medication usually helps to confirm the diagnosis. However, a number of other disorders also feature degeneration of the substantia nigra and may therefore both mimic idiopathic PD and exhibit a positive response to anti-parkinsonian drugs. The term 'Parkinson's plus' has been introduced to cover disorders such as progressive supranuclear palsy (PSP) and multiple systems atrophy (MSA). Brain injuries occasioned by infarction, infection and injury are all also capable of producing a parkinsonian syndrome if the injuries involve the substantia nigra. These confounds to the process of diagnosing idiopathic PD mean that the false-positive diagnosis rate can run as high as 25% (see postmortem studies by Hughes et al[28]). A second interesting issue is the presence of pathomnemonic Lewy bodies in the substantia nigra of approximately 10% of control brains at postmortem. Last, it is possible that cognitive change occurs early in the disease process before the cardinal signs that drive most patients to find medical advice. This means that a number of elderly controls may be further confounding our results, as they may have 'preclinical' PD with associated cognitive change.

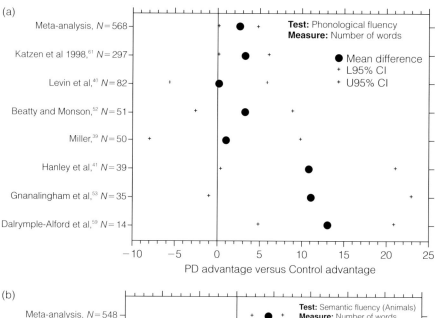

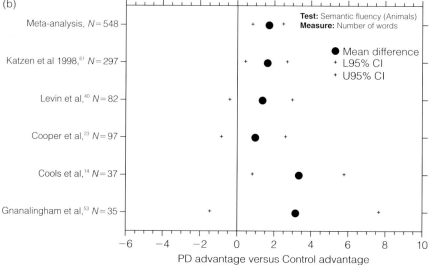

Figure 10.1a-d

Each panel shows a 'tree' or 'funnel' plot showing a summary of both published and unpublished performance on the tasks described in the text. Along the ordinate (x axis) is the difference in means between controls and PD patients, together with a 95% confidence interval, calculated using the standard error of the difference (SED). The abscissa (y axis) shows the studies from which data have been taken. The studies have been ordered according to sample size, with the largest study at the top and the smallest at the bottom. As the SEM is partially a function of sample size, smaller studies tend to have large confidence intervals. Thus ordering the studies by size leads to wider confidence intervals at the bottom with narrower ones at the top, giving the plot its 'tree' shape. The meta-analysis combining all the data is shown at the top of the graph and, as the largest sample, has the smallest confidence interval. This graphical representation of data has a number of useful characteristics. First, it is clear from the plot which are the statistically significant results, as any confidence interval that does not include the 'zero' point illustrates a 'real'

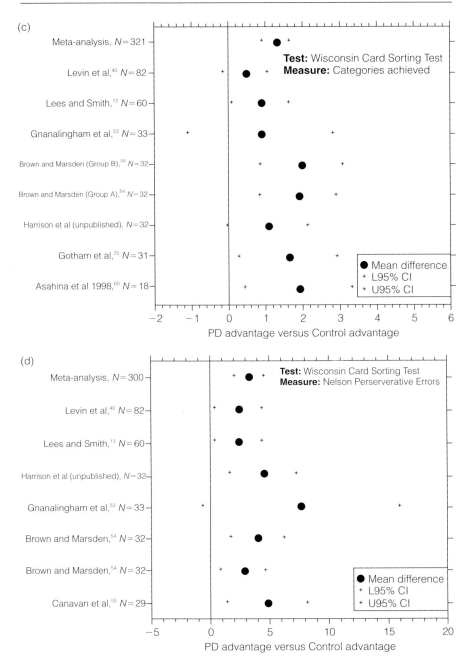

effect. Second, the width of the confidence interval gives a good account of the power of the study to detect an effect. Third, it is a good way to illustrate reporter bias in the form of unreported non-significant results. If the real effect is not large, that is to say is close to the zero difference, then the expected pyramid shape of the tree plot may become lop-sided. This is because small sample size studies at the base of the pyramid are omitted, because they overlap the zero line and therefore indicated no significant difference. However, the meta-analysis reveals that, with smaller sample sizes, studies of these sizes should on occasion report non-significant results.

L: lower limit; U: upper limit.

Depression

The incidence of depression in PD patients is inflated compared to the general population and also compared to other groups of terminally ill patients. The estimates of the incidence of depression vary considerably from nearly 50%[29] to 23% in an early-in-course untreated sample.[23] The presence of depression is acknowledged to impair a variety of cognitive functions; for example, Beats et al[30] reported impairments in a variety of cognitive domains in elderly depressed patients, including attentional set-shifting and recognition memory.

Dementia

The incidence of dementia is also significant in PD patients, being between 10% and 15%.[31] The concept of subcortical dementia had recently become more accepted (see Cummings and Benson[32] for a review). However, this definition has not been accepted in all circles and it is clear that when comparing between disease groups it is important to take the level of functioning into account. There is also the possibly of comorbid Alzheimer's disease, given the age of many patients.

Drug induced cognitive changes

Anticholinergic medication has been found to be efficacious in the management of tremor in PD. However, it follows that anticholinergic medication may well compromise the functional integrity of cognitive skills dependent upon cholinergic neurotransmitter systems. The British National Formulary (BNF) states that anticholinergic therapy can cause confusion, an observation supported by a wealth of empirical evidence.[33–36] However, other investigators have looked at the specific effect of taking anticholinergic drugs on tests of cognitive function comparing subgroups taking and not taking anticholinergic drugs, and concluded that there was no effect; some of these investigations are discussed later.

In the following two sections, we will examine some of these issues more closely in the context of specific deficits that have been reported in PD in verbal fluency and attentional set-shifting performance, respectively.

Verbal fluency

Verbal fluency tasks assess the retrieval of semantic information under a time constraint. One type is where subjects have to produce words beginning with certain letters of the alphabet (phonological fluency) and the other is where patients have to name members of a given category (semantic fluency). Typically, subjects are given 1 min for each letter (F,

A and S are commonly used) or category (typical categories are animals and fruit); for phonological fluency, patients are asked to avoid proper nouns and alternative forms of the same word.

Verbal fluency is often used in cognitive assessments because it is known to be sensitive to frontal dysfunction, as patients with frontal lobe damage perform poorly on this task relative to controls.[37] In this way, the interpretation of poor performance as indicating 'frontal impairment' is somewhat circular. Although some investigators have used verbal fluency tasks specifically as a measure of 'frontal' or executive function,[21,38,39] others have used it as a test of language.[23,40] Both interpretations of the skills needed to perform the task are backed up by experimental findings and to some extent overlap, as while the test does require verbal abilities in order to perform the task subjects have to be able to plan and initiate search strategies. Therefore, as Jacobs et al[38] hypothesized, the deficits observed may reflect problems in planning and initiating strategic searches rather than a specific word-finding difficulty. However, Hanley[48] also showed that in non-dementing PD there was a significant relationship between verbal ability as assessed by the Mill Hill test and verbal fluency, indicating that this test does measure language abilities.

The performance of PD patients on verbal fluency tasks varies considerably from study to study. This may be partly due to small sample sizes and different exclusion criteria. In order to get a clear picture, we will now present two meta-analyses of PD patients' performance on the 'FAS' phonological fluency task and the 'animal' category semantic fluency task. In each case, studies comparing people with PD and controls were used, and no studies that selected patients on the basis of dementia or depression status were used, so the incidence of these possibly coexisting disorders was not inflated in the overall sample.

Figure 10.1a is a tree plot which shows the difference in performance between controls and PD patients on the 'FAS' fluency task for seven different studies and the meta-analysis combining these results. Figure 10.1b is a similar tree plot which shows the difference in performance between controls and PD patients on the 'animal' fluency tasks for five different studies and the meta-analysis which combined the results from these studies. In both cases, where the 95% confidence interval lines overlap the zero difference point the study found no significant difference between the control and PD groups.

The meta-analyses show relatively small but significant impairments of the PD group relative to the controls on both verbal fluency tasks. There is a mean difference of 2.64 ± 2.30 words for the 'FAS' version of the phonological fluency task, and a mean difference of 1.77 ± 0.82 words for the 'animal' version of semantic fluency task. The difference for FAS is only just significant, an unsurprising result given that four of the studies showed no significant difference between PD patients and controls.

Figure 10.1a also appears to reveal a degree of 'reporter' bias. The expected shape of such a plot is a pyramid shape. The studies with smaller numbers of subjects having large variances (and hence confidence intervals) make the base of the pyramid, and as the studies increase in power, the confidence intervals shorten so the that lines appear to be converging towards a point creating the triangular shape. What we can see on Figure 10.1a is a lack of studies in the bottom left-hand corner of the graph that would be consistent with the overall finding of a significant difference between controls and PD patients. As these studies would overlap the 'zero' difference line, they may not have been published, due to the lack of a significant difference. Looking at Figure 10.1b, we can see that although three of the five studies found no difference between controls and PD patients on animal fluency, increasing the power by increasing the number of subjects led to the difference becoming significant. Therefore, in both cases there is a modest effect of PD on fluency performance, but when the number of patients is relatively small, i.e. 40 or less, a significant difference between controls and PD patients will not be consistently found.

One constraint of the analysis above is that it only includes data published in sufficient numerical detail to be included. Other studies did not always report their 'raw' data and therefore could not be included; this means that many studies were left out, so we will now discuss the above findings in this wider context. First, variations in the task will be considered to see how they may contribute to these different findings, and then different intersubject variables will also be examined, as they may also explain some of the differences between studies.

Several researchers have noted that semantic and phonological fluency do not have a similar degree of difficulty; both healthy controls and PD patients find that phonological fluency tasks are harder than semantic fluency tasks.[41,42] This said, Bayles et al[43] have demonstrated that the specific category used may be of greater importance then the type of fluency task. They showed that healthy adults found that the category 'animals' was easier than 'S', which in turn was easier than 'F', 'A', 'vegetables' and 'fruit' (in increasing order of difficulty). These differences in task difficulty could explain the category-specific deficits found, for example, by Levin et al[40] and Cooper et al,[23] who both found impairments on one semantic category (food and objects respectively) but not with the 'animals' category. This means that certain categories may be more effective at detecting subtle deficits, as they are harder to start with. Downes et al[44] made one of the most concerted efforts to control for the difference in difficulty of categories by using seven different letters and seven semantic categories and counterbalancing their use. Using these averaged scores, they found no significant differences in either type of verbal fluency between PD and control groups.

Some papers have subgrouped PD populations on the basis of intersubject variables and used verbal fluency as one of a number of tests to look for any evidence of cognitive impairment, either by directly comparing subgroups or by correlating disease severity measures with test performance. One important intersubject variable is depression status, as previously mentioned. Two papers that address this issue are by Kuzis et al[45] and Hanley et al.[47] The first directly compared depressed patients with and without PD, and non-depressed PD patients and healthy controls. The second investigated whether the variation in verbal fluency performance can be explained by scores on a depression rating scale. Kuzis et al[45] found that depressed status, independently of PD status, impaired fluency performance, but Hanley et al[41] found that the depression rating scale did not account for a significant amount of subject variation on verbal fluency tasks. One difference is that the former used a very carefully rated measure of depression, determining status by using DSM III criteria and the Hamilton depression scale, while the second used a self-rating scale (Geriatric Depression Scale). This means that subjects in the Hanley et al[47] study did not receive a diagnosis of depression and therefore, while possibly exhibiting depressed symptomatology, cannot be unequivocally said to be depressed. This suggests that depression may be detrimental to verbal fluency performance but self-rating scales may not be a sufficiently sensitive means of subgrouping patients. Other studies have tried to avoid the possibly deleterious effect of depression by excluding depressed patients, however, given the rate of depression in PD, it is not clear that this is the most thorough approach, as the remaining patients are then not typical of a PD sample.

Dementia is another important variable to consider, given the increased incidence of dementia in PD patients. Troster et al[46] divided their PD group into demented and non-demented on the basis of Cummings and Benson's criteria. Bayles et al[42] also favored this approach, splitting the group on the basis of Mini-Mental State Examination, with <27 being classified as demented. Bayles et al[42] found that non-dementing PD patients were worse than controls on verbal fluency tasks, even when age and MMSE status were taken into account. The Troster study by contrast, with its stricter measure of dementia found that non-demented PD patients were unimpaired on verbal fluency tasks. Jacobs et al,[38] in a longitudinal study, found that poor verbal fluency predicts the onset of dementia in PD patients a year later suggesting that poor test performance can indicate preclinical dementia. This means that even when PD groups are screened for dementia to avoid the confounding effects of dementia on verbal fluency performance, the impairments found in so called 'undemented' groups could be caused by patients with preclinical dementia. This may explain the impairment of the 'non-dementing' PD group in the Bayles et al[42] study. Given the increased risk of dementia in PD patients, it is clearly worthwhile when trying to exclude dementing patients to use criteria liable to pick up any signs of dementia at the earliest possible stage; for this, the MMSE may not be sufficiently sensitive.

Rate of speech production also differs between patients with PD and healthy controls, and it is important to consider the possibility that this may confound differences found between the two groups. Gurd and Ward[47] demonstrated that there is no significant relationship between verbal output rate and verbal fluency, either for controls or PD patients. Therefore, although PD patients do have a slower rate of speech compared to controls, it is not this that is impairing their verbal fluency performance. Age also influences test performance[42]; increasing age is linked with poorer verbal fluency performance. Careful matching of controls and PD patients for age is therefore important for ruling out any possibility of the difference being to due to having an older patient group; Hanley et al[41] criticized a study for this very reason.

In general, the effects of disease status on both phonological and semantic fluency are small. PD patients as a group perform worse than controls, but this is only reliably detected in large samples. When looking at the effect of disease status, excluding other variables, it is important to exclude depressed patients, and those with dementia, and to carefully match groups for age, as all these factors can and do influence performance. Finding a difference in verbal fluency performance then presents the investigator with an interpretation problem; is the deficit due to 'storage' problems, language deficits or an inability to search successfully for words? To address this issue, some investigators have used modifications of the basic task to look at a specific aspect of verbal fluency, that is 'attentional set-shifting'.[44,47] In these instances, the patients switch between letters, categories or both, still under a time constraint, to see how efficient they are at reorganizing their behavior according to changing task demands. This type of attentional set-shifting task will be described below, together with other examples outside of the domain of fluency tasks.

Attention set-shifting

Attentional set-shifting tasks look at the ability to change behavior according to task demands, to literally shift from one type of response to another. Many different types of task can be used, including block-sorting, card-sorting, verbal fluency tasks, Stroop word-reading tasks and reaction time tasks. Attentional set-shifting tasks are used with PD patients for two main reasons. The first is that some of these tasks, the Wisconsin Card Sorting Task (WCST) in particular, have been shown to be sensitive to frontal dysfunction. Milner[48] showed that patients with dorsolateral frontal lesions achieved fewer categories and made more errors than lesion controls (including patients with temporal, parietalotemporooccipital, orbitofrontal and temporal lobe lesions). Therefore, investigators have used the test to look for signs of 'frontal-like' impairment in PD. The second reason is that animal work suggests that basal ganglia dysfunction disrupts learning and adaptive behavior[14] and therefore by analogy we would expect PD patients to be impaired on some forms of learning.

Suggesting that PD patients may have 'frontal-like' impairments does not imply that they have the same type of damage as 'frontal' patients. Since the early 1980s, the relationship between the striatal and frontal cortex has been increasingly well characterized[49] and this work clearly suggests that striatal dysfunction can influence behavior dependent on frontal lobe integrity via frontostriatal loops connecting these areas. The WCST and other attentional set-shifting tasks have also been used to look at the relative importance of internal and external cues in this process of adapting behavior.

One of the most widely used tests of 'attentional set-shifting' in PD patients is the WCST, originally used by Grant and Berg.[50] During the test, the subject has to sort cards into piles according to certain rules, and at various points (when the rule has been acquired) they then have to shift to sorting by a new rule. The cards vary on three 'dimensions', shape, color and number; therefore, the three rules are simply matching by number, color or shape. The two most widely used versions of the WSCT test are the Milner[48] and the Nelson[51] versions; the Nelson is a simplification of the Milner, shortened from 128 to 48 cards. It is also simplified by explicitly telling the subject to change rules and by ensuring that no card in the pack shares more than one dimension with each of the four key cards that form the basis of the sorting piles.

The WCST aims to assess the patient's ability to form concepts or sets (i.e. select a sorting dimension), maintain set (continue sorting by that dimension) and shift set (sort by a new dimension). Different outcome measures assess these abilities; the key measures used are 'categories achieved', 'perseverative errors' and 'non-perseverative errors'. Hence, 'categories achieved' looks at the ability to form concepts, and 'perseverative errors' looks at the subject's ability to shift set. The two versions of the WCST have different definitions for 'perseverative errors'. Some studies have been known to use other measures, such as 'number of trials until the first category is achieved'[21] and 'failures to maintain set'.[52] 'Number of trials to the first category' is an interesting measure, in that it is designed to examine whether subjects have problems learning the task in the first place. 'Failure to maintain set' was used by Beatty and Monson,[52] as they claim that poor task performance can result from an inability to *maintain* set as well as an inability to shift set.

In order to look at the effect of PD, we conducted a meta-analysis of eight studies using the more commonly used Nelson version of the task. All the studies compared PD performance to control performance on the two measures, categories achieved and perseverative errors, except that one of these studies did not report perseverative errors. Figures 10.1c and 10.1d show these findings in the form of tree plots. Figure 10.1c illustrates the differences found between controls and PD patients on categories achieved, and Figure 10.1d illustrates the differences found between controls and PD patients on number of perseverative errors made. The meta-analysis for category achieved shows that, on average, PD patients produce 1.33 ± 0.36 less categories than controls.

Figure 10.1d shows that in all but one of the studies a significant difference was found between PD patients and controls; this is reflected in the meta-analysis that shows that PD patients produce on average 3.43 ± 1.24 more errors than controls. The only study that did not show a significant effect is the Gnanalingham et al study,[53] where the number of PD patients was much smaller than in the other studies, being only 12. This means that the confidence interval is much larger than in the other studies. As before, this represents only those studies including data that could be meaningfully interpreted, and thus a further discussion of different factors that affect performance follows.

One point made by a number of papers is the fact that when a significant difference is found between controls and the PD group, this is often the result of a specific subset of patients performing badly. For example, Lees and Smith[13] found an impairment consistent with frontal dysfunction in only 11/30 patients (37%) and Brown and Marsden[54] found that only 5/16 (31%) patients made more than four perseverative errors. This represents about a third of patients being impaired on the WCST; a substantial minority, but a minority nonetheless.

Dubois et al[34] used this task to look at the effect of anticholinergic medication, comparing two PD groups, one on medication and one not. They found a significant additional impairment effect of taking anticholinergic medication on top of the impairment already observed in the PD population. However, it is not clear what metric is being used. Other studies using patients both on and off anticholinergic medication compared the subgroups and found no differences between them.[40,55]

Reports differ on the relationship between motor dysfunction and WSCT performance. Both Pillon et al[56] and Canavan et al[55] found that WCST performance correlated with rigidity; Levin et al,[40] on the other hand, found a relationship between WCST shifts and bradykinesia. Cooper et al,[23] in a study of early untreated PD, found no relationship between WSCT and motor control, although in this study the PD group members were only impaired on 'cards to first category', and none of the other standard measures. This somewhat unclear picture makes it impossible to conclude that the same deficits are responsible for motor dysfunction and problems in attentional set-shifting.

Several studies have used WCST to look at changes in cognition at different stages of the disease. Levin,[40] Cooper,[23] Lees and Smith[13] and Canavan[55] all compared patients in the early stages of disease with matched controls. Of these four studies, only one found an impairment on number of categories achieved.[13] Two found an impairment relative to controls on 'perseverative errors',[40,55] although Cooper et al report that they found a non-significant trend for perseverative errors, and Lees and Smith[13] found an impairment on the Milner-type perseverative errors. On this basis, it could be concluded that there is some impairment on WCST (albeit in a specific subset of patients) at the early stage of the disease, but that this is not easy to detect using the relatively insensitive measure of categories achieved and is better investigated using perseverative errors.

Both Taylor et al[21] and Cooper et al[23] found PD patients to be impaired on the number of cards taken to achieve the first category. This increased time taken to achieve the first category supports Beatty and Monson's[52] idea that PD patients have problems in maintaining set. Kuzis et al[45] and Cooper et al[23] looked at the effect of depression on WSCT. Cooper et al found that the subgroup of PD patients scoring >14 on the Beck Depression Inventory were impaired on number of cards to first category. Kuzis et al[45] also found that the depressed PD patients performed significantly different from PD and depressed subjects and controls on categories achieved. However, the depressed PD patients did not differ significantly from PD patients in terms of perseverative errors.

Canavan et al[55] found no significant effect of age on WCST performance, although they found that the more impaired PD patients were older.

Many studies using WCST to look at PD excluded dementing patients; however, some studies have looked at the effect of mental status on task performance.[52] Beatty and Monson[52] found that only those impaired on MMSE produced more perseverative errors than controls.

Attention set-shifting using verbal fluency tasks

Several papers have addressed the issue of attentional set-shifting by asking patients to alternate between letters or semantic categories during verbal fluency tasks. For example, Gurd and Ward[47] found no additional impairment for patients switching from generating words starting with a given letter or switching categories, although they were already impaired on the verbal fluency tasks relative to controls. Cooper et al,[24] however, found that patients were impaired relative to controls in switching between categories, specifically from 'birds' to 'colors'. Downes et al,[44] found that verbal fluency was essentially unimpaired in their patient group versus their control group, except for when patients had to switch 'domains', that is from letters to categories. This is seen as analogous to deficits in extradimensional set-shifting when a subject has to shift from responding to one 'concept' to another, and Downes et al[16] conclude that patients exhibit a specific problem in extradimensional set-shifting. By this definition, all WCST shifts are extradimensional; however, in another type of set-shifting task, the types of shift required are varied from intradimensional to extradimensional to look at what part of the process patients are impaired on. This intra–extradimensional set-shift task is discussed below.

Intradimensional and extradimensional (IDED) shifting tasks

Downes et al[16] first used a paradigm derived from the animal and human learning literature to assess attentional set-shifting and reversal shifting in both medicated and non-medicated patients with PD. The test was devised to decompose the WCST, in which set-shifting is supposed to be a central component of performance. Performance on the WCST, they argued, involves, among others, the following cognitive abilities: (1) matching to sample; (2) conditional visuospatial learning contingencies (set-formation); and (3) inhibition in responding to a particular dimension and shifting to respond to another dimension. In their paradigm, discrimination learning, reversal shifting, intradimensional shifting (IDS) (in which shifts are made to different exemplars of the same rule or perceptual dimension) and extradimensional shifting (EDS) (in which shifts are to different perceptual dimensions) can be separately investigated. The IDED task has been extensively described in previous papers,[16,57] and we refer the reader to those descriptions. Downes et al[16] provided evidence for a specific EDS deficit in PD, relative to other forms of shift, such as reversal and the IDS. Non-medicated mild PD patients also showed difficulties in learning a compound discrimination (CD). Owen et al[6] replicated the finding of a parkinsonian deficit on the IDED task. However, in this study, impairments for non-medicated PD were not specifically limited to the EDS stage, also being evident in earlier stages of the task. In both studies, non-medicated patients performed more poorly, but not significantly so, than medicated PD patients, hinting at a beneficial effect of dopaminergic medication on attentional set-shifting. A study by Lange et al[18] provided further evidence for such an effect. Nine out of ten PD patients reached a later stage in the IDED shift task when on medication, as compared to their off-medication state. However, it is unclear from this study whether the deficit was specific to the EDS stage, because many patients failed earlier stages in their off-medication state.

A pooling of results from these studies compared to control performance by means of a chi-squared analysis reveals significant differences in performance at the EDS (seen as analogous to WCST shifts).

In a recent study,[58] further support was found for a *specific* EDS deficit, in terms of both percentage of failures and number of errors, in mild PD patients. No impairments were found at other stages. These patients were divided into three groups according to their Hoehn and Yahr scores (I, II and III). Results from that study showed an improvement in EDS performance with increased severity of PD. The more severe the symptoms of the patients, the better they performed on the task, and particularly at the EDS stage. At first glance, these findings seem to contradict results from Owen et al.[6] They found severe PD patients to be much more impaired than milder patients (although this effect did not reach significance). However, it must be noted that all patients in the Cools study[58] were still in relatively mild stages of their disease (Hoehn and Yahr I–III). Furthermore, the duration of the disease correlated significantly with Hoehn and Yahr ratings. Thus, such PD patients would have been taking medication for a longer period. It is therefore hypothesized that the seemingly severity-related improvement in performance on the IDED task actually may reflect an effect of medication. The notion that medication improves shifting performance is consistent with previous findings.[6,11,16,18] It must be noted that sample sizes were small when the PD group was subdivided according to severity. Nevertheless, it can be concluded that, in the context of previous results, this study supports the above-mentioned hypothesis.

Owen et al[7] directly compared medicated and non-medicated PD patients with patients with frontal lobe excisions. They designed a different version of the IDED task, in which they distinguished a 'perseveration condition' and a 'learned irrelevance condition'. They defined perseveration as 'the inability to shift from a perceptual dimension which has previously been irrelevant'. In the 'learned irrelevance condition', the previously *relevant* dimension was substituted for a novel dimension. Thus, in this condition any impairment could not be a consequence of perseveration. The authors argue, therefore, that any impairment can only be a consequence of learned irrelevance. In the 'perseveration condition', the previously *irrelevant* dimension was substituted for a novel one. Therefore, any impairment must be due to perseveration and not learned irrelevance. Non-medicated patients with PD were equally impaired in both conditions. Medicated PD patients were only impaired in the 'learned irrelevance condition', but not in the 'perseveration condition'. Patients with frontal lobe damage showed the opposite pattern of deficits: increased levels of 'perseveration', but normal levels of 'learned irrelevance'. These differences were found exclusively at the EDS (+ED reversal) stages.

All patients were unimpaired at the IDS and ID reversal stages. The authors suggest that the deficit in medicated PD patients (the 'learned irrelevance' deficit), which is opposite to the deficit seen in patients with frontal lobe damage, involves a dysfunctioning of circuitry *not* involving the prefrontal cortex. Furthermore, non-medicated patients with PD also showed a 'frontal-like' perseverative tendency, as well as enhanced learned irrelevance. On this basis, it was suggested that L-DOPA medication ameliorated the perseveration deficit in the medicated PD group relative to the non-medicated group but not the learned irrelevance deficit.

References

1. Warburton JW. Memory disturbance and the Parkinson syndrome. *Br J Med Psychol* (1967) **40:** 169–71.

2. Wilson RS, Kaszniak AW, Klawans HL et al. High speed memory scanning in parkinsonism. *Cortex* (1980) **16:** 67–71.

3. Tweedy JR, Langer KG, McDowell FH et al. The effect of semantic relations on the memory deficit associated with Parkinson's disease. *J Clin Neuropsychol* (1982) **4:** 235–47.

4. Flowers KA, Pearce I, Pearce JMS et al. Recognition memory in Parkinson's disease. *J Neurol Neurosurg Psychiatry* (1984) **47:** 1174–81.

5. Sullivan EV, Sagar HJ. Double dissociation of short-term and long-term memory for non verbal material in Parkinson's disease and global amnesia. A further analysis. *Brain* (1991) **114:** 893–906.

6. Owen AM, James M, Leigh PN et al. Fronto-striatal cognitive deficits at different stages of Parkinson's disease. *Brain* (1992) **115:** 1727–51.

7. Owen AM, Roberts AC, Hodges JR et al. Contrasting mechanisms of impaired attentional set-shifting in patients with frontal lobe damage or Parkinson's disease. *Brain* (1993) **116:** 1159–79.

8. Bowen FP, Hoehn MM, Yahr MD et al. Parkinsonism: alterations in spatial orientation as determined by a route-walking test. *Neuropsychologia* (1972) **10:** 355–61.

9. Bowen FP. Behavioural alterations in patients with basal ganglia lesions. *Research Publications: Assoc Res Nerv Ment Dis* (1976) **55:** 169–80.

10. Boller F, Passafiume D, Keefe N et al. Visuospatial impairment in Parkinson's disease. The role of perceptual and motor factors. *Arch Neurol* (1984) **41:** 485–90.

11. Bowen FP, Kamienny MA, Burns MM et al. Parkinsonism: effects of Levodopa treatment on concept formation. *Neurology* (1975) **25:** 701–4.

12. Flowers KA. Frontal lobe signs as a component of parkinsonism. *Behav Brain Res* (1982) **5:** 100.

13. Lees AJ, Smith E. Cognitive deficits in the early stages of Parkinson's disease. *Brain* (1983) **106:** 257–70.

14. Cools AR, Van den Bercken JHL, Horstink MWI et al. Cognitive and motor shifting aptitude disorder in Parkinson's disease. *J Neurol Neurosurg Psychiatry* (1984) **47:** 443–53.

15. Flowers KA, Robertson C. The effects of Parkinson's disease on the ability to maintain a mental set. *J Neurol Neurosurg Psychiatry* (1985) **48:** 517–29.

16. Downes JJ, Roberts AC, Sahakian BJ et al. Impaired extra-dimensional shift performance in medicated and unmedicated Parkinson's disease: evidence for a specific attentional dysfunction. *Neuropsychologia* (1989) **27:** 1329–43.

17. Owen AM, Beksinska M, James M et al. Visuo-spatial memory deficits at different stages of Parkinson's disease. *Neuropsychologia* (1993) **31(7):** 627–44.

18. Lange KW, Robbins TW, Marsden CD et al. L-Dopa withdrawal in Parkinson's disease selectively impairs cognitive performance in tests sensitive to frontal lobe dysfunction. *Psychopharmacology* (1992) **107:** 394–404.

19. Morris RG, Downes JJ, Sahakian

BJ et al. Planning and spatial working memory in Parkinson's disease. *J Neurol Neurosurg Psychiatry* (1988) **51:** 757–66.

20. Owen AM, Sahakian BJ, Hodges JR et al. Dopamine-dependent fronto-striatal planning deficits in early Parkinson's disease. *Neuropsychology* (1995) **9:** 126–40.

21. Taylor AE, Saint-Cyr JA, Lang AE et al. Frontal lobe dysfunction in Parkinson's disease: the cortical focus of neostriatal outflow. *Brain* (1986) **109:** 845–83.

22. Bradley VA, Welch JL, Dick DJ et al. Visuospatial working memory in Parkinson's disease. *J Neurol Neurosurg Psychiatry* (1989) **52:** 1228–35.

23. Cooper JA, Sagar HJ, Jordan N et al. Cognitive impairment in early, untreated Parkinson's disease and its relationship to motor disability. *Brain* (1991) **114:** 2095–122.

24. Cooper JA, Sagar H, Doherty SM et al. Different effects of dopaminergic and anticholinergic therapies on cognitive and motor function in Parkinson's disease: a follow-up study of untreated patients. *Brain* (1992) **115:** 1701–25.

25. Gotham AM, Brown RG, Marsden CD et al. 'Frontal' cognitive functions in patients with Parkinson's disease 'on' and 'off' levodopa. *Brain* (1988) **111:** 299–321.

26. Postle BR, Corkin S, Growdon JH et al. Dissociation between two kinds of visual working memory in Parkinson's disease. *Soc Neurosci Abstr* (1993) **409(10):** 1002.

27. Owen AM, Iddon JL, Hodges JR et al. Spatial and non-spatial working memory at different stages of Parkinson's disease. *Neuropsychologia* (1997) **35:** 519–32.

28. Hughes AJ, Daniel SE, Kilford L et al. Accuracy of clinical diagnosis of idiopathic Parkinson's disease, a clinico-pathological study of 100 cases. *J Neurol Neurosurg Psychiatry* (1992) **55:** 181–4.

29. Mayeux R, Stern Y, Rosen J et al. Depression, intellectual impairment and Parkinson's disease. Neurology (1981) **31:** 645–50.

30. Beats BC, Sahakian BJ, Levy R. Cognitive performance in tests sensitive to frontal lobe dysfunction in the elderly depressed. *Psychol Med* (1996) **26:** 591–603.

31. Brown RG, Marsden CD. How common is dementia in Parkinson's disease? *Lancet* (1984) **ii:** 1262–5.

32. Cummings JL, Benson DF. Psychological dysfunction accompanying subcortical dementia. *Annu Rev Med* (1988) **39:** 53–61.

33. De Smet Y, Ruberg M, Serdaru M et al. Confusion, dementia and anticholinergics in Parkinson's disease. *J Neurol Neurosurg Psychiatry* (1982) **45:** 1161–4.

34. Dubois B, Pillon B, Llhermitte F et al. Cholinergic deficiency and frontal dysfunction in Parkinson's disease. *Ann Neurol* (1990) **28:** 117–21.

35. Sadeh M, Braham J, Modan M et al. Effects of anticholinergic drugs on memory in Parkinson's disease. *Arch Neurol* (1982) **39:** 666–7.

36. Syndulko K, Gilden ER, Hansch EC et al. Decreased verbal memory associated with anti-cholinergic treatment in Parkinson's disease patients. *Int J Neurosci* (1982) **14:** 61.

37. Benton AL. Differential behavioural effects of frontal lobe disease. *Neuropsychologia* (1968) **6:** 53–60.

38. Jacobs DM, Marder K, Cote LJ et al. Neuropsychological characteristics of preclinical dementia in Parkinson's disease. *Neurology* (1995) **45:** 1691–6.

39. Miller E. Possible frontal impairments in Parkinson's disease: a test using a measure of verbal fluency. *Br J Clin Psychol* (1985) **24:** 211–12.

40. Levin BE, Llabre MM, Weiner WJ et al. Cognitive impairments associated with early Parkinson's disease. *Neurology* (1989) **39:** 557–61.

41. Hanley JR, Dewick HC, Davies AD et al. Verbal fluency in Parkinson's disease. *Neuropsychologia* (1990) **28:** 737–41.

42. Bayles KA, Trosset MW, Tomoeda CK et al. Generative naming in Parkinson disease patients. *J Clin Exp Neuropsychol* (1993) **15:** 547–62.

43. Bayles KA, Salmon DP, Tomoeda CK. Semantic and letter naming in Alzheimer's patients: a predictable difference. *Dev Neuropsychol* (1989) **5:** 335–47.

44. Downes JJ, Sharp HM, and Costall BM et al. Alternating fluency in Parkinson's disease. *Brain* (1993) **116:** 887–902.

45. Kuzis G, Sabe L, Tiberti C et al. Cognitive functions in major depression and Parkinson disease. *Arch Neurol* (1997) **54(8):** 982–6.

46. Troster AI, Fields JA, Testa JA et al. Cortical and subcortical influences on clustering and switching in the performance of verbal fluency tasks. *Neuropsychologia* (1998) **36:** 295–304.

47. Gurd JM, Ward CD. Retrieval from semantic and letter-initial categories in patients with Parkinson's disease. *Neuropsychologia* (1989) **27:** 743–6.

48. Milner B. Effects of different brain lesions on card sorting: the role of the frontal lobes. *Arch Neurol* (1963) **9:** 90–100.

49. Alexander GE, DeLong MR, Strick PL et al. Parallel organisation of functionally segregated circuits linking basal ganglia and cortex. *Annu Rev Neurosci* (1986) **9:** 357–81.

50. Grant DA, Berg EA. A behavioural analysis of degree of reinforcement and ease of shifting to new responses in a Weigl-type card-sorting problem. *J Exp Psychol* (1948) **38:** 404–11.

51. Nelson HE. A modified card sorting test sensitive to frontal lobe defects. *Cortex* (1976) **12:** 313–24.

52. Beatty WW, Monson N. Picture and motor sequencing in Parkinson's disease. *J Geriatr Psychiatry Neurol* (1990) **3:** 192–7.

53. Gnanalingham KK, Byrne EJ, Thorton A et al. Motor and cognitive in Lewy body dementia: comparison with Alzheimer's and Parkinson's diseases. *J Neurol Neurosurg Psychiatry* (1997) **62:** 243–52.

54. Brown RG, Marsden CD. Internal versus external cues and the control of attention in Parkinson's disease. *Brain* (1988) **111:** 323–45.

55. Canavan AGM, Passingham RE, Marsden CD et al. The performance on learning tasks of patients in the early stages of Parkinson's disease. *Neuropsychologia* (1989) **27:** 141–56.

56. Pillon B, Dubois B, Cusimano G et al. Does cognitive impairment result from non-dopaminergic lesions? *J Neurol Neurosurg Psychiatry* (1989) **52:** 201–6.

57. Owen AM, Roberts AC, Polkey CE et al. Extra-dimensional versus intra-dimensional set shifting performance following frontal lobe excisions, temporal lobe excisions or amygdalo-hippocampectomy in man. *Neuropsychologia* (1991) **29:** 993-1006.

58. Cools R. Mechanisms of task-set switching in Parkinson's disease. M Phil thesis, University of Cambridge, 1999.

59. Dalrymple-Alford JC, Kalders AS, Jones RD et al. A central executive deficit in patients with Parkinson's disease. *J Neurol Neurosurg Psychiatry* (1994) **57:** 360–7.

60. Asahina M, Suhara T, Shinotoh H et al. Brain muscarinic receptors in progressive supranuclear palsy and Parkinson's disease: a positron emission tomographic study. *J Neurol Neurosurg Psychiatry* (1988) **65(2):** 155–63.

61. Katzen HL, Levin BE, Llabre ML. Age of disease onset influences cognition in Parkinson's disease. *J Int Neuropsychol Soc* (1997) **4(3):** 285–90.

11
Schizophrenia

Christos Pantelis, Stephen J Wood, and Paul Maruff

I can still only too well remember the perplexity with which I faced, throughout very many years, the vast number of states of mental weakness harboured by every large asylum. Their manifold manifestations were to a certain extent grouped together, but, in spite of all variety in outward form, definite characteristic features recurred with surprising uniformity.

(Kraepelin,[1] p. 200)

Summary

Schizophrenia is a relatively common and often severe psychiatric disorder. Recent notions consider the disorder to have a neurodevelopmental basis and to be characterized by deficits in neuropsychological functioning, particularly in attention, executive function and memory. However, while such deficits have often been characterized using batteries of neuropsychological tests, few studies have approached the problem from within a theoretical framework. Further, the component cognitive processes that may account for cognitive dysfunction have not been fully examined. Therefore, it has proved difficult to assess the relevance of observed deficits and to relate these to underlying neurobiological substrates. The dorsolateral prefrontal cortex has been consistently implicated in schizophrenia, as shown by deficits on tasks of executive function. However, there is evidence that other regions within the prefrontal cortex are also dysfunctional. While such deficits are particularly severe, the nature and extent of deficits in other domains such as memory have not been adequately characterized. Recent brain–behavior models of schizophrenia have extended these observations to propose that the cognitive deficits and symptomatology observed in the disorder reflect disturbances of corticocortical and corticosubcortical connectivity. The relevant neural networks proposed include 'prefrontal–basal ganglia–thalamic' and 'prefrontal–medial temporal lobe' circuits. In this chapter we examine the neuropsychological evidence for these models and we also review the limited available literature that implicates 'prefrontal–parietal' circuitry. The main theme that emerges is that dysfunction of the prefrontal cortices is central to the disorder, and the involvement of other brain structures almost always relates to their connections with prefrontal cortices. Such models provide potentially testable hypotheses, which can be addressed using recent technological advances in neuroimaging and cognitive neuropsychology and can be interpreted with respect to anatomical connectivity between the areas of interest.

Introduction

Schizophrenia is a serious psychiatric disorder presenting in the late teens and early twenties, with a lifetime prevalence of greater than 1% (review: Jablensky[2]). It is characterized clinically by abnormal experiences and beliefs, disturbances of emotion and affect, and behavioral disturbances and impaired social functioning. These symptoms usually include abnormal experiences, termed 'positive symptoms', such as prominent auditory and/or other sensory hallucinations, experiences of alien control, delusional ideas, and a characteristic disorder of thinking. There is also a loss of normal functioning, often termed 'negative symptoms', characterized by avolition and apathy, blunting of affect, and poverty of speech. The latter are particularly difficult to manage and treat and have been associated with neuropsychological deficits and a poorer prognosis. Up to 50% of patients have a severe illness with a relatively poor outcome, with about 5–10% having progressive, treatment-resistant illness.[3,4]

Despite the high heritability of the disorder,[5] other etiological factors are apparent and have been considered relevant to a neurodevelopmental pathogenesis.[6] Thus, the prevailing current view is that schizophrenia is a neurodevelopmental disorder in which structural brain changes, caused by an early antenatal or perinatal insult, confer a predisposition to the development of schizophrenia, but are not progressive beyond the onset of symptoms.[7–9] These authors draw on various sources of evidence, such as the higher incidence of obstetric complications, winter births, minor physical abnormalities and soft neurological signs in schizophrenia, to support their arguments. Furthermore, the motor, cognitive, social and emotional changes which have been described in children who go on to develop schizophrenia may be subtle, early manifestations of such a lesion.[10,11] According to the neurodevelopmental model, the lesion produced by an early insult will interact with normal post-pubertal brain maturation to produce the clinical symptoms of schizophrenia. A number of factors have been proposed as causative, including intrauterine events around the 4th to 5th month of gestation, such as viruses, malnutrition, or hypoxia.[6,12] Others consider that a neurodegenerative course is also apparent,[13] and may result from a vulnerability consequent on a neurodevelopmental lesion.[14]

Researchers had previously conceptualized schizophrenia as having a predominantly psychological or sociological origin, but more recently the illness has been thought to have a neurological basis.[15] This conceptual shift has led to numerous neurobiological studies of schizophrenia, partly stimulated by technological advances providing in vivo information about brain structure and function (e.g. magnetic resonance imaging (MRI);[16] MR spectroscopy (MRS);[17] functional MR (fMRI);[18] and positron emission tomography (PET)[19]). Together with improved methodologies in neuropathology and neurochemistry, these studies have begun to improve our understanding of the neurobiological basis of this multifaceted disorder.

Neuropsychological studies have also informed our understanding of the neurobiology of schizophrenia. The most pronounced and consistent deficits occur in attention, executive function and memory (reviews: Pantelis,[11] Elliot and Sahakian,[20] and Heinrichs and Zakzanis[21]). In addition, they are present from illness onset (and perhaps earlier) and the available longitudinal studies indicate that they are not progressive.[22–24] Recently, investigators have attempted to understand these deficits as disturbances of interconnected cortical–subcortical or corticocortical neural networks. Three models are discussed below which all include prefrontal dysfunction as central to this disorder.

The neuropsychological evidence implicates the involvement of the prefrontal cortex and its connections with medial temporal lobe and subcortical structures.[25–27] Recent work implicates the parietal cortex in schizophrenia,[28–30] although this would also seem to be in the context of associated prefrontal lobe involvement.[31]

The main theme that emerges is that dysfunction of the prefrontal cortices is central to the disorder, and the involvement of other brain structures almost always relates to their connections with prefrontal cortices. Thus, schizophrenia has been conceptualized as a disorder of connectivity involving prefrontal–thalamic–striatal systems,[32–35] prefrontal–temporal lobe (especially medial temporal) circuits[36,37] or prefrontal–thalamic–cerebellar systems.[38,39] Prefrontal–parietal networks have also been implicated.[40,41] The notion here is that disconnection of these neural networks explains the features of schizophrenia, including neuropsychological deficits and the findings from functional imaging studies. An interesting hypothesis that attempts to unify the available evidence suggests that schizophrenia is a disorder of cognitive networks involving heteromodal association neocortex (dorsolateral prefrontal cortex, superior temporal and inferior parietal cortices), which are interconnected and have extensive connections with limbic and subcortical structures.[30]

In this chapter, we will consider how the neuropsychological deficits can be understood in the context of these brain systems. The focus will be on the involvement of the prefrontal cortex and its connections with other regions, particularly subcortical and limbic structures, and we will discuss the neuropsychological evidence that supports disruption of these networks in schizophrenia. We will argue that such disturbances provide a basis for understanding the underlying neurobiology of the disorder.

Schizophrenia as a disturbance of frontal–striatal–thalamic systems

The most common cognitive deficits reported in schizophrenia are observed on neuropsychological tests of executive function. These tests assess the ability to plan, organize or generate novel problem-solving strategies. Each of these different cognitive processes has been shown to depend upon the normal function of the prefrontal cortex in studies of both human and non-human primates.[42] Accordingly, in schizophrenia, deficits in executive function are also inferred to reflect dysfunction of prefrontal brain regions. These inferences are consistent with the results of functional neuroimaging studies that find hypofunctioning of the prefrontal cortex in patients during rest and when challenged using cognitive activation tasks.[19] In addition, MRS studies have identified compromise of prefrontal neurons in schizophrenia.[17] Despite this evidence, it has been difficult to prove that this dysfunction can be attributed to pathology within, and restricted to, the prefrontal cortex. In this context, recent models suggest that impairments in executive function in schizophrenia arise from dysfunction of prefrontal–striatal–thalamic circuitry,[32–35,43] or, more recently, of prefrontal–thalamic–cerebellar circuits.[38,39] For example, we have suggested previously that, in schizophrenia, deficits in executive function may be secondary to disturbed pathophysiology in subcortical areas such as the basal ganglia or thalami.[33,44] This is consistent with neuroimaging and postmortem findings of changes in neuronal structure and function in the basal ganglia and thalami.[33–35,39,45–50]

Neuroanatomy of frontal–striatal–thalamic circuits

The proposal that schizophrenia arises from dysfunction of neurocognitive circuits that are distributed across frontal and subcortical brain regions is consistent with the neuroanatomical organization of prefrontal–subcortical circuits.[51] These circuits form parallel and segregated cortical–subcortical feedback systems that include at least five prefrontal cortical regions (dorsolateral prefrontal cortex (DLPFC), orbitofrontal cortex (OFC), anterior cingulate (AC), frontal eye fields (FEF), and supplementary motor area (SMA)).

The anatomical connectivity of these regions suggests that each of the circuits subserves a separable function. While there is debate about whether the frontal lobes can be modularized in terms of their function, this anatomical organization would tend to favor such fractionation (review: Roberts et al[42]). This is consistent with the notion that each of the prefrontal cortical areas (together with their subcortical and allocortical connections) is associated with specific patterns of cognition and behavior.[52] We have previously reviewed this evidence, and suggested that prefrontal syndromes related to each circuit[53,54] can be related to particular symptomatic, behavioral and cognitive features of schizophrenia.[34,35]

Neuropsychological evidence for prefrontal–striatal–thalamic circuit disturbance in schizophrenia

In schizophrenia, there is evidence that all five frontal–striatal–thalamic circuits are disrupted[34,35] This is in contrast with other psychiatric disorders, such as obsessive-compulsive disorder and depression, in which more limited deficits involving these circuits are suggested (Chapter 12).[55] Thus, the DLPFC, OFC and AC are involved in mediating cognitive processes that are disturbed in schizophrenia, while the FEF has been implicated in the eye movement disturbances observed.[56,57] The SMA may be important in mediating certain symptoms of schizophrenia, including delusions of passivity in which patients believe they are being controlled by external forces or agencies.[58,59] In this section we will focus particularly on the three circuits implicated in cognition.

DLPFC–striatal–thalamic circuit

In schizophrenia, the most consistent findings from functional neuroimaging studies have been hypofunctioning in the DLPFC.[60-63] (review: Velakoulis and Pantelis[19]). Data from MRS have identified lower N-acetylaspartate (NAA) levels in the DLPFC, implying reduced neuronal integrity in this region (review: Vance et al[17]). In a recent study, Bertolino et al[64]). found an association between MRS evidence for neuronal pathology in the DLPFC (decreased NAA) and striatal dopamine activity, thereby implicating this circuit in schizophrenia.

Disruption to the DLPFC or its subcortical connections has been associated with deficits in executive function and motor programming abnormalities, which result in impairments in temporal and sensory integration, planning and maintenance of goal-directed behavior and behavioral flexibility. Neuropsychologically, deficits are observed on attentional set-shifting tasks, working memory and strategic ability, verbal fluency tasks, and other tasks that require cognitive flexibility and complex problem-solving.

Working memory

Working memory may be defined as a limited-capacity memory system for the temporary storage and manipulation of information (e.g. verbal material, visuospatial images).[65] Deficits in working memory are prominent features of schizophrenia. However, a problem in the literature[65] is that few studies have operationalized the definition of working memory or used specific working memory tasks. The studies are further complicated because many cognitive tasks have components of working memory and few investigators have examined their contribution to task performance. Despite these difficulties, the neural systems mediating working memory have been well studied. The evidence from animal work, lesion studies in humans[66,67] and human PET studies[68–70] has demonstrated that working memory tasks involve the DLPFC and the basal ganglia,[66,67,71–78] regardless of the modality of the information.[79]

Patients with schizophrenia are impaired on visuospatial working memory tasks, such as delayed-response (DR) tasks,[80–86] the 'self-ordered' spatial working memory task[87,88] and the 'N-back' task.[89] Impairments in verbal working memory have also been described in schizophrenia using Brown–Peterson paradigms, in which verbal stimuli are followed by a distraction task before subjects are asked to recall the original stimuli.[90,91] The specificity of sensory modality was examined by Park and Holzman,[81] who identified deficits on both oculo-motor DR and a haptic DR task in schizophrenia compared with normals or bipolar patients. These data demonstrated that working memory deficits were not modality specific but were diagnosis specific.

While many of these studies have relied on tasks that only require the holding of information 'on-line' (i.e. short-term memory), the notion of working memory also includes the active manipulation of information, particularly as memory load increases. The 'self-ordered' spatial working memory task (part of the CANTAB computerized battery[92]) addresses both components. The task has been utilized in a number of neurological groups, and performance has been shown to be impaired in patients with frontal lesions and patients with basal ganglia disorders.[73–78,93] Further, PET studies using this task have demonstrated that DLPFC and ventrolateral prefrontal areas are involved in different aspects of the task.[70] In their study of spatial working memory, Pantelis et al[87] directly compared patients with chronic schizophrenia with other neurological groups. Patients with schizophrenia were similar to patients with Parkinson's disease (PD) in showing impaired short-term memory capacity, and were similar to both PD patients and patients with frontal lesions in showing deficits in spatial working memory and impaired ability to generate a systematic strategy. In contrast, patients with temporal lobe lesions were unimpaired on this task.[75] The results were consistent with Petrides'[94] notion that different regions of the dorsal prefrontal cortex are involved in working memory, providing support for the notion that both ventrolateral and dorsolateral frontal circuits (as well as their interaction) are compromised in schizophrenia.[87]

Attentional set-shifting tasks

In set-shifting paradigms, subjects are required to shift attention between different stimulus dimensions on the basis of reinforcing feedback. Patients with frontal lesions are impaired in their ability to inhibit previously learned responses and, as a consequence, are unable to shift their attention to the relevant stimulus, thus making errors of perseveration.[95] Several studies have confirmed that patients with schizophrenia perform poorly on such tasks, as exemplified by performance on the Wisconsin Card Sorting Test (WCST).[60,96–98] In general, the results indicate that patients with schizophrenia achieve fewer sorting categories than controls and display significantly more perseverative errors. The common explanation provided for this performance is that patients with schizophrenia fail to inhibit inappropriate responses. While it is inferred that set-shifting deficits are indicative of frontal lobe dysfunction, the cognitive deficit underlying failure in patients with schizophrenia may differ from that in patients with frontal lobe damage. Indeed, the WCST is not specific to dysfunction of the frontal lobe, with patients with hippocampal lesions committing significantly more perseverative errors than patients with frontal damage.[99] In order to examine this issue, three studies have examined attentional set-shifting in schizophrenia, using a computerized task that examines the component cognitive processes involved.[88,100,101] This task derives from the Cambridge Neuropsychological Test Automated Battery (CANTAB) computerized battery[102] and examines two types of set-shifting; intradimensional (ID) shifts, which involve the transfer of a rule within the same stimulus dimension (e.g. choosing circles instead of squares), and extradimensional (ED) shifts, which require a transfer of attention across different stimulus dimensions (e.g. choosing on the basis of color rather than the previous category of shape). In essence, ED shifting is the core component of the WCST, and is the basis for the achievement of novel sorting categories. ID shifting is a more basic element of the WCST and is related to the ability of the subject to be aware of the conceptual category within which they are responding. A successful ID shift requires a generalization of learning or the ability to 'learn set'. A modification of this task (abbreviated as IDED shifting task) has also been used to examine whether poor performance is due to perseveration (i.e. continuing to respond inappropriately to a previously reinforced dimension) rather than to learned irrelevance (i.e. ignoring a previously irrelevant dimension). Previous studies have demonstrated that patients with frontal lesions and basal ganglia disorders show impairments on this task; further, while frontal lesion patients demonstrated perseverative errors, PD patients fail because of learned irrelevance.[93]

Using this task, Hutton et al[88] found that first-episode patients were relatively unimpaired in set-shifting ability, while Elliott et al[100] found that patients with moderately severe schizophrenia fail at the ED stage due to a tendency to perseverate, akin to frontal lesion patients. In their study, Pantelis et al[101] directly compared a more chronic group of patients with schizophrenia with a cohort of patients with frontal lobe lesions, and found more severe deficits, with failure at both ID and ED. Taken together, these studies suggest progressive deterioration on this task, although there are no published longitudinal studies available. Such progression is observed also in patients with Huntington's disease, which has been attributed to progressive neuropathology seen in the caudate.[103] While these findings in schizophrenia are suggestive of the involvement of prefrontal–striatal–thalamic circuits, there are no available imaging studies using this task to validate this notion.

OFC–striatal–thalamic circuit

Disruption of the OFC is characterized clinically by marked changes in personality, including irritability, disinhibition, inappropriate self-indulgence and lack of concern for others, which have been described as the 'pseudo-psychopathic' personality.[104] Cummings further states that this syndrome is characterized by an 'enslavement to environmental cues with automatic imitation of the gestures and actions of others, or enforced utilisation of objects in the environment'.[52] Such 'utilization' behavior was described by Lhermitte,[105] who termed it the 'environmental dependency syndrome'. This has also been described with lesions of the caudate.[106] Such phenomena are also observed in schizophrenia, with changed personality, disinhibition, and reliance on external cues to guide action.[107,108] More recently, the OFC has been considered to be important in the ability to make decisions between equally compelling contingencies, such that the OFC is involved in emotional aspects of decision-making.[109]

Neuropsychologically, patients with lesions of the OFC circuit are impaired on 'Go–No Go' tasks, indicating an inability to suppress inappropriate responses,[110] while they have been found to perform normally on card-sorting tasks.[111] Impairments have also been described on delayed–alternation tasks,[112,113] as well as object alternation.[114,115] There are limited data, however, on such tasks in schizophrenia.[35,84] The most robust probes of the integrity of functioning of this area are olfactory identification ability (review: Pantelis et al[116]) and performance on a gambling task,[117,118] both of which have been examined in schizophrenia. While patients with schizophrenia performed poorly on tests of olfactory identification,[116] their performance on a gambling task has been reported as normal in one small study.[119]

AC–striatal–thalamic circuit

The AC circuit is linked to the hippocampus (HC) and forms part of the paralimbic cortex. It also has close connections with other prefrontal areas, such as the DLPFC and OFC circuits, and has important connections to the parietal cortex (considered later).[120-122] As might be expected, there is an overlap of function,[123] with these areas acting in concert when engaged in tasks requiring initiation, motivation, selection and inhibition. The AC circuit enables the intentional selection of external stimuli based upon the internal relevance that these stimuli have for the organism. Input about the internal relevance is provided by the activity of the OFC circuit, while the DLPFC is involved in developing novel strategies and appropriate response selection. Lesions to the AC circuit result in akinesis, impaired ability to inhibit inappropriate responses, and apathy. Bilateral lesions of the AC result in akinetic mutism and impairments in the ability to express and experience affect,[124] these phenomena being very similar to the negative symptoms of schizophrenia. Interestingly, pathological investigations have identified alterations of the circuitry of the AC of patients with schizophrenia,[122] while recent morphological studies have also shown differences in the degree of folding of this structure in first-episode and chronic schizophrenia.[125,126]

Like patients with lesions of the OFC, patients with dysfunction of the AC are also impaired on 'Go–No Go' tasks. Of relevance are the PET studies of the Stroop task in normal subjects,[127,128] a task that requires 'attention for action' and inhibition of inappropriate responses but not novel responses (such as in card-sort tasks). In this task, patients are asked to name the color of the ink that words are written in when the letters spell the name of a different color (incongruent condition) versus when they spell the name of the same color (congruent condition). These studies identified activation of the AC circuit during performance of this task.

Neuropsychological studies have shown that patients with schizophrenia perform poorly on the Stroop task.[129,130] In agreement with the findings of Liddle and colleagues, Joyce et al[130] found that impaired Stroop performance was associated with increased severity of the 'disorganization syndrome', which includes thought disorder and inappropriate affect.[129] This was supported by a resting PET study[131] which found that scores for the disorganization syndrome were correlated with increased activity in the AC. Only one published study has examined patients with schizophrenia using the Stroop task under PET activation conditions. In this study, patients with schizophrenia showed significantly less AC gyrus activation while naming the color of color-incongruent stimuli during the Stroop task.[132]

The evidence above supports the notion that frontal–subcortical neuronal systems are involved in schizophrenia. However, studies that have specifically examined the structural and functional relationships between prefrontal cortex, basal ganglia and thalami are few. Neuropsychological studies are limited in their ability to examine the functioning of each node within these circuits, but more sophisticated statistical techniques for the analysis of functional imaging data that examine networks of anatomically interconnected areas may be successful in this regard.[133]

Schizophrenia as a disturbance of frontal–temporal systems

Along with the basal ganglia, several lines of investigation implicate dysfunction or pathology in other areas with which the frontal lobes also connect, such as the temporal lobes. Medial temporal disturbance in schizophrenia has been suggested by clinical observations of the relationship between temporal lobe epilepsy and schizophrenia as well as by recent neuroimaging,[16] neuropsychological[134] and neuropathological[135] research. Further, medial temporal lobe structures have been considered as important regions for a proposed neurodevelopmental lesion of schizophrenia[7] because of their role in cognitive and emotional functioning, vulnerability to early insults and connections to other relevant brain structures.[136,137] In addition, the reported deficits in frontal lobe function may be attributable to structural abnormalities in other regions such as temporal lobe areas, a notion proposed by Weinberger[36] and by Goldman-Rakic.[138] These authors have drawn on animal literature studying working memory[139] to suggest that the consistent findings of deficits of frontal lobe functioning may result from disruption of the circuitry connecting with limbic structures. Specifically, they argue that the neuropsychological dysfunction in schizophrenia results from disruption of the circuitry connecting the HC with prefrontal cortical areas. While these authors have focused particularly on the DLPFC, they acknowledge that other regions, such as the OFC, may be equally important.[140]

Neuroanatomy of frontal–temporal circuits

While there is some evidence for a dysfunctional relationship between the DLPFC and the HC, which is outlined below, there is little anatomical evidence for connectivity between the two. Despite strong connections between the rostral HC and the medial and orbital prefrontal cortices, there are only sparse ones with the DLPFC.[141,142] One explanation is that the hippocampal influence on the DLFPC is mediated by the 'caudomedial lobule', which is situated at the caudoventral tip of the cingulate gyrus, and is well connected with both the HC and DLPFC.[139] However, it seems that the most important site within the prefrontal cortex for hippocampal influence is the medial prefrontal cortex, with additional projections to the OFC.[142] This region is known to play a role in affect, aggression and motivation as well as olfactory ability (described earlier), changes to which are features of schizophrenia. In addition, the medial prefrontal cortex is activated by tasks such as the Tower of London

(TOL)[143] and the Stroop test,[144] tasks on which patients with schizophrenia perform abnormally.[87,145,146] It therefore seems likely that a discussion of the role of prefrontal–hippocampal connections should not be limited to the DLPFC. In particular, the direct connections with the orbital and medial prefrontal regions suggest that the hippocampal abnormalities recently described in schizophrenia may have direct effects on the integrity of this circuitry, with consequent disruption of its function.

Functional imaging studies of frontal–hippocampal dysfunction in schizophrenia

The frontal–hippocampal hypothesis was first examined in a study of monozygotic twins discordant for schizophrenia.[137] All subjects had their cerebral blood flow (CBF) measured using the ^{133}Xe inhalation technique during performance on the WCST. The differences between twin pairs in prefrontal blood flow during the task were significantly correlated with the difference in left hippocampal size between these twins, after covarying whole brain CBF. Further, an inverse correlation was also observed between the left HC and the difference between twins in parietal CBF.[137] It was concluded that these regions were coupled during tasks such as the WCST, and that abnormal coupling was apparent in schizophrenia, which is consistent with the notion that schizophrenia involves disruption of a distributed neocortical–limbic neural network involving these regions. However, as acknowledged by the authors, while these correlational analyses might imply a functional deficit secondary to anatomical disconnectivity, they do not necessarily imply direct connection between these structures. There may be other areas within the network that provide paths from medial temporal lobe structures to the prefrontal cortex, including ventral–anterior thalamus.[147] The use of ^{133}Xe inhalation, however, precluded examination of ventral and medial prefrontal areas, or subcortical structures. Further, the relationship with parietal lobe function may implicate the network proposed by Mesulam,[120] which is discussed further below.

   In order to address some of these methodological issues, functional imaging studies that examine all brain areas are necessary, using PET or fMRI techniques.[18,19] One PET study of conscious recollection of studied words[148] found that control subjects activated the superior dorsal prefrontal area (Brodmann's area (BA) 8) bilaterally during a shallow-encoding (low-recall) task compared with a baseline task. The only additional areas activated during a deep-encoding task (high-recall) were the right hippocampus/parahippocampus and right superior temporal gyrus (BA 22/42). In contrast, patients with schizophrenia, while strongly activating prefrontal regions (BA 9, 10, 11) in the shallow-encoding task, were unable to recruit the HC during the semantically encoded task. The authors concluded that in normals the DLPFC was involved in effortful retrieval of poorly encoded material, while the HC was involved in the conscious recollection of well-encoded material. Further, they suggested that the findings in schizophrenia reflected 'the functional correlate of an abnormal corticohippocampal interaction'.[148] It should be noted, however, that the DLPFC has more strictly been considered to include BA 46/9. Further, those prefrontal areas activated by the patient group were more anterior and included the OFC (areas 9, 10 and 11 rather than area 8). Interestingly, the inferior parietal lobule (area 40) was also activated in the patients, which was interpreted as secondary to the failure to activate the HC in these patients. Therefore, the main finding from this study is of inability to activate the HC in patients with schizophrenia during the recall of semantically encoded verbal information. Although the findings in prefrontal cortex were in keeping with impaired prefrontal–hippocampal connectivity, the prefrontal areas implicated were not necessarily those considered to be part of the DLPFC. Instead, they included the OFC, suggesting that the problem may be a failure of OFC–hippocampal connectivity, which is more in keeping with the anatomical connectivity of these areas. In support of this notion, Malaspina et al[149] also found a failure of normal hippocampal activation in response to an odor-identification task.

As suggested by these studies, the notion that the reduced CBF in the DLPFC described in schizophrenia is related to structural abnormalities in the medial temporal lobe receives limited support. Further studies using MRS provide another means to examine this hypothesis. The available studies have identified lower levels of NAA in the HC and prefrontal areas in patients with schizophrenia compared to controls, implying neuronal loss or dysfunction,[17] although few studies have used MRS to examine the inter-relationship between these areas. In a recent study, Bertolino et al[150] compared 12 medication-free (5 neuroleptic-naive) patients with 12 normals matched for sex and age, using ^{1}H-MRSI (magnetic resonance spectroscopic imaging) to obtain data from all brain regions. They found that patients had lower NAA levels in hippocampal and DLPFC regions. However, examination of their data in the patient group did not reveal any significant correlation between these two measures, raising the possibility that abnormalities in these regions occurred independently (data from normals were not presented). Further, they did not find any correlations between metabolite ratios and either frontal lobe or hippocampal volumes, although the prefrontal lobe specifically was not included in the analysis.

Neuropsychological studies implicating frontal–temporal areas in schizophrenia

In their correlational study of 29 patients with first-episode psychosis, Bilder et al[151] directly set out to examine the hypothesis that deficits in executive function could be understood as a dysfunction of prefrontal–temporal connectivity. A composite measure of executive function, made up of tests such as Trails B, perseverative responses on the WCST and Picture Arrangement, was found to correlate well with the volume of the anterior HC. This supported the findings of Weinberger et al,[137] described above, in that functional deficits were associated with structural changes. However, it does not follow that this has demonstrated the importance of the DLPFC, but rather the prefrontal lobe as a whole. Indeed, even WCST performance, which is regarded as the best test of DLPFC function, has been shown to be affected more by hippocampal than by frontal lobe lesions.[100]

Few studies have investigated the relationship of olfactory deficits to other tasks which have been deemed specific to prefrontal or medial temporal areas. Seidman et al[152] found no association between performance with the WCST and the olfactory deficits and suggested that the deficits in schizophrenia could be subdivided into subtypes of DLPFC, OFC and generalized prefrontal impairment. In a study comparing normals and patients with chronic schizophrenia, Brewer et al[84] found that patients had olfactory identification deficits and demonstrated impaired performance on tasks of memory, and on DR and WCST tasks. Olfactory identification deficits were associated with impaired performance on tasks of executive function rather than poor memory ability. In controls but not patients, olfactory identification was significantly associated with a verbal memory index. This suggested that, in this group, putative function of the prefrontal cortex was not related to measures of left medial temporal lobe function. In support of these findings, the relationship between measures of frontal lobe function and olfactory identification ability remained significant after partialling out the performance on measures of memory. Thus, though identification ability in normal subjects was related to indices of medial temporal lobe function, the deficits of identification found in schizophrenia were not related to medial temporal lobe function. However, a significant association was found between identification ability and measures of frontal lobe function. One possibility is that this reflects impaired connections between OFC and medial temporal regions in schizophrenia.

In summary, it is not entirely clear what the relationship is between structural abnormalities in the medial temporal lobe and impairments of frontal lobe function. While the DLPFC has been implicated, it now seems that OFC and medial prefrontal cortex may be equally important.

Neuropsychological evidence for dysfunction of temporal lobe and limbic structures in schizophrenia

While the frontal–hippocampal model provides a possible explanation for some of the profound deficits of executive function observed in schizophrenia, it does not discuss other possible ramifications of lesions in the HC or other medial temporal structures. Thus, while there is now good evidence to implicate pathological involvement of the temporal lobe in schizophrenia,[135,153] the studies that have examined neuropsychological functions directly relevant to the medial temporal lobe have paid little attention to the cognitive demands of the tasks and their neuroanatomical basis. Thus, these areas are critically important to normal episodic memory function,[154] and are also likely to play a role in semantic,[155] topographic[156] and recognition memory.[157] In addition, neuroimaging and neuropathological studies have implicated the involvement of other medial temporal lobe areas, including the parahippocampal gyrus and fusiform gyrus,[158] further suggesting that memory function would be impaired in schizophrenia.

The numerous studies of memory in schizophrenia have generally concluded that memory function is impaired both in chronically unwell patients[159] and in those in their first episode of a psychotic illness.[160,161] By and large, verbal memory deficits appear to be more robust than visuospatial ones, and verbal memory shows little improvement over the first few years of illness.[24] Nonetheless, a recent meta-analysis of 70 studies of memory in schizophrenia provided strong support for a deficit in recall and recognition for both verbal and visual material, as well as forward and backward digit span.[134] Surprisingly, negative symptoms were associated with memory deficits, which are usually thought to be related to impairments of prefrontal function, especially involving the DLPFC.[131] However, the analysis did not investigate whether the impairment of memory was over and above the recognized impairments of global cognitive function (as measured by IQ), attention or working memory.

Investigators have speculated about whether these findings implicate medial temporal lobe regions[160,162] or frontal lobe dysfunction.[161,163] However, to date most studies have relied on general tests of memory, have not been hypothesis-driven and have not considered the various neurocognitive components of memory tasks that may have guided interpretation of the results. In particular, the early studies[159,163] were undertaken in the context of limited data being available from neuropathology or neuroimaging studies to inform such hypotheses, while more recent studies have utilized large batteries of neuropsychological tests rather than employing experimental designs.[23,164]

In addition, the construct of memory has rarely informed the selection of neuropsychological tests used. For example, there are three different forms of verbal memory frequently assessed in neuropsychological studies; list-learning, memory for prose, and paired-associate learning. These are likely to be subsumed by different temporal lobe regions, and some may not involve the medial temporal lobe. List-learning was found to be related to oral word association and visual naming, and was not associated with the integrity of medial temporal structures.[165] Prose recall is highly context-dependent, and the use of context is known to be impaired in schizophrenia, which has been related to frontal dysfunction.[166] Verbal paired-associate learning is much more clearly a task that is mediated by temporal rather than frontal lobe structures. However, the precise neural substrate is critically dependent on the nature of the pairs, such that semantically related ('easy') pairs are mediated by lateral temporal neocortex, while semantically unrelated ('hard') pairs are mediated by the medial temporal lobe (most probably the HC).[167,168] Unfortunately, almost all studies in schizophrenia to date have combined both kinds of pairs to produce a single score. One study which used only hard pairs[169] found that although patients with schizophrenia recalled fewer pairs, they were able to learn over repeated presentations at the same rate as control subjects. Similarly, Goldberg et al[170] noted that the schizophrenic twin of discordant pairs learnt hard pairs as well as the unaffected twin. These findings seem to suggest that the verbal memory deficit in schizophrenia does not concord with the pattern observed following damage to the HC.[167] Instead, these deficits may result from impaired strategic abilities or other executive functions,[161] thereby implicating prefrontal areas.

The investigation of non-verbal memory has also been problematic because of the use of inappropriate tests which are either easily verbalized or which may not involve the temporal lobe at all.[171] In an attempt to overcome these problems, Rushe et al[162] used a visuospatial paired-associate learning test to examine the modality-specific nature of the hippocampal finding on the verbal form of the test. Although patients with schizophrenia were impaired relative to controls, the task still combined 'easy' and 'hard' pairs, and the stimuli were simple and easy to verbalize. In addition, the authors did not compare the learning curves of the two groups. Another visual paired-associate learning test is that from the CANTAB,[172] which pairs patterns to spatial locations. This task appears sensitive to early dementia of the Alzheimer type[173] and is a good candidate for a test of right hippocampal integrity. We have used this test to investigate 67 patients with first-episode psychosis and 30 with chronic schizophrenia, and compared them to 41 healthy controls. When the effects of global cognitive function, spatial span, age and pattern recognition were removed, only the chronic patients were impaired when compared to controls (Wood, Pantelis, McGorry et al, unpublished data). This implies that in patients with chronic schizophrenia there may be a true hippocampal memory deficit for visuospatial information, possibly explained by the bilateral hippocampal atrophy observed in these patients.[14]

To date, the findings of memory impairment have not been placed in the context of the neurodevelopmental hypothesis of schizophrenia. The HC is seen as a likely candidate for a neurodevelopmental lesion because it is selectively vulnerable to hypoxia,[174] hypoglycemia,[175] undernutrition[176] and hypothyroidism.[177] Depending on the nature and extent of this putative early hippocampal pathology, memory function will be forced to develop in abnormal circumstances. This may result in atypical relationships between measures of memory and medial temporal lobe integrity.[167,178]

Despite this, the investigation of the relationship between memory function and early hippocampal pathology in schizophrenia has been confined to animal studies.[179] This research has confirmed that neonatal hippocampal lesions produce a similar memory impairment to that seen following the same lesions acquired in adulthood, namely impaired relational learning.[180] However, only these early lesions also produce behavioral abnormalities such as locomotor stereotypies and fewer social interactions.[181] While this clearly has implications for the etiology of schizophrenia, it should be borne in mind that the sort of hippocampal pathology produced by these lesions is totally different to that seen in the disorder itself, where subtle changes in neuronal size, shape and orientation are seen.[135] In this regard, the neuropsychological study of developmental dysplasia may prove fruitful.

In summary, while there is some evidence for an impaired relationship between prefrontal cortex and medial temporal lobe, its exact nature is unclear. The anatomical evidence indicates that the OFC and medial frontal cortex, rather than the DLPFC, are the major targets of hippocampal neurons projecting to the prefrontal lobe. However, there are few studies which have directly tested the integrity of this axis in schizophrenia. It is also uncertain what findings of structural abnormalities in the medial temporal lobe mean in terms of memory function. That there are 'memory' impairments is unquestionable, but to what extent these are due to medial temporal lobe dysfunction, to altered lateral temporal or frontal lobe abilities, or to more general cognitive dysfunction, is unclear. In part this is because the precise functions of the HC and surrounding neocortex are matters of energetic debate, but it is also the case that there are very few studies which have approached the concept of memory impairment in schizophrenia from a theoretical standpoint. In addition, it is clearly critical to our understanding both of frontal–hippocampal connectivity and memory dysfunction in schizophrenia to have some idea of the normal developmental trajectory of hippocampal memory, and how this is altered by neurodevelopmental lesions.

Evolving evidence of frontal–parietal system disturbance in schizophrenia

As stated above, it is commonly observed in schizophrenia that abnormally low levels of CBF in the DLPFC are associated with abnormally high CBF in the parietal lobe.[19] Given the strong interconnections between frontal and parietal areas, this association is not surprising.[120,139] However, brain–behavior models of schizophrenia rarely consider the pathological significance of abnormal activity in parietal lobe areas. Neuropsychological studies of human and non-human primates show that the right parietal lobe is important to the representation of space and the programming of actions within spatiotopic reference frames. The left parietal lobe is necessary for skilled and purposive movement and gestures.[96] Many studies have shown that the representation of space is disrupted in patients with schizophrenia. This manifests as the subtle neglect of left hemispace during cancellation, covert attentional and motor tasks.[108,182] Interestingly, this neglect is most robust in patients with high levels of positive symptoms and often resolves following brief periods of treatment with antipsychotic medication.[182] Importantly, these cognitive impairments are qualitatively similar but quantitatively less severe than impairments found when patients with focal lesions of the parietal lobe perform the same tasks.

Neuroanatomy of frontal–parietal circuits

The parietal lobe consists of the post-central gyrus (BA 1, 2 and 3), the superior parietal lobule (BA 5 and 7), the inferior parietal lobule (BA 40 and 43) and the angular gyrus (BA 39). These are considered as two functional zones that consist of an anterior zone comprising BA 1, 2, 3 and 43 as well as anterior aspects of BA 5 and 7, and a posterior zone that comprises the posterior aspects of BA 5 and 7 and areas 39 and 40. The anterior zone consists of primary and secondary somatosensory cortex and the posterior zone association cortex. Major inputs to parietal lobe association areas project from the lateral and posterior thalamus and primary and secondary sensory areas. Major outputs from parietal lobe association areas to subcortical areas that include the lateral and posterior thalamus, the posterior regions of the striatum, the midbrain (superior colliculus) and spinal cord and to the temporal and frontal cortices. Interconnections between the parietal and frontal cortex also follow the anterior–posterior distinction, with regions in the anterior parietal zone projecting to premotor areas in the frontal cortex, and association areas 39 and 40 projecting to the principal sulcus (BA 46) or DLPFC (review: Goldman-Rakic[71]).

Evidence for parietal lobe involvement in schizophrenia

Few studies have sought to investigate the role of the parietal cortex in schizophrenia directly. Four reasons for this follow. First, few similarities have been noted between the symptoms of schizophrenia and the behavioral consequences of parietal lobe lesions (e.g. compared with those found between patients with schizophrenia and those with focal lesions of the frontal lobe or with temporal lobe epilepsy). Second, conventional neuropsychological models of parietal lobe function, based mainly on disturbances of spatial cognition such as those associated with neglect, produce tests that are inappropriate for the investigation of the more subtle deficits in integrative cognitive processes that occur in schizophrenia. Third, because of the lack of obvious morphological landmarks, volumetric studies using MRI in schizophrenia have difficulty in defining a region of interest (ROI) within the parietal lobe. Fourth, these previous three points have led researchers away from considering tasks of parietal lobe function as activation tasks in functional neuroimaging studies; indeed, early neuroimaging studies used the parietal cortex as a reference point.[19]

Despite these limitations, there is now converging neuroscientific evidence for the involvement of the parietal lobe in schizophrenia. There is evidence to show that patients with focal lesions of the parietal cortex also report significant symptoms of alienation, neglect, anosagnosia and distortions of body image.[183–186] Furthermore, these symptoms are qualitatively similar to some of the Schneiderian first-rank symptoms observed in patients with schizophrenia.[183] There are also similarities in the neurobehavioral deficits of patients with schizophrenia and patients with lesions of the parietal cortex (described above), and there is some neuroanatomical evidence indicating that neuronal density in the parietal lobe is abnormal in schizophrenia.[30,187,188] Finally, direct evidence for involvement of the parietal cortex in schizophrenia comes from Spence et al,[40] who examined regional cerebral blood flow (rCBF) in patients with schizophrenia with and without passivity delusions using PET. During the scan, the patients were required to move a joystick voluntarily and to freely select the direction of the movement. Most of the passivity group reported vivid experiences of alien control when performing this motor task. When compared to the non-passivity schizophrenia group, the passivity group showed increased rCBF in a cortical network that included the left premotor cortex and the right inferior parietal lobule.

In our laboratory, we have found neuropsychological evidence for parietal lobe dysfunction in a study that required patients with schizophrenia to perform simple saccade tasks. Patients with schizophrenia failed to correct inaccuracies in the endpoint of hypometric saccades when those saccades were made on the basis of an internal representation of target location. Control subjects always corrected hypometric saccades spontaneously, and both groups corrected spontaneously any inaccuracies in the endpoint of visually guided saccades.[189] In normal subjects and alert primates, the spontaneous correction of hypometric saccades is hypothesized to occur because the sensory feedback of eye position does not match the forward model of the saccade goal. In primates, the forward modeling of saccade-related information occurs in neurons in the lateral intraparietal sulcus.[190,191] Accordingly, patients with focal lesions of the parietal lobe cannot plan saccades on the basis of forward models of saccade goals when those saccades must be made in a contralesional direction. Patients with unilateral lesions of the FEF, DLPFC and SMA show no such impairment.[192] Impairment in the ability to anticipate the effects of movements on the basis of internal models of those movements is also seen in the impaired motor imagery of patients with lesions of the parietal cortex. Normally, actual and imagined movements are constrained by the same biomechanical or environmental factors, activate the same regions in functional neuroimaging studies and are disrupted in the same way by lesions at different levels of the motor system. On the basis of this information, it has been proposed that the imagination of motor acts is based on forward models of the efference copy of actual but unexecuted movements.[193,194] In patients with schizophrenia characterized by passivity delusions, imagined performance on a motor task did not conform to conventional speed/accuracy trade-offs, whereas actual movements did.[41] This pattern of performance was similar to that observed in patients with focal lesions of the parietal lobe but not the motor cortex, basal ganglia or cerebellum (review: Maruff and Currie[41]), supporting further the involvement of the parietal lobe in schizophrenia.

These data suggest that dysfunction of the parietal lobe occurs in at least a subgroup of patients with schizophrenia. In functional neuroimaging studies of healthy individuals performing executive function tasks, reliable inverse correlations between activity in the frontal and parietal cortices suggest reciprocal interaction between the two areas. Such correlations are not observed in the patterns of rCBF when patients with schizophrenia perform similar tasks, suggesting that functional connectivity within frontal–parietal neurocognitive networks is disrupted in schizophrenia.[148] On this basis, Frith has suggested that positive symptoms such as passivity phenomena arise from disconnection between prefrontal association cortex, where intentions to act are generated, and parietal association cortex, where the sensory consequences of motor actions are modeled.[195] The next challenge is to understand the relationship between structural and functional abnormalities in the frontal and parietal lobe association areas in patients with schizophrenia.

A unifying hypothesis

The evidence presented above suggests that a number of neurocognitive networks are dysfunctional in schizophrenia and help to explain the range of deficits observed neuropsychologically. It is apparent that the most profound deficits are observed on cognitive tasks of executive function, thereby implicating prefrontal cortical regions. However, impairments in function are also observed in cognitive domains that can be attributed to other regions with which the prefrontal cortex has direct connections, including the basal ganglia and thalami, medial temporal lobe structures such as the HC, and the parietal lobe. These findings are consistent with schizophrenia being a disorder of connectivity[196] involving prefrontal–striatal-thalamus disconnection[33] and prefrontal–temporal disconnection,[36,138] and there is emerging evidence for the involvement of circuits that link with the parietal lobe.

The way forward is to constrain brain–behavior models of schizophrenia with reference to the known corticocortical and corticosubcortical anatomical interconnectivity. These relationships can be specified further by referring to studies that have investigated the correlation between two or more nodes within such networks simultaneously, as observed in animal studies.[197] In humans, a similar approach, as used in epilepsy, has been to model relative changes in blood flow in different brain regions using PET or fMRI, or by correlating single neuronal firing rates within complex structures such as the HC with depth electrodes.[198] While the latter approach is not feasible in schizophrenia, the recording of surface activity using electro- or magneto-encephalography may provide some ability to examine correlated activity in different but interconnected areas of the cortex (review: Reite et al[199]). The source generators in these studies could be correlated with findings from functional imaging studies using the same activation tasks.[200] Further, as neurochemical processes are relatively well understood within specific neural pathways, the application of radiolabeled ligands specific to relevant neurotransmitter systems (e.g. dopamine, GABA, serotonin) may also help us to elucidate functional relationships between distributed but interconnected brain areas.[201] Finally, novel methods in structural neuroimaging can now examine white matter tracts (e.g. with diffusion-weighted imaging), thereby providing an additional tool with which to directly assess structural connectivity between different brain regions.[18] If schizophrenia is a disorder of connectivity, the application of two or more of these approaches simultaneously is clearly necessary to advance our understanding of the nature of brain dysfunction in this disorder.

Acknowledgements

This work was supported by NH&MRC Grants 970598 and 981112.

References

1. Kraepelin E. *Lectures in Clinical Psychiatry* (New York: Macmillan, 1899).

2. Jablensky A. Schizophrenia: the epidemiological horizon. In Hirsch SR, Weinberger DR (eds) *Schizophrenia* (Oxford: Blackwell Science, 1995): 206–52.

3. Moller H-J, von Zerssen D. Course and outcome of schizophrenia. In Hirsch SR, Weinberger DR (eds) *Schizophrenia*

(Oxford: Blackwell Science, 1995): 106–27.

4. Pantelis C, Barnes TRE. Drug strategies and treatment-resistant schizophrenia. *Aust NZ J Psychiatry* (1996) **30:** 20–37.

5. Asherson P, Mant R, McGuffin P. Genetics and schizophrenia. In Hirsch SR, Weinberger DR (eds) *Schizophrenia* (Oxford: Blackwell Science, 1995): 253–74.

6. McGrath J, Murray R. Risk factors for schizophrenia: from conception to birth. In Hirsch SR, Weinberger DR (eds) *Schizophrenia* (Oxford: Blackwell Science, 1995): 187–205.

7. Weinberger DR. Implications of normal brain development for the pathogenesis of schizophrenia. *Arch Gen Psychiatry* (1987) **44:** 660–9.

8. Jones P, Murray RM. The genetics of schizophrenia is the genetics of neurodevelopment. *Br J Psychiatry* (1991) **158:** 615–23.

9. Murray RM. Neurodevelopmental schizophrenia: the rediscovery of dementia praecox. *Br J Psychiatry Suppl* (1994) **165:** 6–12.

10. Walker E, Savoie T, Davis D. Neuromotor precursors of schizophrenia. *Schizophr Bull* (1994) **20:** 441–51.

11. Pantelis C. Overview: towards a neuropsychology of schizophrenia. In Pantelis C, Nelson HE, Barnes TR (eds) *Schizophrenia: A Neuropsychological Perspective* (London: John Wiley & Sons, 1996): 3–18.

12. McGrath J. Hypothesis: is low prenatal vitamin D a risk-modifying factor for schizophrenia? *Schizophr Res* (1999) **40:** 173–7.

13. DeLisi LE. Defining the course of brain structural change and plasticity in schizophrenia. *Psychiatry Res Neuroimaging Section* (1999) **92:** 1–9.

14. Velakoulis D, Wood SJ, McGorry PD, Pantelis C. Evidence for progression of brain structural abnormalities in schizophrenia: beyond the neurodevelopmental model. *Aust NZ J Psychiatry* (2000) **34:** S113–26.

15. Rogers DGC. The cognitive disorder of psychiatric illness: a historical perspective. In Pantelis C, Nelson HE, Barnes TR (eds) *Schizophrenia: A Neuropsychological Perspective* (Chichester: John Wiley & Sons, 1996): 19–29.

16. Wright IC, Rabe-Hesketh S, Woodruff PW et al. Meta-analysis of regional brain volumes in schizophrenia. *Am J Psychiatry* (2000) **157:** 16–25.

17. Vance AL, Velakoulis D, Maruff P et al. Magnetic resonance spectroscopy and schizophrenia: what have we learnt? *Aust N Z J Psychiatry* (2000) **34:** 14–25.

18. Fu CH, McGuire PK. Functional neuroimaging in psychiatry. *Philos Trans R Soc Lond B* (1999) **354:** 1359–70.

19. Velakoulis D, Pantelis C. What have we learned from functional imaging studies in schizophrenia? The role of frontal, striatal and temporal areas. *Aust NZ J Psychiatry* (1996) **30:** 195–209.

20. Elliott R, Sahakian BJ. The neuropsychology of schizophrenia: relations with clinical and neurobiological dimensions. *Psychol Med* (1995) **25:** 581–94.

21. Heinrichs RW, Zakzanis KK. Neurocognitive deficit in schizophrenia: a quantitative review of the evidence. *Neuropsychology* (1998) **12:** 426–45.

22. Rund BR. A review of longitudinal studies of cognitive functions in schizophrenia patients. *Schizophr Bull* (1998) **24:** 425–35.

23. Gold S, Arndt S, Nopoulos P et al. Longitudinal study of cognitive function in first-episode and

recent-onset schizophrenia. *Am J Psychiatry* (1999) **156:** 1342–8.

24. Hoff AL, Sakuma M, Wieneke M et al. Longitudinal neuropsychological follow-up study of patients with first-episode schizophrenia. *Am J Psychiatry* (1999) **156:** 1336–41.

25. Lawrie SM, Whalley H, Kestelman JN et al. Magnetic resonance imaging of brain in people at high risk of developing schizophrenia. *Lancet* (1999) **353:** 30–3.

26. Kuperberg G, Heckers S. Schizophrenia and cognitive function. *Curr Opin Neurobiol* (2000) **10:** 205–10.

27. Gold JM, Harvey PD. Cognitive deficits in schizophrenia. *Psychiatr Clin North Am* (1993) **16:** 295–312.

28. Frederikse M, Lu A, Aylward E et al. Sex differences in inferior parietal lobule volume in schizophrenia. *Am J Psychiatry* (2000) **157:** 422–7.

29. Kirkpatrick B, Conley RC, Kakoyannis A et al. Interstitial cells of the white matter in the inferior parietal cortex in schizophrenia: an unbiased cell-counting study. *Synapse* (1999) **34:** 95–102.

30. Ross CA, Pearlson GD. Schizophrenia, the heteromodal association neocortex and development: potential for a neurogenetic approach. *Trends Neurosci* (1996) **19:** 171–6.

31. Buchanan RW, Strauss ME, Kirkpatrick B et al. Neuropsychological impairments in deficit vs nondeficit forms of schizophrenia. *Arch Gen Psychiatry* (1994) **51:** 804–11.

32. Robbins TW. The case for frontostriatal dysfunction in schizophrenia. *Schizophr Bull* (1990) **16**(3): 391–402.

33. Pantelis C, Barnes TR, Nelson HE. Is the concept of frontal–subcortical dementia relevant to schizophrenia? *Br J Psychiatry* (1992) **160:** 442–60.

34. Pantelis C, Brewer WJ. Neuropsychological and olfactory dysfunction in schizophrenia: relationship of frontal syndromes to syndromes of schizophrenia. *Schizophr Res* (1995) **17:** 35–45.

35. Pantelis C, Brewer WJ. Neurocognitive and neurobehavioural patterns and the syndromes of schizophrenia: role of frontal–subcortical networks. In Pantelis C, Nelson HE, Barnes TR (eds) *Schizophrenia: A Neuropsychological Perspective* (Chichester: John Wiley & Sons, 1996): 317–43.

36. Weinberger DR. Anteromedial temporal-prefrontal connectivity: a functional neuroanatomical system implicated in schizophrenia. In Carroll B, Barrett J (eds) *Psychopathology and the Brain* (New York: Raven Press, 1991): 25–43.

37. Fletcher PC. The missing link: a failure of fronto-hippocampal integration in schizophrenia. *Nature Neurosci* (1998) **1:** 266–7.

38. Andreasen NC, O'Leary DS, Cizadlo T et al. Schizophrenia and cognitive dysmetria: a positron-emission tomography study of dysfunctional prefrontal–thalamic–cerebellar circuitry. *Proc Natl Acad Sci USA* (1996) **93:** 9985–90.

39. Andreasen NC, Paradiso S, O'Leary DS. 'Cognitive dysmetria' as an integrative theory of schizophrenia: a dysfunction in cortical–subcortical–cerebellar circuitry? *Schizophr Bull* (1998) **24:** 203–18.

40. Spence SA, Brooks DJ, Hirsch SR et al. A PET study of voluntary movement in schizophrenic patients experiencing passivity

phenomena (delusions of alien control). *Brain* (1997) **120:** 1997–2011.

41. Maruff P, Currie J. Abnormalities of motor imagery associated with passivity phenomena in patients with schizophrenia. *Schizophr Res* (2001) (in press).

42. Roberts AC, Robbins TW, Weiskrantz L. *The Prefrontal Cortex* (Oxford: Oxford University Press, 1998).

43. Buchsbaum MS. The frontal lobes, basal ganglia, temporal lobes as sites for schizophrenia. *Schizophr Bull* (1990) **16:** 379–90.

44. Collinson SL, Pantelis C, Barnes TR. Abnormal involuntary movements in schizophrenia and their association with cognitive impairment. In Pantelis C, Nelson HE, Barnes TR (eds) *Schizophrenia: A Neuropsychological Perspective* (London: John Wiley & Sons, 1996): 237–58.

45. Early TS, Reiman EM, Raichle ME, Spitznagel EL. Left globus pallidus abnormality in never medicated patients with schizophrenia. *Proc Natl Acad Sci USA* (1987) **84:** 561–3.

46. Frith CD, Done DJ. Towards a neuropsychology of schizophrenia. *Br J Psychiatry* (1988) **153:** 437–43.

47. Buchsbaum MS, Potkin SG, Siegel BV Jr et al. Striatal metabolic rate and clinical response to neuroleptics in schizophrenia. *Arch Gen Psychiatry* (1992) **49:** 966–74.

48. Siegel BV, Buchsbaum MS, Bunney WE et al. Cortical–striatal–thalamic circuits and brain glucose metabolic activity in 70 unmedicated male schizophrenic patients. *Am J Psychiatry* (1993) **150:** 1325–36.

49. Andreasen NC, Ehrhardt JC, Swayze VW et al. Magnetic resonance imaging of the brain in schizophrenia. The pathophysiologic significance of structural abnormalities. *Arch Gen Psychiatry* (1990) **47:** 35–44.

50. Andreasen NC, Arndt S, Swayze V et al. Thalamic abnormalities in schizophrenia visualized through magnetic resonance image averaging. *Science* (1994) **266:** 294–8.

51. Alexander G, DeLong M, Strick P. Parallel organization of functionally segregated circuits linking basal ganglia and cortex. *Annu Rev Neurosci* (1986) **9:** 357–81.

52. Cummings JL. Frontal–subcortical circuits and human behaviour. *Arch Neurol* (1993) **50:** 873–80.

53. Duffy JD, Campbell JJ. The regional prefrontal syndromes: a theoretical and clinical overview. *J Neuropsychiatry Clin Neurosci* (1994) **6:** 379–87.

54. Mega MS, Cummings JL. Frontal–subcortical circuits and neuropsychiatric disorders. *J Neuropsychiatry Clin Neurosci* (1994) **6:** 358–70.

55. Purcell R, Maruff P, Kyrios M, Pantelis C. Neuropsychological deficits in obsessive-compulsive disorder: a comparison with unipolar depression, panic disorder and normal controls. *Arch Gen Psychiatry* (1998) **55:** 415–23.

56. Henderson L, Crawford T, Kennard C. Neuropsychology of eye movement abnormalities in schizophrenia. In Pantelis C, Nelson HE, Barnes TR (eds) *Schizophrenia: A Neuropsychological Perspective* (Chichester: John Wiley & Sons, 1996): 259–77.

57. Maruff P, Currie J. Neuropsychology of visual attentional deficits in schizophrenia. In Pan-

telis C, Nelson HE, Barnes TR (eds) *Schizophrenia: A Neuropsychological Perspective* (Chichester: John Wiley & Sons, 1996): 87–105.

58. Frith C. *The Cognitive Neuropsychology of Schizophrenia* (Lawrence Erlbaum Associates, 1993).

59. Cahill C, Frith C. A cognitive basis for the signs and symptoms of schziophrenia. In Pantelis C, Nelson HE, Barnes TR (eds) *Schizophrenia: A Neuropsychological Perspective* (Chichester: John Wiley & Sons, 1996): 373–95.

60. Weinberger DR, Berman KF, Zec RF. Physiologic dysfunction of dorsolateral prefrontal cortex in schizophrenia. I. Regional cerebral blood flow evidence. *Arch Gen Psychiatry* (1986) **43:** 114–24.

61. Berman KF, Zec RF, Weinberger DR. Physiologic dysfunction of dorsolateral prefrontal cortex in schizophrenia. II. Role of neuroleptic treatment, attention, and mental effort. *Arch Gen Psychiatry* (1986) **43:** 126–35.

62. Berman KF, Illowsky BP, Weinberger DR. Physiological dysfunction of dorsolateral prefrontal cortex in schizophrenia. IV. Further evidence for regional and behavioral specificity. *Arch Gen Psychiatry* (1988) **45:** 616–22.

63. Weinberger DR, Berman KF, Illowsky BP. Physiological dysfunction of dorsolateral prefrontal cortex in schizophrenia. III. A new cohort and evidence for a monoaminergic mechanism. *Arch Gen Psychiatry* (1988) **45:** 609–15.

64. Bertolino A, Knable MB, Saunders RC et al. The relationship between dorsolateral prefrontal N-acetylaspartate measures and striatal dopamine activity in schizophrenia. *Biol Psychiatry* (1999) **45:** 660–7.

65. Keefe RSE. Working memory dysfunction and its relevance in schizophrenia. In Sharma T, Harvey PD (eds) *Cognition in Schizophrenia: Characteristics, Correlates, and Treatment* (Oxford: Oxford University Press, 2000): 16–49.

66. Partiot A, Verin M, Pillon B et al. Delayed response tasks in basal ganglia lesions in man: further evidence for a striato-frontal cooperation in behavioural adaptation. *Neuropsychologia* (1996) **34:** 709–21.

67. Verin M, Partiot A, Pillon B et al. Delayed response tasks and prefrontal lesions in man — evidence for self generated patterns of behaviour with poor environmental modulation. *Neuropsychologia* (1993) **31:** 1379–96.

68. Owen AM, Stern CE, Look RB et al. Functional organization of spatial and nonspatial working memory processing within the human lateral frontal cortex. *Proc Natl Acad Sci USA* (1998) **95:** 7721–6.

69. Stern CE, Owen AM, Tracey I et al. Activity in ventrolateral and mid-dorsolateral prefrontal cortex during nonspatial visual working memory processing: evidence from functional magnetic resonance imaging. *NeuroImage* (2000) **11:** 392–9.

70. Owen AM, Evans AC, Petrides M. Evidence for a two-stage model of spatial working memory processing within the lateral frontal cortex: a positron emission tomography study. *Cereb Cortex* (1996) **6:** 31–8.

71. Goldman-Rakic PS. Circuitry of primate prefrontal cortex and regulation of behavior by representational memory. In Blum F (ed.) *Handbook of Physiology:*

The Nervous System (Bethesda MD: American Psychological Society, 1987): 373–417.

72. Goldman-Rakic PS, Friedman HR. The circuitry of working memory revealed by anatomy and metabolic imaging. In Levin HS, Eisendberg HM, Benton AL (eds) Frontal Lobe Function and Dysfunction (Oxford: Oxford University Press, 1991): 72–91.

73. Owen AM, Downes JJ, Sahakian BJ et al. Planning and spatial working memory following frontal lobe lesions in man. Neuropsychologia (1990) 28: 1021–34.

74. Owen AM, James M, Leigh PN et al. Fronto-striatal cognitive deficits at different stages of Parkinson's disease. Brain (1992) 115: 1727–51.

75. Owen AM, Morris RG, Sahakian BJ et al. Double dissociations of memory and executive functions in working memory tasks following frontal lobe excisions, temporal lobe excisions or amygdalo-hippocampectomy in man. Brain (1996) 119: 1597–615.

76. Owen AM, Iddon JL, Hodges JR et al. Spatial and non-spatial working memory at different stages of Parkinson's disease. Neuropsychologia (1997) 35: 519–32.

77. Robbins TW, James M, Lange KW et al. Cognitive performance in multiple system atrophy. Brain (1992) 115: 271–91.

78. Robbins TW, James M, Owen AM et al. Cognitive deficits in progressive supranuclear palsy, Parkinson's disease, and multiple system atrophy in tests sensitive to frontal lobe dysfunction. J Neurol Neurosurg Psychiatry (1994) 57: 79–88.

79. Frith C, Dolan R. The role of the prefrontal cortex in higher cognitive functions. Brain Res Cogn Brain Res (1996) 5: 175–81.

80. Raine A, Lencz T, Reynolds GP et al. An evaluation of structural and functional prefrontal deficits in schizophrenia: MRI and neuropsychological measures. Psychiatry Res (1992) 45: 123–37.

81. Park S, Holzman PS. Schizophrenics show spatial working memory deficits. Arch Gen Psychiatry (1992) 49: 975–82.

82. Partiot A, Jouvent R, Dubois B et al. Cortical dysfunction and schizophrenic deficit: preliminary findings with the delayed reaction paradigm. Eur Psychiatry (1992) 7(4): 171–5.

83. Keefe RS, Roitman SE, Harvey PD et al. A pen-and-paper human analogue of a monkey prefrontal cortex activation task: spatial working memory in patients with schizophrenia. Schizophr Res (1995) 17: 25–33.

84. Brewer WJ, Edwards J, Anderson V et al. Neuropsychological, olfactory, and hygiene deficits in men with negative symptom schizophrenia. Biol Psychiatry (1996) 40: 1021–31.

85. Keefe RS, Lees-Roitman SE, Dupre RL. Performance of patients with schizophrenia on a pen and paper visuospatial working memory task with short delay. Schizophr Res (1997) 26: 9–14.

86. Fleming K, Goldberg TE, Binks S et al. Visuospatial working memory in patients with schizophrenia. Biol Psychiatry (1997) 41: 43–9.

87. Pantelis C, Barnes TRE, Nelson HE et al. Frontal-striatal cognitive deficits in patients with chronic schizophrenia. Brain (1997) 120: 1823–43.

88. Hutton SB, Puri BK, Duncan LJ et al. Executive function in first-episode schizophrenia. Psychol Med (1998) 28: 463–73.

89. Bertolino A, Esposito G, Callicott JH et al. Specific relationship between prefrontal neuronal N-acetylaspartate and activation of the working memory cortical network in schizophrenia. *Am J Psychiatry* (2000) **157:** 26–33.

90. Randolph C, Gold JM, Carpenter CJ et al. Release from proactive interference: determinants of performance and neuropsychological correlates. *J Clin Exp Neuropsychol* (1992) **14:** 785–800.

91. Fleming K, Goldberg TE, Gold JM, Weinberger DR. Verbal working memory dysfunction in schizophrenia: use of a Brown–Peterson paradigm. *Psychiatry Res* (1995) **56:** 155–61.

92. Robbins TW, James M, Owen AM et al. Cambridge Neuropsychological Test Automated Battery (CANTAB): a factor analytic study of a large sample of normal elderly volunteers. *Dementia* (1994) **5:** 266–81.

93. Owen AM, Roberts AC, Hodges JR et al. Contrasting mechanisms of impaired attentional set-shifting in patients with frontal lobe damage or Parkinson's disease. *Brain* (1993) **116:** 1159–75.

94. Petrides M. Frontal lobes and working memory: evidence from investigations of the effects of cortical excisions in nonhuman primates. In Boller F, Grafman J (eds) *Handbook of Neuropsychology* (Amsterdam: Elsevier, 1994): 59–82.

95. Milner B. Effects of different brain lesions on card sorting. *Arch Neurol* (1963) **9:** 307–16.

96. Kolb B, Whishaw IQ. Performance of schizophrenic patients on tests sensitive to left or right frontal temporal, or parietal function in neurological patients. *J Nerv Ment Dis* (1983) **171:** 435–43.

97. Goldberg TE, Weinberger DR, Berman KF et al. Further evidence for dementia of the prefrontal type in schizophrenia? A controlled study of teaching the Wisconsin Card Sorting Test. *Arch Gen Psychiatry* (1987) **44:** 1008–14.

98. Morice R, Delahunty A. Frontal/executive impairments in schizophrenia. *Schizophr Bull* (1996) **22:** 125–37.

99. Corcoran R, Upton D. A role for the hippocampus in card sorting? *Cortex* (1993) **29:** 293–304.

100. Elliott R, McKenna PJ, Robbins TW, Sahakian BJ. Neuropsychological evidence for frontostriatal dysfunction in schizophrenia. *Psychol Med* (1995) **25:** 619–30.

101. Pantelis C, Barber FZ, Barnes TR et al. Comparison of set-shifting ability in patients with chronic schizophrenia and frontal lobe damage. *Schizophr Res* (1999) **37:** 251–70.

102. Downes JJ, Roberts AC, Sahakian BJ et al. Impaired extra-dimensional shift performance in medicated and unmedicated Parkinson's disease: evidence for a specific attentional dysfunction. *Neuropsychologia* (1989) **27:** 1329–43.

103. Lawrence AD, Sahakian BJ, Hodges JR et al. Executive and mnemonic functions in early Huntington's disease. *Brain* (1996) **119:** 1633–45.

104. Blumer D, Benson DF. Personality changes with frontal and temporal lobe lesions. In Benson DF, Blumer D (eds) *Psychiatric Aspects of Neurologic Disease* (New York, Grune & Stratton, 1975): 151–70.

105. Lhermitte F. Human autonomy and the frontal lobes. Part II: Patient behavior in complex and

social situations: the 'environmental dependency syndrome'. *Ann Neurol* (1986) **19:** 335–43.

106. Rudd R, Maruff P, MacCupsie-Moore C et al. Stimulus relevance in eliciting utilisation behaviour case study in a patient with a caudate lesion. *Cogn Neuropsychiatry* (1998) **3:** 287–98.

107. Maruff P, Pantelis C, Danckert J et al. Deficits in the endogenous redirection of covert visual attention in chronic schizophrenia. *Neuropsychologia* (1996) **34:** 1079–84.

108. Downing ME, Phillips JG, Bradshaw JL et al. Cue dependent right hemineglect in schizophrenia: a kinematic analysis. *J Neurol Neurosurg Psychiatry* (1998) **65:** 454–9.

109. Damasio AR. *Descartes' Error: Emotion, Reason, and the Human Brain* (New York: Grosset/Putnam, 1994).

110. Malloy P, Bihrle A, Duffy J, Cimino C. The orbitomedial frontal syndrome. *Arch Clin Neuropsychol* (1993) **8:** 185–201.

111. Laiacona M, De Santis A, Barbarotto R et al. Neuropsychological follow-up of patients operated for aneurysms of anterior communicating artery. *Cortex* (1989) **25:** 261–73.

112. Oscar-Berman M, McNamara P, Freedman M. Delayed-response tasks: parallels between experimental ablation studies and findings in patients with frontal lesions. In Levin HS, Eisenberg HM, Benton AL (eds) *Frontal Lobe Function and Dysfunction* (New York: Oxford University Press, 1991): 230–55.

113. Oscar-Berman M. Clinical and experimental approaches to varieties of memory. *Int J Neurosci* (1991) **58:** 135–50.

114. Mishkin M, Vest B, Waxler M, Rosvold HE. A re-examination of the effects of frontal lesions on object alternation. *Neuropsychologia* (1969) **7:** 357–63.

115. Freedman M. Object alternation and orbitofrontal system dysfunction in Alzheimer's and Parkinson's disease. *Brain Cogn* (1990) **14:** 134–43.

116. Pantelis C, Brewer WJ, Maruff P. Olfactory cortex. In Craighead WE, Nemeroff C (eds) *Encyclopedia of Psychology and Neuroscience* (Chichester: John Wiley & Sons, 2000).

117. Bechara A, Damasio H, Damasio AR. Emotion, decision making and the orbitofrontal cortex. *Cereb Cortex* (2000) **10:** 295–307.

118. Bechara A, Damasio H, Damasio AR, Lee GP. Different contributions of the human amygdala and ventromedial prefrontal cortex to decision-making. *J Neurosci* (1999) **19:** 5473–81.

119. Wilder KE, Weinberger DR, Goldberg TE. Operant conditioning and the orbitofrontal cortex in schizophrenic patients: unexpected evidence for intact functioning. *Schizophr Res* (1998) **30:** 169–74.

120. Mesulam MM. Spatial attention and neglect: parietal, frontal and cingulate contributions to the mental representation and attentional targeting of salient extrapersonal events. *Philos Trans R Soc Lond B* (1999) **354:** 1325–46.

121. Benes FM, Sorensen I, Vincent SL et al. Increased density of glutamate-immunoreactive vertical processes in superficial laminae in cingulate cortex of schizophrenic brain. *Cereb Cortex* (1992) **2:** 503–12.

122. Benes FM. Emerging principles of altered neural circuitry in schizophrenia. *Brain Res Rev* (2000) **31:** 251–69.

123. Devinsky O, Morrell MJ, Vogt

BA. Contributions of anterior cingulate cortex to behaviour. *Brain* (1995) **118:** 279–306.

124. Damasio AR, van Hoesen GW. Focal lesions of the limbic frontal lobe. In Heilman KM, Satz P (eds) *Neuropsychology of Human Emotion* (New York: Guilford Press, 1983): 85–110.

125. Yucel M, Stuart G, Velakoulis D et al. Hemispheric asymmetries and gender differences in the organisation of the anterior cingulate cortex in normal volunteers: a neuroimaging study. *Cereb Cortex* (2000) (in press).

126. Yucel M, Stuart G, Velakoulis D et al. Morphological organisation in the anterior cingulate cortex: lack of hemispheric asymmetry differences in chronic schizophrenia versus normal control subjects. *Schizophr Res* (1999) **36:** 215 (abstract).

127. Pardo J, Pardo P, Janer K, Raichle ME. The anterior cingulate mediates processing selection in the Stroop attentional conflict syndrome. *Proc Nat Acad Sci* (1990) **87:** 256–9.

128. Bench CJ, Frith CD, Grasby PM et al. Investigations of the functional anatomy of attention using the Stroop test. *Neuropsychologia* (1993) **31:** 907–22.

129. Liddle PF, Morris DL. Schizophrenic syndromes and frontal lobe performance. *Br J Psychiatry* (1991) **158:** 340–5.

130. Joyce EM, Collinson SL, Crichton P. Verbal fluency in schizophrenia: relationship with executive function, semantic memory and clinical alogia. *Psychol Med* (1996) **26:** 39–49.

131. Liddle PF, Friston KJ, Frith CD, Frackowiak RS. Cerebral blood flow and mental processes in schizophrenia. *J R Soc Med* (1992) **85:** 224–7.

132. Carter CS, Mintun M, Nichols T, Cohen JD. Anterior cingulate gyrus dysfunction and selective attention deficits in schizophrenia: [^{15}O]H$_2$O PET study during single-trial Stroop task performance. *Am J Psychiatry* (1997) **154:** 1670–5.

133. Horwitz B, Tagamets MA, McIntosh AR. Neural modeling, functional brain imaging, and cognition. *Trends Cogn Sci* (1999) **3:** 91–8.

134. Aleman A, Hijman R, de Haan EH, Kahn RS. Memory impairment in schizophrenia: a meta-analysis. *Am J Psychiatry* (1999) **156:** 1358–66.

135. Harrison PJ. The neuropathology of schizophrenia: a critical review of the data and their interpretation. *Brain* (1999) **122:** 593–624.

136. Suddath RL, Christison GW, Torrey EF et al. Anatomical abnormalities in the brains of monozygotic twins discordant for schizophrenia. *N Engl J Med* (1990) **322:** 789–94.

137. Weinberger DR, Berman KF, Suddath RL, Torrey EF. Evidence of dysfunction of a prefrontal–limbic network in schizophrenia: an MRI and regional cerebral blood flow study of discordant monozygotic twins. *Am J Psychiatry* (1992) **149:** 890–7.

138. Goldman-Rakic PS. Prefrontal cortical dysfunction in schizophrenia: the relevance of working memory. In Carroll B, Barrett J (eds) *Psychopathology and the Brain* (New York: Raven Press, 1991): 1–23.

139. Goldman-Rakic PS. Circuitry of the prefrontal cortex and the regulation of behaviour by representational knowledge. In Plum F, Mountcastle V (eds) *Handbook of Physiology*, Vol. 5 (Bethesda, MD: American Physiological Society, 1987): 373–417.

140. Goldman-Rakic PS, Selemon LD. Functional and anatomical aspects of prefrontal pathology in schizophrenia. *Schizophr Bull* (1997) **23:** 437–58.

141. Barbas H, Blatt GJ. Topographically specific hippocampal projections target functionally distinct prefrontal areas in the rhesus monkey. *Hippocampus* (1995) **5:** 511–33.

142. Carmichael S, Price J. Limbic connections of the orbital and medial prefrontal cortex in macaque monkeys. *J Comp Neurol* (1995) **363:** 615–41.

143. Andreasen NC, Rezai K, Alliger R et al. Hypofrontality in neuroleptic-naive patients and in patients with chronic schizophrenia: assessment with [133]xenon single-photon emission computed tomography and the Tower of London. *Arch Gen Psychiatry* (1992) **49:** 943–58.

144. Taylor SF, Kornblum S, Lauber EJ et al. Isolation of specific interference processing in the Stroop task: PET activation studies. *NeuroImage* (1997) **6:** 81–92.

145. Barch DM, Carter CS, Perlstein W et al. Increased stroop facilitation effects in schizophrenia are not due to increased automatic spreading activation. *Schizophr Res* (1999) **39:** 51–64.

146. Perlstein WM, Carter CS, Barch DM, Baird JW. The Stroop task and attention deficits in schizophrenia: a critical evaluation of card and single-trial Stroop methodologies. *Neuropsychology* (1998) **12:** 414–25.

147. Friedman H, Goldman-Rakic PS. Coactivation of prefrontal cortex and inferior parietal cortex in working memory tasks revealed by 2DG functional mapping in the rhesus monkey. *J Neurosci* (1994) **14:** 2775–88.

148. Heckers S, Rauch SL, Goff D et al. Impaired recruitment of the hippocampus during conscious recollection in schizophrenia. *Nature Neurosci* (1998) **1:** 318–23.

149. Malaspina D, Perera G, Lignelli A et al. SPECT imaging of odor identification in schizophrenia. *Psychiatry Res* (1998) **82:** 53–61.

150. Bertolino A, Callicott JH, Elman I et al. Regionally specific neuronal pathology in untreated patients with schizophrenia: a proton magnetic resonance spectroscopic imaging study. *Biol Psychiatry* (1998) **43:** 641–8.

151. Bilder RM, Bogerts B, Ashtari M et al. Anterior hippocampal volume reductions predict frontal lobe dysfunction in first episode schizophrenia. *Schizophr Res* (1995) **17:** 47–58.

152. Seidman LJ, Talbot N, Kalinowski A et al. Neuropsychological probes of fronto-limbic dysfunction in schizophrenia: olfactory identification and Wisconsin Card Sorting performance. *Schizophr Res* (1992) **6:** 55–65.

153. Lawrie SM, Abukmeil SS. Brain abnormality in schizophrenia: a systematic and quantitative review of volumetric magnetic resonance imaging studies. *Br J Psychiatry* (1998) **172:** 110–20.

154. Squire LR, Knowlton BJ. Memory, hippocampus and brain systems. In Gazzaniga MS (ed.) *The Cognitive Neurosciences* (London: MIT Press, 1995): 825–37.

155. Vargha-Khadem F, Gadian DG, Watkins KE et al. Differential effects of early hippocampal pathology on episodic and semantic memory. *Science* (1997) **277:** 376–80.

156. Maguire EA. Hippocampal involvement in human topographical memory: evidence

from functional imaging. *Philos Trans R Soc Lond B* (1997) **352:** 1475–80.

157. Manns JR, Squire LR. Impaired recognition memory on the Doors & People Test after damage limited to the hippocampal region. *Hippocampus* (1999) **9:** 495–9.

158. McDonald B, Highley JR, Walker MA et al. Anomalous asymmetry of fusiform and parahippocampal gyrus gray matter in schizophrenia: a postmortem study. *Am J Psychiatry* (2000) **157:** 40–7.

159. Saykin AJ, Gur RC, Gur RE et al. Neuropsychological function in schizophrenia. Selective impairment of memory and learning. *Arch Gen Psychiatry* (1991) **48:** 618–24.

160. Saykin AJ, Shtasel DL, Gur RE et al. Neuropsychological deficits in neuroleptic naïve patients with first-episode schizophrenia. *Arch Gen Psychiatry* (1994) **51:** 124–31.

161. Riley EM, McGovern D, Mockler D et al. Neuropsychological functioning in first-episode psychosis — evidence of specific deficits. *Schizophr Res* (2000) **43:** 47–55.

162. Rushe T, Woodruff PW, Murray RM, Morris RG. Episodic memory and learning in patients with chronic schizophrenia. *Schizophr Res* (1999) **35:** 85–96.

163. Goldberg TE, Weinberger DR, Pliskin N et al. Recall memory deficit in schizophrenia. A possible manifestation of prefrontal dysfunction. *Schizophr Res* (1989) **2:** 251–7.

164. Bilder RM, Goldman RS, Robinson D et al. Neuropsychology of first-episode schizophrenia: initial characterization and clinical correlates. *Am J Psychiatry* (2000) **157:** 549–59.

165. Hermann BP, Wyler AR, Steenman H, Richey E. The interrelationship between language function and verbal learning/memory performance in patients with complex partial seizures. *Cortex* (1988) **24:** 245–53.

166. Manschreck TC, Maher BA, Candela SF et al. Impaired verbal memory is associated with impaired motor performance in schizophrenia: relationship to brain structure. *Schizophr Res* (2000) **43:** 21–32.

167. Wood AG, Saling MM, O'Shea MF et al. Components of verbal learning and hippocampal damage assessed by T2 relaxometry. *J Int Neuropsychol Soc* (2000) **6:** 525–34.

168. Saling MM, Weintrob D. The functional neuroanatomy of verbal memory in focal epilepsy. *J Int Neuropsychol Soc* (1999) **5:** 274 (abstract).

169. Smith D, Savage G, Saling MM et al. Relational learning and hippocampal volume in chronic schizophrenia. *Schizophr Res* (2000) **41:** 119–20 (abstract).

170. Goldberg TE, Torrey EF, Gold JM et al. Learning and memory in monozygotic twins discordant for schizophrenia. *Psychol Med* (1993) **23:** 71–85.

171. Barr WB. Examining the right temporal lobe's role in nonverbal memory. *Brain Cogn* (1997) **35:** 26–41.

172. Owen AM, Sahakian BJ, Semple J et al. Visuo-spatial short-term recognition memory and learning after temporal lobe excisions, frontal lobe excisions or amygdalo-hippocampectomy in man. *Neuropsychologia* (1995) **33:** 1–24.

173. Fowler KS, Saling MM, Conway EL et al. Computerized neuropsychological tests in the early detection of dementia: prospec-

tive findings. *J Int Neuropsychol Soc* (1997) **3:** 139–46.

174. Schmidt-Kastner R, Freund T. Selective vulnerability of the hippocampus in brain ischemia. *Neuroscience* (1991) **40:** 599–636.

175. Fujioka M, Okuchi K, Hiramatsu K et al. Specific changes in human brain after hypoglycaemic injury. *Stroke* (1997) **28:** 584–7.

176. Katz H, Davies C, Dobbing J. Effects of undernutrition at different ages early in life and later environmental complexity on parameters of the cerebrum and hippocampus in rats. *J Nutr* (1982) **112:** 1362–8.

177. Madeira M, Sousa N, Lima-Andrade M et al. Selective vulnerability of the hippocampal pyramidal neurons to hypothyroidism in male and female rats. *J Comp Neurol* (1992) **322:** 501–18.

178. Wood AG, Saling MM, O'Shea MF et al. Reorganization of verbal memory and language: a case of dissociation. *J Int Neuropsychol Soc* (1999) **5:** 69–74.

179. Bachevalier J, Alvarado MC, Malkova L. Memory and socioemotional behaviour in monkeys after hippocampal damage incurred in infancy or in adulthood. *Biol Psychiatry* (1999) **46:** 329–39.

180. Bachevalier J, Mishkin M. Effects of selective neonatal temporal lobe lesions on visual recognition memory in rhesus monkeys. *J Neurosci* (1994) **14:** 2128–39.

181. Malkova L, Mishkin M, Suomi S, Bachevalier J. Socioemotional behaviour in adult rhesus monkeys after early versus late lesions of the medial temporal lobe. *Ann NY Acad Sci* (1997) **807:** 538–40.

182. Maruff P, Hay D, Malone V, Currie J. Asymmetries in the covert orienting of visual spatial attention in schizophrenia. *Neuropsychologia* (1995) **33:** 1205–23.

183. Cutting J. Evidence for right hemisphere dysfunction in schizophrenia. In Cutting J, David A (eds) *The Neuropsychology of Schizophrenia* (London: Lawrence Erlbaum, 1994).

184. Nasrallah HA. The unintegrated right cerebral hemispheric consciousness as alien intruder: a possible mechanism for Schneiderian delusions in schizophrenia. *Compr Psychiatry* (1985) **26:** 273–82.

185. Mesulam MM. Dissociative states with abnormal temporal lobe EEG. Multiple personality and the illusion of possession. *Arch Neurol* (1981) **38:** 176–81.

186. Critchely M. *The Parietal Lobes* (New York: Hafner Press, 1953).

187. Lieberman J, Bogerts B, Degreef G et al. Qualitative assessment of brain morphology in acute and chronic schizophrenia. *Am J Psychiatry* (1992) **149:** 784–94.

188. Schlaepfer TE, Harris GJ, Tien AY et al. Decreased regional cortical gray matter volume in schizophrenia. *Am J Psychiatry* (1994) **151:** 842–8.

189. Maruff P, Danckert J, Pantelis C, Currie J. Saccadic and attentional abnormalities in patients with schizophrenia. *Psychol Med* (1998) **28:** 1091–100.

190. Colby C, Goldberg ME. Space and attention in parietal cortex. *Annu Rev Neurosci* (1999) **22:** 349

191. Anderson RA, Synder LH, Bradley DC, Xing J. Multimodal representation of space in the posterior parietal cortex and its use in planning movements. *Annu Rev Neurosci* (1997) **20:** 303–30.

192. Heide W, Blankenburg M, Zimmermann E, Kompf D. Cortical control of double-step saccades: Implications for spatial orientation. *Ann Neurol* (1995) **38:** 748

193. Crammond DJ. Motor imagery: never in your wildest dream. *Trends Neurosci* (1997) **20:** 54–7.

194. Jeannerod M. *The Cognitive Neuroscience of Action: Fundamentals of Cognitive Neuroscience* (Oxford: Blackwell, 1997).

195. Frith CD, Blakemore S, Wolpert DM. Explaining the symptoms of schizophrenia: abnormalities in the awareness of action. *Brain Res Rev* (2000) **31:** 357–63.

196. McGuire PK, Frith CD. Disordered functional connectivity in schizophrenia. *Psychol Med* (1996) **26:** 663–7.

197. Sommer MA, Wurtz RH. Composition and topographic organization of signals sent from the frontal eye field to the superior colliculus. *J Neurophysiol* (2000) **83:** 1979–2001.

198. Heit G, Smith ME, Halgren E. Neural encoding of individual words and faces by the human hippocampus and amygdala. *Nature* (1988) **333:** 773–5.

199. Reite M, Teale P, Rojas DC. Magnetoencephalography: applications in psychiatry. *Biol Psychiatry* (1999) **45:** 1553–63.

200. Bush G, Luu P, Posner MI. Cognitive and emotional influences in anterior cingulate cortex. *Trends Cogn Sci* (2000) **4:** 215–22.

201. Ball S, Busatto GF, David AS et al. Cognitive functioning and GABAA/benzodiazepine receptor binding in schizophrenia: a 123I-iomazenil SPET study. *Biol Psychiatry* (1998) **43:** 107–17.

12
Obsessive-compulsive disorder

Paul Maruff, Rosemary Purcell, and Christos Pantelis

Summary

Like most neuropsychiatric disorders, the development of brain–behavior models of obsessive-compulsive disorder (OCD) has been characterized by variability. The variable results are most likely to be due to the small sample sizes that characterize most studies, the large number of comparisons made without adjustment of Type I error rates, and poor inclusion and exclusion criteria. These factors are common in psychiatric research, and their effects in obscuring true differences between the population of patients with OCD and healthy controls are exacerbated by the variability in the presentation of the psychiatric illness itself. However, when the field is viewed from a broader perspective, a convergence of neuropsychological, psychopharmacological, neuroimaging and behavioral approaches becomes evident. The disorder appears to involve both the basal ganglia (specifically the caudate nucleus) and the orbitofrontal cortex (OFC), and probably the direct and indirect interconnections between these two regions. Both the serotonergic and dopaminergic systems are involved in OCD, although, as with the functional neuroimaging studies, it is still difficult to disentangle the relationship between abnormal function, obsessive–compulsive symptoms and general anxiety. Cognitive impairment is subtle in OCD and, in the main, is not characterized by perseverative responding or general failures of inhibition. These impairments can be described parsimoniously as an inability to guide behavior on the basis of an internal and non-verbal representation of the task information. Cognitive impairments become greater and more reliable when neuropsychological task performance depends upon function in the OFC. Interestingly, these tasks also generally contain an emotional or social dimension. Therefore, these factors must be taken into account before more complete brain–behavior models of OCD can be developed. However, advances in the cognitive neuroscience and neuropsychology of emotion and social cognition provide a sound foundation for this endeavor.

Introduction

Obsessive-compulsive disorder is characterized by persistent, unwanted and intrusive thoughts, ideas, impulses or images (obsessions), and repetitive or ritualized behaviors (compulsions), which are performed usually to neutralize the distress associated with obsessive concerns. The American Psychiatric Association's *Diagnostic and Statistical Manual of Mental Disorders* (4th revision)[1] diagnoses OCD by the presence of persistent obsessions and/or compulsions that are ego-dystonic, cause marked distress and are sufficiently severe to interfere with the individual's occupational, social or interpersonal functioning.

Obsessive-compulsive disorder was once considered to be a relatively rare, 'hidden' syndrome,[2] but data from the Epidemiologic Catchment Area (ECA) study indicated the 6-month prevalence of OCD to be 1.6%, with the lifetime prevalence estimated to be as high as 2–3%.[3,4] On the basis of these figures, OCD has been recognized as the fourth most common psychiatric disorder, after substance abuse, simple phobias and major depression.[5] It has recently been suggested, however, that the ECA data may overestimate the true prevalence of the disorder, with data from other epidemiological studies showing that the temporal stability of the OCD diagnosis is low,[6] particularly upon clinical reappraisal of subjects.[7]

Obsessive-compulsive disorder is a heterogeneous disorder in terms of its pattern of onset, symptom presentation, course and response to treatment. The modal age of onset is typically during adolescence and early adulthood, with symptoms developing before the age of 25 in 65% of cases.[8] The majority of patients present with both obsessive and compulsive phenomena,[2] though some experience primary obsessional symptoms in the absence of overt compulsive behaviors. The most common obsessions associated with OCD include thoughts of contamination, disease or illness, and repeated doubts (e.g. wondering whether the door has been locked, or whether an accident has befallen a loved one). Less frequently encountered but no less distressing are obsessions involving aggressive or sexual themes (e.g. physically or sexually abusing one's child), scrupulosity, violent or horrific images (e.g. vivid visual images of oneself being mutilated) and the need for symmetry or perfection. Compulsive behaviors can be both overt and covert in nature, with patients often engaging in surreptitious cognitive rituals (e.g. silent counting or praying), in order to neutralise or suppress obsessional thoughts.[9] Commonly encountered compulsions consist of repeated checking and washing or cleaning behaviors (both of the self and other objects), though counting, repeating actions and ordering rituals also frequently occur.

In addition to obsessions and compulsions, patients often present with phobic avoidance of the situations or stimuli that trigger these phenomena, to the extent that severe anxiety and agoraphobic reactions typically emerge as secondary psychological difficulties.[10] The incidence of major mood disorder associated with OCD has also been noted,[11] with 85% of patients in one study also meeting the criteria for a major depressive episode or dysthymia during their lifetime.[5]

Towards a brain–behavior model of OCD

Although psychoanalytic, cognitive-behavioral and learning theories of OCD abound,[2,12] four lines of evidence indicate that OCD is a brain disorder. First, obsessive and compulsive symptoms can arise following focal brain lesions of the frontal lobes or with neurodegenerative disease involving the basal ganglia. Second, neuroimaging studies have identified abnormalities of brain structure and function in patients with OCD. Third, pharmacological agents such as selective serotonin reuptake inhibitors (SSRIs) reduce the severity of symptoms in patients with OCD, while animal and human studies also suggest a role for dopamine in the disorder. Fourth, neuropsychological studies of OCD demonstrate impairment in cognitive functions that depend upon neurocognitive networks that are distributed across the frontal lobes and basal ganglia. These are now considered in turn.

OCD symptoms in neurological disorders

As early as 1917, Von Ecomono (translated in 1931)[13] reported compulsive behaviors similar to those observed in 'obsessional neurosis' in patients with post-encephalitic Parkinson's disease (PD), an association subsequently replicated by Schilder.[14] Obsessive and compulsive symptoms have also consistently been reported in patients with Gilles de la Tourette's syndrome[15,16] (review: Sheppard et al[17]), Sydenham's chorea,[18] Huntington's disease (HD)[19] and PD.[20] That obsessive or compulsive phenomena are observed in disorders with basal ganglia dysfunction suggests strongly that structural or functional impairment in subcortical regions may also be present in otherwise healthy patients with OCD (review: Rapoport[21]).

The qualitative similarity between the obsessions and compulsions of OCD and the perseverative and stereotypic behaviors that can follow focal lesions of the prefrontal cortex has been noted.[22,23] Typically, patients with OCD know that their thoughts and related actions are inappropriate, illogical or irrational but report that they are unable to inhibit them. Intrusive thoughts and compulsive behaviors have been observed in patients with both diffuse frontal lobe damage and focal lesions of the prefrontal cortex,[23] while stereotaxic lesions of the anterior cingulate (AC) have been found to alleviate OCD symptoms for a significant proportion of patients.[24–26] Soft neurological signs are also increased in these patients. For example, patients with obsessional slowness show hesitancy in movement initiation, a loss of motor fluency and abnormalities of gait.[27] Hollander et al[28,29] also noted abnormalities in fine motor coordination, involuntary and mirror movements and visuospatial function in clinically diagnosed patients relative to matched controls. On the basis of these findings, the frontal cortex and striatum have consistently been proposed as candidate sites of dysfunction in OCD.[30–32]

Neuroimaging studies of OCD

Despite variability in the location, direction (e.g. increase or reduction) and magnitude of structural and functional brain abnormalities identified, two brain regions are continually shown to be involved in OCD. These are the caudate nucleus and the orbitofrontal cortex (OFC). An early study using computerized tomography (CT) identified reduced volume of the caudate nucleus in patients with OCD.[33] More recent studies using magnetic resonance imaging (MRI) have provided inconsistent results regarding the caudate, with reports of both increased[34,35] and reduced[36] volumes. Other structural abnormalities identified have included diffuse reductions in white matter[37,38] and increased ventricular brain ratio.[39] Nonetheless, at least two structural imaging studies have found no differences in overall brain structure between patients and healthy controls.[40,41] Advances in MRI field strength, acquisition sequences and data analytic methods have enabled more fine-grain analysis of brain structure in OCD. A recent MRI study, which used a parcellation analysis based on the sulcal anatomy of the frontal cortex, identified specific volume reductions in orbitofrontal lobes bilaterally in patients with OCD. Interestingly, this orbitofrontal reduction was associated with a reduction in the volume of the amygdala.[42]

Numerous functional neuroimaging studies have investigated cerebral metabolism and regional cerebral blood flow (rCBF) in OCD. One approach has been to determine the distribution of rCBF while patients are 'at rest'. Studies using this paradigm have reported increased activation of the OFC,[43,44] although decreased activation of the OFC and dorsolateral prefrontal cortex (DLPFC) has been reported by others.[45,46] In the study by Lucey et al, increased severity on an 'obsessive and compulsive symptom' dimension was correlated with decreased activation in the left inferior and medial frontal lobes, whereas an 'anxiety and avoidance symptom' dimension was associated with increased activation of the right inferior, right superior, medial frontal and bilateral caudate nuclei.[46] Perani et al[47] found increased activation in the globus pallidus, putamen and AC gyrus. Furthermore, activation of the AC was reduced following successful treatment of OCD symptoms using SSRIs, although there was no change in basal ganglia activity. Similarly, successful treatment with an SSRI was associated with a decrease in levels of activation in the anterolateral OFC and the right caudate nucleus.[48] However, at least one study reported no change in metabolism of any prefrontal region in medicated patients with OCD.[49] Therefore, despite variation in the precise location and laterality of differences, most 'resting state' studies report abnormal metabolism in the prefrontal (especially orbitofrontal) and striatal brain regions when compared to controls. These studies are limited, however, to the extent that they cannot control the mental state of subjects during the imaging procedure. Individual recordings may thus reflect subject idiosyncrasies rather than reflecting illness-related differences. Furthermore, PET images of OCD patients at rest cannot address whether identified abnormalities reflect the presence of OCD phenomena or enduring features of the condition, that is, state or trait abnormalities.[50]

One method used to control the mental state of patients and also to relate patterns of rCBF to specific OCD symptoms is to stimulate individual obsessions or compulsions during the scanning procedure. To date, several studies have used symptom provocation paradigms to study OCD,[50–53] most reporting increased activation in the OFC, AC and striatum. However, similar patterns of activation are observed in patients with simple phobia when exposed to feared stimuli, suggesting that increased OFC and AC activation is associated with anxiety per se rather than OCD specifically. Further, such provocation studies cannot address whether changes in cerebral activation are related to patients' attempts to resist the urge to obsess or reflect their attempts to suppress thoughts of the feared object during the scanning procedure. For example, in response to tactile stimulation with subject-specific contaminants, patients showed increased activation of the inferior frontal lobe, the AC and striatum.[50,51] Such activation may reflect increased anxiety and/or subjects' cognitions in their attempts to cope with the overwhelming stimuli.

Another approach is to challenge patients with a cognitive activation task that has been found previously to activate brain regions hypothesized to be involved in OCD. One study investigated the functional neuroanatomy associated with the implicit acquisition of a motor skill, a process shown in neuropsychological studies to depend upon the integrity of the basal ganglia. Behavioral data indicated that patients and controls acquired the implicit sequence at the same rates. In controls, this learning was associated with increased rCBF in inferior striatum (bilaterally), whereas the patients showed no striatal activation. Instead, the motor sequence acquisition was associated with increased rCBF in the medial temporal lobe (bilaterally). Thus, patients with OCD could not recruit corticostriatal motor systems for task acquisition and had to rely instead on systems associated with declarative memory and conscious learning.[54] A second study investigated function in the frontal lobe using a phonologically guided word-generation task. Once again, this cognitive task was chosen because of its demonstrated ability to activate frontal lobe areas. Compared to controls, patients with OCD showed a significantly increased bold signal when required to generate words and also when they were required to rest. This suggested that patients with OCD had greater difficulty with the generation of responses as well as in inhibiting these responses once they were no longer required.[55] These data suggest that much will be learned about the neurocognitive basis of OCD through the use of cognitive tasks which challenge the function of brain regions hypothesized to be involved in OCD.

Finally, the number of functional imaging studies completed with this patient population is noteworthy, given the difficulties inherent in scanning patients with OCD, many of whom suffer contamination fears or obsessions regarding illness (eg. cancer), and for whom the prospect of exposure to radiation can be intensely fear-provoking. It is therefore unlikely that the patient groups who have participated in these studies are representative of the general OCD population, given the under-representation of those with contamination fears.

Role of serotonin and dopamine in OCD

Current evidence suggests that serotonin (5-HT) systems are dysfunctional in OCD. Thus, symptoms of OCD are reduced following treatment with SSRIs (e.g. fluvoxamine), but not by drugs that primarily inhibit the reuptake of dopamine or noradrenaline.[56–59] In addition to the SSRIs, the severity of both obsessive and compulsive symptoms is reduced following treatment with the tricyclic antidepressant clomipramine, which has activity at serotonin sites.[59,60] OCD symptoms have been shown to be exacerbated by the serotonin agonist *m*-chlorophenylpiperazine (m-CPP).[61,62] Furthermore, the effects of serotonin agonists on symptoms can be blocked by serotonin antagonists with actions on the $5-HT_1$ and $5-HT_2$ receptors (e.g. metergoline).[63]

Despite the clinical efficacy of SSRIs, there is still debate about the role of serotonin in OCD. For example, despite adequate trials of SSRIs, the clinical profile of 40–60% of patients remains unchanged. In addition, most patients who do respond are left with residual symptoms. Some studies have been unable to replicate the exacerbation of OCD symptoms following administration of m-CPP,[64] while administration of m-CPP to healthy controls increases *anxiety* symptoms but does not induce obsessive or compulsive behaviors.[62,65] Serotonin may therefore underlie anxiety processes, which are related to the exaggerated response of patients with OCD to m-CPP.[66] This hypothesis is supported by data showing that SSRIs alleviate symptoms in individuals with anxiety disorders as well as OCD.[66] Finally, markers of the function of serotoninergic systems are generally within normal limits in unmedicated patients with OCD.[31,67] The partial efficacy of SSRIs in OCD suggests that the main effect may be through modulation of other neurotransmitter systems. Based on known interactions between the dopamine and serotonin neurotransmitter systems, dopamine has emerged as a candidate. Dopamine was originally implicated in OCD following the observation that OCD symptoms are frequently present in neuropsychiatric disorders involving dopamine-rich regions of the basal ganglia and its frontal connections. Since then, a number of lines of evidence have confirmed its involvement. These include animal models of OCD based on hoarding behavior, which has been linked to dopamine systems,[68] worsening of OCD symptoms following administration of the dopamine agonists cocaine and amphetamine,[69] the finding of elevated platelet levels of the dopamine enzyme sulfotransferase in patients with OCD,[70] increased urinary excretion of the dopaminergic metabolite homovanillic acid in unmedicated OCD patients,[71] and blunted growth hormone response to apomorphine in OCD.[72] Further, neurophysiological studies of sensory gating mechanisms have found reduced prepulse inhibition in OCD,[73] which also occurs in healthy humans following administration of dopamine agonists.[74] However, while these studies suggest a role for dopamine in the etiology of OCD, they do not indicate which subfamily of dopamine receptors (D1 or D2) may be involved. Further, known interactions between dopamine and serotonin systems would implicate both neurotransmitter systems as important in this disorder and its treatment. The involvement of dopaminergic neurotransmitter systems may have direct implications for understanding the neuropsychological profile of deficits seen in OCD, particularly the findings of visuospatial working memory deficits described below.

Neuropsychological studies of OCD

Neuropsychological studies inform brain–behavior models of OCD in two ways. First, patterns of impaired performance can suggest or confirm the involvement of specific brain areas or functional networks in the pathophysiology of OCD. Second, neuropsychological tests can elucidate information-processing characteristics which may contribute to the maintenance of the disorder.[75] Like neuroimaging and neuropharmacological studies, neuropsychological investigations of OCD have also provided variable results with respect to precisely what functions are impaired in OCD and to what extent any such functions are impaired. However, when these studies are considered together, two consistent deficits are evident. These are impairments on tests that require visual memory and cognitive set-shifting.

Table 12.1 summarizes the findings from most neuropsychological studies of OCD conducted to date. The results of earlier studies, such as those by Flor-Henry et al,[76] Insell et al,[77] Behar et al,[39] and Head et al,[78] were inconsistent in many cases in terms of both the nature and laterality

Table 12.1 Summary of neuropsychological studies of OCD

Study	Sample	Neuropsychological tests	Main finding in OCD	Inference
Flor Henry et al (1979)[76]	11 OCD 11 Control (6 OCD patients with depression or anxiety)	Halstead–Reitan Battery WAIS-R	Bilateral frontal, temporal and parietal dysfunction (L>R). Impairment on Digit Symbol and Digit Span tests	Dominant (left) hemisphere dysfunction, predominantly frontal lobe
Insel et al (1983)[77]	18 OCD No control group (depression/anxiety present in OCD group)	Halstead–Reitan Battery WAIS-R	Impairment on non-visuospatial task. WAIS verbal scores > performance scores in 9 patients	Right-hemisphere dysfunction. Also effect of anxiety and depression
Behar et al (1984)[39]	16 OCD 16 matched controls 3/17 MDD	MRMT, SM, list-learning ROCFT, diphatic testing, reaction time, 2 Flash Threshold	Deficits in SM learning, MRMT. 'Immature' approach on ROCF. No memory deficits	Frontal lobe dysfunction
Malloy (1987)[80]	17 OCD No control group	WCST, FAS, Letter Vigilance, WAIS-R, WMS-R, Boston Naming Test, LOT	Impairment on WCST, above-average scores on attention and intelligence measures	Frontal lobe dysfunction
Head et al (1989)[78]	15 OCD (all unmedicated) 15 matched controls	LOT, BD, WCST, WF, MRMT, SPOT, SMT	Impairments on WCST, MRMT, WF and Block Design, no impairment in spatial, intellectual or attentional functions	Inability to shift cognitive set and difficulties in manipulating information due to frontal lobe dysfunction
Martinot et al (1990)[45]	14 OCD 17 controls	FAS, Mental Control, Stroop, ROCFT, RAVLT, SCT, GAST, DSF, DSB, TMT	Impairment on attentional and memory tasks (require more time). Impairment in naming colors and color words on Stroop task	Frontal lobe dysfunction. Restricted capacity to inhibit immediate but inappropriate response

Study	Sample	Tests	Findings	Conclusion
Hollander et al (1990)[28]	41 OCD 20 matched controls	Motor and sensory tasks Visuospatial tasks	Neurological soft signs evident. These correlate with severity of obsession	Right-hemisphere dysfunction
Boone et al (1991)[86]	20 OCD (all unmedicated) 16 matched controls	WAIS-R, WMS, ROCFT, WCST, Stroop, ACT, FAS, DFT, HVOT, Rey Tangled Lines	Subtle impairment in visuospatial function and visual memory. No deficits in executive functions, verbal memory, attention or intellect	Basal ganglia and right-hemisphere dysfunction
Zelinski et al (1991)[87]	21 OCD (pure obsessionals excluded) 21 matched controls	CVLT, CPT, RFT, WCST, Corsi Blocks, DFT, Raven's Progressive Matrices, FAS	Impairments in visuospatial recall, recognition and sequencing. No deficits in verbal or executive functions	Visuospatial and memory deficits due to orbitofrontal dysfunction
Christensen et al (1992)[88]	18 OCD (all unmedicated) 18 matched controls	WAIS-R, WMS, CPAT, Booklet memory test, Porteus Maze, WCST, FAS, DFT, Corsi Blocks, MAB, Purdue Pegboard, TPT	Impairment in reproducing designs, word fluency, category test, recent visual memory. General impairment in response speed. No impairments in verbal functions	Right medial temporal lobe dysfunction + E16
Aronowitz et al (1994)[79]	31 OCD (all unmedicated) 22 matched controls Anxiety/depression NR	WAIS-R, DRST, Memory for Designs Test	Impairments on BVRT, TMT and MFFT. Attentional and intellectual functions normal. Impairments greater in males	Impairments in visual perceptual and visuospatial functions. Impaired set-shifting
Dirson et al (1995)[89]	26 OCD (?medication) 20 matched controls Included patients with depression if secondary to OCD	Raven's Progressive Matrices, Halters KT, SMEB, word stem completion (with free recall)	Impairment in visual short-term memory, verbal memory normal. General response slowing	Impaired visual memory and attention
Martin et al (1995)[92]	18 OCD (all unmedicated) 18 matched controls	Spatial and non-spatial conditional learning task, self-ordered pointing task	Impairments in response latency but not accuracy	Frontostriatal dysfunction

(Contd.)

Table 12.1 continued

Study	Sample	Neuropsychological tests	Main finding in OCD	Inference
Galderesi et al (1995)[91]	22 OCD 22 matched controls	Conditional associative learning task, self-ordered pointing task, block tapping, digit recurring sequences	Impairments on speed but not accuracy of most tasks	Frontostriatal dysfunction
Veale et al (1996)[81]	40 OCD 40 matched controls Anxiety/depression NR	NART, CANTAB: TOL and attentional set-shifting tasks	Normal accuracy on TOL but slowed movement times. Impairment in attentional set-shifting	Frontostriatal dysfunction
Gross-Iseroff et al (1996)[93]	15 OCD (all female) 15 matched controls	Delayed-alternation tests WCST	Increased time and errors on WCST. Increase errors on alternation tasks (correlated with Y-BOCS)	Orbitofrontal dysfunction
Purcell et al (1998)[83]	23 OCD (17 medicated) 23 matched controls	NART, CANTAB: Attentional, Memory and Planning batteries	Impairments in spatial working memory, spatial span and spatial recognition memory Slowed movement times on TOL	Frontostriatal dysfunction
Purcell et al (1998)[82]	30 OCD (23 medicated) 30 panic disorder 20 depression 30 matched controls	NART, CANTAB: Attentional, Memory and Planning batteries	Impairments in spatial working memory, spatial span and spatial recognition memory. Slowed movement times on TOL	Frontostriatal dysfunction
Schmidtke et al (1998)[85]	29 OCD (all unmedicated) 58 matched controls Depression in some OCD patients	Letter and category fluency, Five-point test, DCT, TMT, Stroop, CRT, Concept Formation, TOH, WST, AVLT	Impairments on timed tests of verbal and non-verbal fluency, attentional functions and weight-sorting	Anterior cingulate dysfunction

Study	Sample	Tests	Findings	Conclusion
Savage et al (1999)[95]	20 OCD (all unmediated) 20 matched controls	Rey Figure, WAIS information, vocabulary similarities, visual verbal test, odd man out test, mental rotations test	Immediate non-verbal memory problems in OCD were mediated by impaired organization strategies on initial copy of Rey Figure	Frontostriatal dysfunction
Barnett et al (1999)[94]	20 OCD (13 medicated) 20 matched controls	NART, CANTAB: spatial working memory and spatial recognition test. UPSIT	Impairments in spatial working memory and olfactory identification	Orbitofrontal dysfunction

mNR, not reported; OCD, obsessive compulsive disorder; ? med, medication status not presented; MDD, major depression diagnosed; ACT, Auditory Consonant Trigrams; AVLT, Auditory Verbal Learning Test; BD, Block Design; BVRT, Benton Visual Retention Test; CANTAB, Cambridge Neuropsychological Test Automated Battery; CPAT, Continuous Paired Associate Task; CPT, Continuous Performance Task; CRT, Choice Reaction Time Task; CVLT, California Verbal Learning Task; DCT, Digit Connection Test; DFT, Design Fluency Test; DRST, Delayed Recognition Span Test; FAS, Controlled Word Fluency Test; GAST, Graphic Alternating Sequences Test; HVOT, Hopper Visual Organization Test; Halter's KT, attentional task; LM, Logical Memory subtest from WMS-R; LOT, Bentons Judgment of Line Orientation Test; MAB, Multidimensional Aptitude Test, MFFT, Matching Familiar Figures Test; MRMT, Money Road Map Test; NART, National Adult Reading Test; ROCFT, Rey Osterrieth Complex Figure Test; RFT, Recurring Figures Test; SCT, Stimuli Cancellation Test; SMT, Stylus Maze Test; SMEB, Signoret's Memory Efficiency Battery; SPOT, Semmes Personal Orientation Test; TAT, Thematic Apperception Test; TMT, Trail Making Test; TOH, Tower of Hanoi; TOL, Tower of London; TPT, Tactual Performance Test; VR, Visual Recall; WAIS-R, Weschler Adult Intelligence Scale-Revised; WCST, Wisconsin Card Sorting Test; WF, Word Fluency; WISC, Weschler Intelligence Scale for Children; WMS-R, Weschler Memory Scale-Revised; WST, Weight Sorting Test.

of suggested impairment. Small sample sizes and large test batteries may account for these differences. More recent studies have reported deficits in attentional set-shifting ability, response inhibition, and trial-and-error learning.[45,79–85] Another group of studies, however, has failed to find any evidence of impairments in executive function, instead reporting impairment in visual memory and visuospatial ability.[86–90] Several studies have reported no specific impairment in cognitive function other than a slowing of responses,[91–93] or response-slowing in the presence of other cognitive impairments.[81,83,84]

Although the results of neuropsychological studies have been conflicting, when considered as a group, these studies suggest that the most reliable impairments occur for some executive and visual memory processes, while verbal memory and language remain intact. Inconsistencies in the findings of these studies may be due in part to variations in the methodologies used. For example, many studies have measured performance in only small samples of patients with OCD. This reduces the likelihood of detecting impaired performance in comparison with controls (i.e. reduces statistical power) and thereby decreases the extent to which the results can be generalized to other patients with OCD. Similarly, these studies have also tended to employ large batteries of neuropsychological tests despite small subject groups without adjusting experiment-wise error rates to control for false-positive findings. Other methodological limitations concern the patient groups used. Though major depression is associated with specific neuropsychological impairments, several studies have included patients meeting the clinical criteria for *both* a depressive disorder and OCD. Increased levels of depressive or anxiety symptoms are also associated with poor performance on neuropsychological tests, even if not sufficient to meet clinical diagnostic criteria. Unfortunately, few studies have considered the potential confounding effects of comorbid depression and anxiety symptoms in their OCD cohorts, and therefore the contribution of these symptoms to the pattern of results is unknown. Finally, some studies have failed to specify the exclusion criteria for selecting both the patients and controls. Therefore, in some studies, the pattern of neuropsychological impairment identified in the patients with OCD will have been influenced by some, if not all, of these methodological shortcomings.

In our own series of studies, we have sought to address these limitations by recruiting large groups of patients with OCD, measuring levels of comorbid anxiety and depression in these patients, and excluding patients who meet clinical criteria for any axis I diagnosis. We have also used a series of neuropsychological tests with demonstrated reliability and validity for the assessment of executive function and visual memory, limiting the number of tests employed to protect against false-positive results. The aim of our studies has been to assess whether the cognitive impairment associated with OCD could provide evidence of dysfunction of brain systems and the extent to which the same impairments occurred in other psychiatric patient groups. In one study,[82] performance on a battery of tests measuring attentional set-shifting, planning, spatial working memory and visual recognition memory was compared between 30 patients with OCD, 20 patients with unipolar depression, 30 patients with panic disorder and 30 normal controls. These groups were matched on age, gender, education level, and estimated IQ. The patients with OCD showed selective impairments, not observed in the other patient groups, on the tests of spatial working memory, spatial recognition memory, and the speed of motor initiation and execution during problem-solving. Importantly, not all aspects of executive and visual memory function were impaired in the OCD group, with set-shifting, planning and pattern recognition performance intact. The specificity of this impairment was notable when compared to other studies that have investigated neuropsychological performance in patients with lesions of the frontal lobes or degenerative diseases of the basal ganglia. Where impairments in executive function have been identified in these previous studies, they occur across the planning, set-shifting and spatial working memory aspects of executive function. Another important aspect of the OCD performance was that the magnitude of the deficits detected was mild when compared to the considerable impairment found when patients with lesions of the frontal lobe or basal ganglia have been compared to matched controls. The results of this study have now been replicated in a subsequent neuropsychological investigation using the same test battery in a different group of patients.[94]

An abnormality in forming internal representations in OCD?

Impairments in executive functions in patients with OCD have generally been interpreted as reflecting dysfunction in *inhibitory* areas of the frontal lobes. This is consistent with suggestions that obsessive or compulsive phenomena also reflect a deficit primarily of inhibition.[24,28] However, no studies to our knowledge have attributed poor performance on tests of executive function to an inability to sustain attention, inability to inhibit inappropriate responses or increased distractibility in these patients. Furthermore, the impairments on tests of visual memory and working memory may arise from the same cognitive abnormality. Accordingly, Savage et al[95] have proposed that executive function deficits give rise to impaired visual memory. They argue that impaired executive function decreases the ability of patients to organize non-verbal information during encoding, and, therefore, to recall this information at a later time. An alternative hypothesis proposed by our group[82] is that patients with OCD have difficulty on tasks requiring an internal representation of the task stimuli to achieve the task goal. This hypothesis may account for the selective nature of deficits in executive function observed in patients. For example, on tasks such as the Tower of London planning test or set-shifting tasks, the information necessary to achieve the task goal remains visible throughout. Patients typically have no difficulty in using the stimuli to generate plans or to attend to multiple dimensions simultaneously in order to complete the task. However, success on visual memory tasks requires patients to store a representation of the stimuli (i.e. a memory) and use this to achieve the goal. Similarly, when searching through different locations to find objects on a spatial working memory task, efficiency in achieving the task goal requires that patients form a representation of the locations that they have already searched. There is one important caveat to this hypothesis. As patients with OCD have no difficulty in performing verbal memory or language tasks, the magnitude of performance impairments will decrease or vanish altogether if task stimuli can be stored using verbal representations. Support for the operation of this caveat is found in the report that performance on a non-verbal recognition memory task became impaired in patients with OCD, to a greater extent than in controls, only when verbal mediation was restricted.[86] The notion that forming or using non-verbal internal representations is impaired in OCD is also supported by experiments in which we employed a number of other non-verbal tasks. These include saccade and antisaccade tasks as well as tests of olfactory identification ability, which are described below.

The antisaccade task

One way to determine whether cognitive impairment in OCD arises from deficits in the inhibitory aspects of executive function or reflects difficulties in forming and using internal representations is to challenge patients with a cognitive task that requires both processes. One candidate for this is the antisaccade task. Antisaccades are eye movements made deliberately in the direction opposite to that of a sudden-onset peripheral target. To perform the antisaccade task, subjects must suppress or inhibit a reflexive saccade towards the target, but attend to and use the target's visual information to move their eyes to a symmetrical but unmarked location in the contralateral visual field.[96] Abnormal performance on the antisaccade task is indicated by an increased number of reflexive glances towards the target (antisaccade error rate) or by increased latency in making correct antisaccades. Some of the strongest evidence in support of the hypothesis that patients with OCD have impaired inhibitory function comes from studies using this task.[97,98] These studies found that patients with OCD make an increased number of incorrect reflexive glances towards the peripheral targets.

As antisaccades must be made to a target location that is not visible, impaired performance on the antisaccade task in patients with OCD may reflect difficulties in using an internal representation of the saccade goal, rather than a difficulty in inhibiting reflexive saccades. If this were the case, then impaired performance should occur on any ocular motor task that requires saccades to be executed to goal locations that are represented internally, irrespective of the requirement for inhibition. We tested this hypothesis using three saccadic tasks in patients with OCD.[99] Patients completed: (1) a visually guided saccade task where the target remained visible until the saccade was completed; (2) a volitionally guided saccade task where the target was extinguished soon after it had appeared and subjects had to make a saccade to the location where it had appeared; and (3) an antisaccade task. There were no differences between groups in performance on the visually guided saccade task. However, the OCD group showed reduced latencies on *both* the volitionally guided saccade task and the antisaccade task, although the magnitude of difference in latency between these two tasks was equal in each group. Thus, the OCD group was slower to assemble saccades to locations where targets were not present, irrespective of whether they were also required to inhibit inappropriate saccades. In fact, the patients with OCD showed no more failures of inhibition than controls. These results are consistent with the hypothesis that patients with OCD have an impairment in forming internal representations of task-relevant stimuli and not a general abnormality of executive function.

Olfactory identification ability in OCD

The data from the antisaccade task suggest that inhibitory processes are not impaired in OCD, at least within the ocular motor system. This accords well with the hypothesis that the area of dysfunction in the frontal cortex in OCD is in the OFC and not in the DLPFC, which is necessary for the inhibitory control of saccades. However, focal lesions of the OFC may also give rise to impairments in inhibition, although these impairments appear to be related more to social behaviors. Interestingly, these inhibitory deficits bear some qualitative similarity to the problems of using internal representations to guide cognitive behaviors in OCD (see Damasio[100]). With focal OFC lesions, patients have difficulty in guiding behavior on the basis of implicit social rules or on the basis of emotional experience.[101] Thus, inhibitory deficits in OCD may be difficult to elicit on conventional neuropsycholgical or ocular motor tasks, whose ability to assess cognitive function objectivity depends on their impersonal or even irrelevant nature. In addition, neuropsychological tasks with sensitivity to OFC function are not well developed. One process that has been associated repeatedly with the normal function of the OFC is olfactory identification. Impairments in olfactory identification are evident in patients with focal lesions of the OFC upon clinical examination using standardized tests.[102–104] Activation of the OFC is observed in normal subjects performing olfactory identification in functional brain imaging experiments.[105,106] Finally, abnormal olfactory identification task performance is correlated with impaired performance on alternation learning tasks, also hypothesized to depend on processing on the OFC.[107] We assessed olfactory identification in patients with OCD and found that this process was considerably impaired. Although patients with OCD could not be classified as having anosmia, the magnitude of the impairment detected was greater than that found in any of our neuropsychological studies.[93] This finding has since been replicated and extended to show that the severity of olfactory impairment identified in this group of patients with OCD was found to correlate with performance on the object alternation task.[108]

Neuropsychology of emotion and OCD

Although brain–behavior models of OCD emphasize dysfunction in frontostriatal networks, the nature of the deficits reported does not necessarily accord with the clinical presentation of the disorder. For example, impaired performance on tests of executive function is qualitatively different to that observed in patients with lesions of the frontal lobes and is not due to perserverative responses, disinhibition or stereotyped responses. In addition, the symptoms of OCD can be so severe that they interfere with an individual's ability to live independently and to maintain employment. However, the magnitude of impaired performance on neuropsychological tasks identified to date has generally been very small. Finally, most studies have failed to find any relationships between the severity of OCD symptoms and the magnitude of impaired performance on neuropsychological tests.

With respect to these points, the recent and dramatic increase in understanding of the neuropsychology of emotion may improve current brain–behavior models of OCD and should also provide a direction for future studies.[100,101] An interesting and important example of this synthesis is found in the studies conducted by Sprenglemeyer and colleagues.[109–111] These studies report that patients with OCD have a specific impairment in the ability to recognize disgust on human faces. They have no difficulty in recognizing expressions of happiness, sadness, fear, anger or surprise and have no problems in understanding the semantic associations of disgust.[109] Surprisingly, patients with HD, a neurodegenerative disorder with a predilection for the caudate nucleus, also showed the specific impairment in recognizing disgust on faces.[110] Even more important for models seeking to link dysfunction of the caudate to OCD was the finding that patients with Huntington's disease are also impaired in olfactory identification.[110] A neuroimaging study by the Sprengelmeyer group, investigating patterns of activation associated with facial expressions of disgust and anger in healthy subjects, reported that, when compared to neutral faces, faces expressing disgust activated the right putamen and left insula cortex specifically. Disgust faces also activated the OFC, although activation of the OFC was also found for facial expressions of anger and fear.[111] The ability to recognize disgust may be part of a common brain system involving the basal ganglia and the OFC.

These findings accord with the impairments in olfactory identification also identified in patients with OCD.[93,108] The control of olfactory identification and disgust recognition by a common brain system is intuitively appealing, as the risk of disease and contamination can be conveyed to individuals both by expressions of disgust on the faces of others and by odors emanating from the source of the risk.[112] Therefore, an abnormality of such a system in OCD also makes intuitive sense, given that contamination is a common feature of OCD symptoms. However, in this context, deficits in recognizing disgust on faces and recognizing odors suggest that there is impaired detection of contamination in OCD, while the increased frequency of cleaning and checking symptoms would suggest a hypersensitivity to such factors. One possible answer for the impairment in recognition of disgust faces is that patients with OCD can feel disgusted when others do not. Therefore, there is little or no correlation between their own feelings of disgust and the facial expressions of disgust in others. This low correlation might then lead to problems in recognizing disgust on the faces of others. Before this explanation can be applied to olfaction, research needs to be performed on emotional responses to different smells. For example, the olfactory identification impairment in OCD may be more acute for disgusting smells than for pleasant smells. Importantly, these data suggest that investigation of emotional and social cognition using cognitive neuroscientific approaches may provide the most complete brain–behavior models for the disorder.

References

1. American Psychiatric Association. *Diagnostic and Statistical Manual of Mental Disorders*, 4th edn. (Washington DC: American Psychiatric Press, 1994): 25–39.

2. Andrews G, Crino R, Hunt C et al. Obsessive compulsive disorder. In Andrews G, Crino R, Hunt C, Lampe L, Page A (eds) *The Treatment of Anxiety Disorders: Clinician's Guide and Patient Manuals* (New York: Cambridge University Press, 1994).

3. Robins LN, Helzer JE, Weissman MM et al. Lifetime prevalence of specific psychiatric disorders in three sites. *Arch Gen Psychiatry* (1984) **41:** 949–58.

4. Reiger DA, Narrow WE, Rae DS. The epidemiology of anxiety disorders: the Epidemiologic

Catchment Area (ECA) experience. *J Psychiatr Res* (1990) **24:** 3–14.

5. Rasmussen SA, Eisen JL. The epidemiology and differential diagnosis of obsessive compulsive disorder. *J Clin Psychiatry* (1992) **53(Suppl):** 4–10.

6. Nelson E, Rice J. Stability of diagnosis of obsessive-compulsive disorder in the Epidemiologic Catchment Area study. *Am J Psychiatry* (1997) **154:** 826–31.

7. Stein MB, Forde DR, Anderson G, Walker JR. Obsessive-compulsive disorder in the community: an epidemiologic survey with clinical reappraisal. *Am J Psychiatry* (1997) **154:** 1120–6.

8. Swoboda KJ, Jenike MA. Frontal abnormalities in a patient with obsessive-compulsive disorder: the role of structural lesions in obsessive-compulsive behavior. *Neurology* (1995) **45:** 2130–4.

9. Foa EB, Tillmans A. The treatment of obsessive compulsive disorder neurosis. In Goldstein A, Foa EB (eds) *Handbook of Behavioral Interventions: A Clinical Guide* (New York: John Wiley, 1980): 173–98.

10. Austin LS, Lydiard RB, Fossey MD, Zealberg JJ. Panic and phobic disorders in patients with obsessive compulsive disorder. *J Clin Psychiatry* (1990) **51:** 456–8.

11. Rasmussen SA, Tsuang MT. Clinical characteristics and family history of DSM-III obsessive compulsive disorder. *Am J Psychiatry* (1986) **143:** 317–22.

12. Salkovskis PM. Obsessions and compulsions. In Scott J, Williams JM, Beck A (eds) *Cognitive Therapy in Clinical Practice* (London: Routledge, 1989): 27–38.

13. von Economo C. *Encephalitis Lethargica, Its Sequellae and Treatment* (London: Oxford University Press, 1931).

14. Schilder P. The organic background of obsessions and compulsions. *Am J Psychiatry* (1938) **94:** 1397–415.

15. Pauls DL, Towbin KE, Leckman JF et al. Gilles de la Tourette's syndrome and obsessive-compulsive disorder: evidence supporting a genetic relationship. *Arch Gen Psychiatry* (1986) **43:** 1180–2.

16. Cummings JL, Frankel M. Gilles de la Tourette syndrome and the neurological basis of obsessions and compulsions. *Biol Psychiatry* (1985) **20:** 1117–26.

17. Sheppard DM, Bradshaw JL, Purcell R, Pantelis C. Tourette's and comorbid syndromes: obsessive-compulsive and attention deficit hyperactivity disorder. A common etiology? *Clin Psychol Rev* (1999) **19:** 531–52.

18. Swedo SE, Rapoport JL, Cheslow DL et al. High prevalance of obsessive-compulsive symptoms in patients with Sydenham's chorea. *Am J Psychiatry* (1989) **146:** 246–9.

19. Cummings JL, Cunningham K. Obsessive-compulsive disorder in Huntington's disease. *Biol Psychiatry* (1992) **31:** 263–70.

20. Tomer R, Levin BE, Weiner WJ. Obsessive-compulsive symptoms and motor asymmetries in Parkinson's disease. *Neuropsychiatry Neuropsychol Behav Neurol* (1993) **6:** 26–30.

21. Rapoport JL. Obsessive compulsive disorder and basal ganglia dysfunction. *Psychol Med* (1990) **20:** 465–9.

22. Ames D, Cummings JL, Wirshing WC et al. Repetitive and compulsive behavior in frontal lobe degenerations. *J Neuropsychiatry Clin Neurosci* (1994) **6:** 100–13.

23. Cummings JL. Frontal–subcortical circuits and human behavior. *Arch Neurol* (1993) **50:** 873–80.

24. Khanna S. Obsessive-compulsive disorder: is there a frontal lobe dysfunction? *Biol Psychiatry* (1988) **24:** 602–13.

25. Baer L, Rauch SL, Ballantine HT et al. Cingulotomy for intractable obsessive-compulsive disorder. Prospective long-term follow-up of 18 patients. *Arch Gen Psychiatry* (1995) **52:** 384–92.

26. Sachdev P, Hay P. Site and size of lesion and psychosurgical outcome in obsessive-compulsive disorder: a magnetic resonance imaging study. *Biol Psychiatry* (1996) **39:** 739–42.

27. Hymas N, Lees A, Bolton D et al. The neurology of obsessional slowness. *Brain* (1991) **114:** 2203–33.

28. Hollander E, Schiffman E, Cohen B et al. Signs of central nervous system dysfunction in obsessive compulsive disorder. *Arch Gen Psychiatry* (1990) **47:** 27–32.

29. Hollander E, Liebowitz MR, Rosen WG. Neuropsychiatric and neuropsychological studies in obsessive compulsive disorder. In Zohar J, Insel T, Rassmussen S (eds) *The Psychobiology of Obsessive Compulsive Disorder* (New York: Springer Publishing, 1991): 201–13.

30. Modell JG, Mountz JM, Curtis GC, Greden JF. Neurophysiologic dysfunction in basal ganglia/limbic striatal and thalamocortical circuits as a pathogenetic mechanism of obsessive-compulsive disorder. *J Neuropsychiatry Clin Neurosci* (1989) **1:** 27–36.

31. Insel TR. Toward a neuroanatomy of obsessive-compulsive disorder. *Arch Gen Psychiatry* (1992) **49:** 739–44.

32. Rauch SL, Jenike MA. Neurobiological models of OCD. *Psychosomatics* (1993) **34:** 20–32.

33. Luxenberg JS, Swedo SE, Flament MF, Friedland RP. Neuroanatomical abnormalities in obsessive-compulsive disorder detected with quantitative X-ray computed tomography. *Am J Psychiatry* (1988) **145:** 1089–93.

34. Calabrese G, Colombo C, Bonfanti G et al. Caudate nucleus abnormalities in obsessive-compulsive disorder: measurements of MRI signal intensity. *Psychiatry Res* (1993) **50:** 89–92.

35. Scarone S, Colombo C, Livian S et al. Increased right caudate nucleus size in obsessive-compulsive disorder: detection with magnetic resonance imaging. *Psychiatry Res* (1992) **45:** 115–21.

36. Robinson D, Wu H, Munne RA, Ashtari M. Reduced caudate nucleus volume in obsessive-compulsive disorder. *Arch Gen Psychiatry* (1995) **52:** 393–8.

37. Brieter HCR, Filipek PA, Kennedy DN et al. Retrocallosal white matter abnormalities in patients with obsessive compulsive disorder. *Arch Gen Psychiatry* (1994) **51:** 663–4.

38. Jenike MA, Breiter HC, Baer L et al. Cerebral structural abnormalities in obsessive compulsive disorder. A quantitative morphometric magnetic resonance imaging study. *Arch Gen Psychiatry* (1996) **53:** 625–32.

39. Behar D, Rapoport JL, Berg CJ et al. Computerized tomography and neuropsychological test measures in adolescents with obsessive-compulsive disorder. *Am J Psychiatry* (1984) **141:** 363–9.

40. Garber HJ, Ananth JV, Chui LC et al. Nuclear magnetic resonance study of obsessive compulsive disorder. *Am J Psychiatry* (1989) **146:** 1001–5.

41. Kellner CH, Jolley RR, Hollgate

RC et al. Brain MRI in obsessive compulsive disorder. *Psychiatry Res* (1991) **36:** 45–9.

42. Szeszko PR, Robinson D, Alvir JMJ et al. Orbital frontal and amygdala volume reductions in obsessive-compulsive disorder. *Arch Gen Psychiatry* (1999) **56:** 913–9.

43. Sawle GV, Hymas NF, Lees AJ, Frackowiak RSJ. Obsessional slowness: functional studies with positron emission tomography. *Brain* (1991) **114:** 2191–202.

44. Rubin RT, Ananth J, Villanueva-Meyer J et al. Regional 133 xenon cerebral blood flow and cerebral 99mTc-HMPAO uptake in patients with obsessive-compulsive disorder before and during treatment. *Biol Psychiatry* (1995) **38:** 429–37.

45. Martinot JL, Allilaire JF, Mazoyer BM et al. Obsessive-compulsive disorder: a clinical, neuropsychological and positron emission tomography study. *Acta Psychiatr Scand* (1990) **82:** 233–42.

46. Lucey JV, Costa DC, Blanes T et al. Regional cerebral blood flow in obsessive-compulsive disordered patients at rest: differential correlates with obsessive-compulsive and anxious-avoidant dimensions. *Br J Psychiatry* (1995) **167:** 629–34.

47. Perani D, Colombo C, Bressi S et al. [18F] FDG PET study in obsessive-compulsive disorder: a clinical/metabolic correlation study after treatment. *Br J Psychiatry* (1995) **166:** 244–50.

48. Saxena S, Brody AL, Schwartz JM, Baxter LR. The neuroimaging of frontal and subcortical circuitry in obsessive compulsive disorder. *Br J Psychiatry* (1998) **173:** 26–37.

49. Edmonstone Y, Austin MP, Prentice N et al. Uptake of TC-99M-Exametazime shown by single photon emission tomography in obsessive compulsive disorder compared with major depression and normal controls. *Acta Psychiatr Scand* (1994) **90:** 298–303.

50. McGuire PK, Bench CJ, Frith CD, Marks IM. Functional anatomy of obsessive-compulsive phenomena. *Br J Psychiatry* (1994) **164:** 459–68.

51. Rauch SL, Jenike MA, Alpert NM et al. Regional cerebral blood flow measured during symptom provocation in obsessive-compulsive disorder using oxygen 15-labeled carbon dioxide and positron emission tomography. *Arch Gen Psychiatry* (1994) **51:** 62–70.

52. Cottraux J, Gerard D, Cinotti L et al. A controlled positron emission tomography study of obsessive compulsive and neutral auditory stimulation in obsessive compulsive disorder with checking rituals. *Psychiatry Res* (1994) **60:** 101–12.

53. Breiter HC, Rauch SL, Kwong KK, Baker JR. Functional magnetic resonance imaging of symptom provocation in obsessive-compulsive disorder. *Arch Gen Psychiatry* (1996) **53:** 595–606.

54. Rauch SL, Savage CR, Alpert NM et al. Probing striatal function in obsessive-compulsive disorder — a PET study of implicit sequence learning. *J Neuropsychiatry Clin Neurosci* (1997) **9:** 568–73.

55. Pujol J, Torres L, Deus J et al. Functional magnetic resonance imaging study of frontal lobe activation during word generation in obsessive-compulsive disorder. *Biol Psychiatry* (1999) **45:** 891–7.

56. Barr LC, Goodman WK, Price LH. The serotonin hypothesis of

obsessive compulsive disorder. *Int J Clin Psychopharmacol* (1993) **8(Suppl 2):** 79–82.

57. Goodman WK, Price LH, Delgardo PL et al. Specificity of serotonin reuptake inhibitors in the treatment of obsessive compulsive disorder: a comparison of fluvozamine and desipramine. *Arch Gen Psychiatry* (1990) **47:** 577–85.

58. Griest JH, Jefferson JW. Pharmacotherapy for obsessive compulsive disorder. *Br J Psychiatry* (1998) **173(suppl 35):** 64–70.

59. Jenicke MA, Baer L, Greist JH. Obsessive compulsive disorder: a double blind trial of clomipramine in 27 patients. *Am J Psychiatry* (1989) **146:** 1328–30.

60. Jenicke MA, Baer L, Greist JH. Clomipramine versus fluoxatine in obsessive compulsive disorder: a retrospective comparison of side effects and efficacy. *J Clin Psychopharmacol* (1990) **10:** 122–4.

61. Hollander E, De Caria CM, Nitescu A et al. Serotoninergic function in obsessive compulsive disorder: Behavioural and neuroendocrine responses to oral m-chlorophenylpiperazine and fenfluramine in patients and healthy volunteers. *Arch Gen Psychiatry* (1992) **49:** 21–8.

62. Zohar J, Insel TR. Obsessive-compulsive disorder: psychobiological approaches to diagnoses, treatment and psychopathology. *Biol Psychiatry* (1987) **22:** 667–87.

63. Piggot TA. Where the serotonin story selectivity story begins. *J Clin Psychiatry* (1996) **57(Suppl 6):** 11–20.

64. Goodman HK, McDougle CJ, Price LH et al. m-Chlorophenylpiperazine in patients with obsessive compulsive disorder. Absence of symptom exacerbation. *Biol Psychiatry* (1995) **38:** 138–49.

65. Mueller EA, Murphy DL, Sunderland T. Further studies of the putative serotonin agonist, m-chlorophenylpiperazine: evidence for a serotonin receptor mediated mechanism of action in humans. *Psychopharmacology* (1986) **89:** 388–91.

66. Crino RD. Obsessive compulsive disorder. *Int Rev Psychiatry* (1991) **3:** 189–201.

67. Thoren P, Asperg M, Bertilsson L et al. Clomipramine treatment of obsessive compulsive disorder, II: Biochemical aspects. *Arch Gen Psychiatry* (1980) **37:** 1289–94.

68. Damecour CL, Charron M. Hoarding: a symptom, not a syndrome. *J Clin Psychology* (1998) **59:** 267–72.

69. McDougle CJ, Goodman WK, Delgado PL, Price LH. Pathophysiology of obsessive-compulsive disorder. *Am J Psychiatry* (1989) **146:** 1350–1.

70. Marazziti D, Hollander E, Lensi P, Ravagli S. Peripheral markers of serotonin and dopamine function in obsessive compulsive disorder. *Psychiatry Res* (1992) **42:** 889–97.

71. Oades RD, Ropcke B, Eggers C. Monoamine activity reflected in the urine of young patients with obsessive compulsive disorder psychosis with and without reality distortion and healthy subjects. *J Neural Transm* (1994) **96:** 143–59.

72. Brambilla F, Bellodi L, Perna G et al. Dopamine function in obsessive compulsive disorder: hormone reponse to apomorphine stimulation. *Biol Psychiatry* (1997) **42:** 889–97.

73. Schall U, Schoen A, Zerbin D et al. Event related potentials dur-

ing an auditory discrimination with prepulse inhibition in patients with schizophrenia, obsessive compulsive disorder and healthy subjects. *Int J Neurosci* (1996) **84:** 15–33.

74. Swerdlow NR, Mansbach RS, Geyer MA et al. Amphetamine disruption of prepulse inhibition of acoustic startle is reversed by depletion of mesolimbic dopamine. *Psychopharmacology* (1990) **100:** 413–6.

75. Otto M. Normal and abnormal information processing: a neuropsychological perspective on obsessive-compulsive disorder. *Psychiatr Clin North Am* (1992) **15:** 825–47.

76. Flor-Henry P, Yeudall LT, Koles KJ, Howarth BG. Neuropsychological and power spectral EEG investigations of the obsessive compulsive syndrome. *Biol Psychiatry* (1979) **14:** 119–29.

77. Insell TR, Donnelly EF, Lalakea ML et al. Neurological and neuropsychological studies of patients with obsessive compulsive disorder. *Biol Psychiatry* (1985) **18:** 741–57.

78. Head D, Bolton D, Hymas N. Deficit in cognitive set shifting ability in patients with obsessive-compulsive disorder. *Biol Psychiatry* (1989) **25:** 929–37.

79. Aronowitz BR, Hollander E, DeCaria C et al. Neuropsychology of obsessive compulsive disorder. *Neuropsychiatry Neuropsychol Behav Neurol* (1994) **7:** 81–6.

80. Malloy P. Frontal lobe dysfunction in obsessive-compulsive disorder. In Perecman F (ed.) *The Frontal Lobes Revisited* (New York: IRBN Press, 1987): 207–23.

81. Veale DM, Sahakian BJ, Owen AM, Marks IM. Specific cognitive deficits in tests sensitive to

frontal lobe dysfunction in obsessive compulsive disorder. *Psychol Med* (1996) **26:** 1216–69.

82. Purcell R, Maruff P, Kyrios M, Pantelis C. Neuropsychological deficits in obsessive compulsive disorder: a comparison with unipolar depression, panic disorder and normal controls. *Arch Gen Psychiatry* (1998) **55:** 415–23.

83. Purcell R, Maruff P, Kyrios M, Pantelis C. Cognitive deficits in obsessive compulsive disorder on tests of frontal–striatal function. *Biol Psychiatry* (1998) **43:** 348–57.

84. Abbruzzese M, Ferri S, Scarone S. Wisconsin Card Sorting Test performance in obsessive-compulsive disorder: no evidence for involvement of dorsolateral prefrontal cortex. *Psychiatry Res* (1995) **58:** 37–43.

85. Schmidtke K, Schorb A, Winkelmann G, Hohagen F. Cognitive frontal lobe dysfunction in obsessive-compulsive disorder. *Biol Psychiatry* (1998) **43:** 666–73.

86. Boone KB, Ananth J, Philpott L et al. Neuropsychological deficits in OCD. *Neuropsychiatry Neuropsychol Behav Neurol* (1991) **4:** 110–21.

87. Zielinski CM, Taylor MA, Juzwin KR. Neuropsychological deficits in obsessive-compulsive disorder. *Neuropsychiatry Neuropsychol Behav Neurol* (1991) **4:** 110–26.

88. Christensen KJ, Kim SW, Dysken MW, Hoover KM. Neuropsychological performance in obsessive-compulsive disorder. *Biol Psychiatry* (1992) **31:** 4–18.

89. Dirson S, Bouvard M, Cottraux J, Martin R. Visual memory impairment in patients with obsessive-compulsive disorder: a

controlled study. *Psychother Psychosomatics* (1995) **63:** 22–31.

90. Savage CR, Keuthen NJ, Jenicke MA et al. Recall and recognition memory in obsessive compulsive disorder. *J Neuropsychiatry* (1996) **8:** 99–103.

91. Galderisi S, Mucci A, Catapano F et al. Neuropsychological slowness in obsessive-compulsive patients: Is it confined to tests involving the fronto-subcortical systems? *Br J Psychiatry* (1995) **167:** 394–8.

92. Martin A, Wiggs CL, Altemus M, et al. Working memory as assessed by subject-ordered tasks in patients with obsessive-compulsive disorder. *J Clin Exp Neuropsychol* (1995) **17:** 786–92.

93. Gross-Isseroff R, Sasson Y, Voet H et al. Alternation learning in obsessive-compulsive disorder. *Biol Psychiatry* (1996) **39:** 733–8.

94. Barnett R, Maruff P, Purcell R et al. Impairment of olfactory identification in obsessive compulsive disorder. *Psychol Med* (1999) **36:** 635–39

95. Savage CR, Baer L, Keuthen NJ et al. Organizational strategies mediate nonverbal memory impairment in obsessive-compulsive disorder. *Biol Psychiatry* (1999) **45:** 905–16.

96. Hallet PE. Primary and secondary saccades to goals defined by instructions. *Vision Res* (1978) **18:** 1279–96.

97. Rosenberg DR, Dick EL, O'Hearn KM, Sweeney JA. Response-inhibition deficits in obsessive compulsive disorder: an indicator of dysfunction in fronto-striatal circuits. *J Psychiatry Neurosci* (1997) **22:** 29–38.

98. Tien AY, Pearlson GD, Machlin SR, Bylsma FW. Oculomotor performance in obsessive-compulsive disorder. *Am J Psychiatry* (1992) **149:** 641–6.

99. Maruff P, Tyler P, Purcell R et al. Abnormalities of internally generated saccades in obsessive compulsive disorder. *Psychol Med* (1999) 11: 342–5.

100. Damasio A. *Descarte's Error: Emotion, Reason and the Human Brain* (New York: Grosset/Putnam, 1994).

101. Adolphs R. Social cognition and the human brain. *Trends Cogn Sci* (1999) **3:** 469–79.

102. Potter H, Butters N. An assessment of olfactory deficits in patients with damage to prefrontal cortex. *Neuropsychologia* (1980) **18:** 621–8.

103. Cicerone KD, Tanenbaum LN. Disturbance of social cognition after traumatic orbitofrontal brain injury. *Arch Clin Neuropsychol* (1997) **12:** 173–88.

104. Varney NR, Bushnell D. Neurospectroscopy findings in patients with posttraumatic anosmia — a quantitative analysis. *J Head Trauma Rehabil* (1998) **13:** 63–72.

105. Sobel N, Prabhakaran V, Desmond JE et al. Sniffing and smelling — separate subsystems in the human olfactory cortex. *Nature* (1998) **392:** 282–6.

106. Levy LM, Henkin RI, Hutter A et al. Functional MRI of human olfaction. *J Computer Assisted Tomography* (1998) **21:** 849–56.

107. Pantelis C, Brewer B. Neuropsychological and olfactory dysfunction in schizophrenia: relationship of frontal syndromes to syndromes of schizophrenia. *Schizophr Res* (1995) **17:** 35–45.

108. Hermesh H, Zohar J, Weizman A et al. Orbitofrontal cortex dysfunction in obsessive-compulsive disorder? II. Olfactory quality discrimination in obsessive-compulsive disorder. *Eur*

Neuropsychopharmacol (1999) **9:** 415–20.

109. Sprengelmeyer R, Young AW, Pundt I et al. Disgust implicated in obsessive-compulsive disorder. *Proc R Soc Lond B* (1997) **264:** 1767–73.

110. Sprengelmeyer R, Young AW, Calder AJ et al. Loss of disgust: perception of faces and emotions in Huntington's disease. *Brain* (1996) **119:** 1647–65.

111. Sprengelmeyer R, Rausch M, Eysel UT, Przuntek H. Neural structures associated with recognition of facial expressions of basic emotions. *Proc R Soc Lond B* (1997) **265:** 1927–31.

112. Rozin P, Lowery L, Ebert R. Varieties of disgust faces and the structure of disgust. *J Personality Social Psychology* (1994) **66:** 870–81.

13
The neuropsychological profile in primary depression

Rebecca Elliott

Summary

This chapter aims to highlight the complexity involved in understanding the neuropsychological profile of depression and to discuss some of the important issues in this area. Evidence suggests that depression is associated with deficits in a range of cognitive domains, including attention, memory and executive function. The impairment tends to be relatively mild compared to that associated with neurological disorders, but is more generalized across domains. However, recent findings have suggested a possible differential sensitivity on effortful executive tasks, dependent on the function of prefrontal cortex. The exact profile of deficit may be influenced by a number of clinical and demographic factors, including severity of depression, patients' age and effects of medication. Neuroimaging evidence, linking neuropsychological deficits to neural substrates, suggests that abnormal functioning of the frontal lobes, and particularly medial prefrontal cortex, may underpin the cognitive impairments, as well as disordered mood, in depression.

Introduction

Ten percent of the population suffers from major depression at some time in their lives, and the disorder is one of the commonest presenting in the primary healthcare sector. Core symptoms of depression are those involving disturbances of mood and affect. DSM-IV[1] lists primary symptoms that include depressed mood, diminished interest and pleasure in most activities, feelings of worthlessness or guilt and various somatic symptoms. Until recently, it was widely believed that even severe depression was associated with only minor neuropsychological impairment.[2] An influential review by Miller[3] challenged this position, concluding that patients showed deficits in a wide range of cognitive domains, a view that is now widely accepted. There is considerable evidence that cognitive function is disrupted; patients presenting with depression frequently list disturbances such as impaired concentration among their symptoms. Systematic neuropsychological investigation has related depression to impairment in many cognitive functions, including attention, memory and executive processing. The majority of these studies reported a generalized profile of impairment, with deficits seen on most tests used. An understanding of these cognitive deficits, and how they relate to mood disorder, has important implications for the study and treatment of depression. In practical terms, impaired cognition may have diagnostic implications, particularly in elderly patients. The cognitive deficits are often very pronounced in elderly patients, affecting everyday social function, and complicating the differential diagnosis of depression and dementia. At a theoretical level, understanding cognitive deficits, and their interaction with affective symptomatology and neural substrates, is essential to a comprehensive understanding of major depression.

Although neuropsychological impairment has been widely studied in unipolar depression, the empirical abundance has not been matched on a theoretical level. There are several fundamental issues with important clinical and theoretical implications. These issues can be subdivided into three general areas. First, it is crucial to try and establish how the neuropsychological deficits in depression may relate to demographic and clinical factors. Second, it remains unclear whether there are specific neuropsychological deficits associated with depression or whether the profile is truly general, perhaps reflecting a basic impairment in, for example, concentration or motivation. Finally, an understanding of how the neuropsychological deficits relate to neuropathology has implications for etiological theories and clinical treatment.

The relationship between symptomatology and neuropsychological performance

Clinical subtypes of depression

It has been argued that depression is not a unitary disorder and it is possible to distinguish various subtypes on the basis of clinical profile. One distinction is between primary depression and depression that is secondary to some other form of disorder. This chapter focuses on the deficits associated with primary depression. Another key distinction is between unipolar (depression alone) and bipolar (depression with mania) depression.

Bipolar patients have been found to show widespread neuropsychological deficits in the manic as well as the depressed phase of their illness.[4–7] In spite of the pronounced differences in clinical presentation, it has in fact proved difficult to distinguish depression and mania on the basis of neuropsychology. Recent evidence, however, suggests that there may be some subtle differences between the two disorders (or two phases of bipolar disorder). Murphy et al[8] confirmed that mania was associated with a generalized profile of impairment similar to that seen in depression. However, they also found that patients with mania were impaired in their ability to inhibit behavioral responses to previously salient stimuli, an impairment also seen in patients with certain forms of frontal lobe damage.[9-10] While this in an interesting finding, further research is necessary to establish the extent to which unipolar and bipolar depression can be neuropsychologically distinguished.

The distinction between unipolar and bipolar depression is universally recognized, but attempts to delineate subtypes within the spectrum of unipolar depression are more controversial. The debate focuses around whether a more severe form of unipolar depression can be clinically distinguished from a milder form. The distinction has been characterized in a number of ways (psychotic/non-psychotic; endogenous/reactive; depression/dysthymia). Attempts to determine the neuropsychological validity of this distinction have been relatively inconclusive, revealing quantitative rather than qualitative differences. For example, Nelson et al[11] demonstrated poorer attentional performance in psychotic depressives than in non-psychotic patients, comparable to that seen in schizophrenia. Similarly, Simpson et al[12] found that psychotic depressives showed more pronounced impairments on tests of executive function and processing speed than non-psychotics. Basso and Bornstein[13] described a similar pattern in younger patients. However, this evidence could be explained in terms of a correlation between neuropsychological impairment and clinical severity rather than a categorical distinction.

Severity of depression

To assess whether clinical severity is an important predictor of neuropsychological impairment, various studies have assessed correlations between the magnitude of cognitive deficits and severity of depression measured on clinical rating scales. Again, the evidence is not conclusive; some studies observe such correlations,[14-16] while others fail to do so.[17] One explanation for these discrepancies is that several different rating scales are routinely used. Questions about cognitive function form an integral component of some scales, and these scales are, inevitably, more likely to correlate with neuropsychological deficits. In a study by Elliott et al,[18] scores on the Hamilton scale[19] did not correlate with any of the neuropsychological variables measured. However, scores on the Montgomery and Asperg scale,[20] which includes several questions related to cognitive function, were significantly correlated with measures of visual memory. Using a somewhat different approach, studies have assessed patients with pronounced diurnal variation in mood and found that the more severe depression, manifest in the mornings, was associated with more significant cognitive impairment than the milder depression of the evenings.[21,22] On balance, it seems that there is some evidence for a relationship between clinical severity and neuropsychological deficits; however, the strength of this relationship may depend on the rating scales used.

Interaction of performance with age

Another important factor in cognitive performance, which may interact with severity, is the age of patients. A crucial question is whether depression in the elderly is a distinct disorder, in either etiological or symptomatological terms. Current theories somewhat favor the existence of this distinction,[23] with cognitive deficits in elderly patients cited as a critical argument. The neuropsychological profile of elderly patients with depression has been compared with that seen in organic dementias, in particular dementia of the Alzheimer type.[24,25] In fact, the term 'pseudodementia' has traditionally been used to characterize the cognitive profile in geriatric depression,[26] and the differential diagnosis of dementia and depression in the elderly is a well-documented problem.[27] The relationship between depression and cognitive decline in the elderly is strengthened by two recent prospective studies of elderly groups.[28,29] Both studies suggested that, while the presence of depressive symptoms may not predict the onset of cognitive decline, there is a relationship between symptoms and *subsequent* cognitive decline in those already exhibiting mild impairments.

An obvious approach to determining whether the neuropsychological profile in elderly depressives is significantly different from that of younger patients is to directly compare populations of different ages. Qualitative comparisons suggest that depression is more reliably related to cognitive impairment in elderly patients[17,30,31] than in patients under 40.[32–34] However, explicit attempts to test whether there is a significant interaction between depression and age in determining cognitive deficits have been less than conclusive. For example, Tarbuck and Paykel[35] compared depressed and recovered patients under and over 60 on various tests. Both depression and age were associated with cognitive impairments; however, there was no interaction between the two.

Studies directly comparing patients of different ages have been rare. However, a recent series of studies using the same computerized test battery[36] in three different age groups also provide interesting comparisons. Patients with a mean age under 40 showed significant impairments, restricted to tests of executive function.[37] By contrast, patients with a mean age around 50 showed more widespread impairments, extending to memory deficits as well as executive dysfunction.[18] Finally, an elderly sample with mean age over 70 showed similar deficits in a

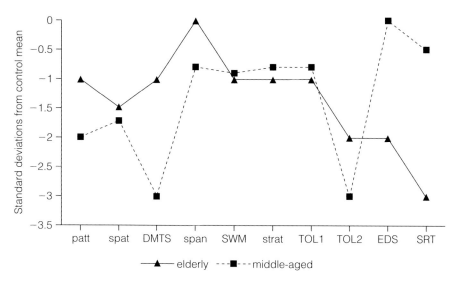

Figure 13.1

Profile of performance of middle aged (mean age 50) and elderly (mean age 70) depressed patients, relative to matched controls, on a variety of tests from the Cambridge Neuropsychological Test Automated Battery (CANTAB).[36] Patt: pattern recognition memory; Spat: Spatial recognition memory; DMTS: delayed matching to sample; Span: spatial memory span; SWM: spatial working memory; Strat: strategy; TOL1 and 2: two versions of the Tower of London task; EDS: attention set shifting; SRT: simple reaction time. Data from Beats et al[30] and Elliott et al.[18]

range of memory and executive tests and, in addition, pronounced cognitive slowing.[30] Figure 13.1 shows the profile of impairment in two age groups. It is tempting to interpret these findings in terms of deficits simply becoming more widespread with age. However, as Figure 13.1 shows, the Beats et al study[30] showed relatively intact performance relative to controls on some measures that were impaired in the middle-aged group. This was actually due to the older control group performing significantly worse than the middle-aged group (consistent with findings by Robbins et al[36] of age-related decline in normal performance on these tests). Thus, the interaction between depression, age and cognitive impairment is a complex one, and the available evidence does not conclusively support the case for a distinct neuropsychological profile in geriatric depression, given the influence of normal aging on cognitive performance. More extensive, and ideally longitudinal, studies may help to clarify this issue in the future.

Effects of treatment factors

The different treatment regimens used to manage depression may be a further significant factor in the neuropsychological profile, and, clearly, treatment factors will interact with both clinical severity and age.

Medication

Probably the most significant treatment variable affecting cognition is medication, and the medication status of patients is an important confound of many neuropsychological studies of depression. Individual medication regimens and histories can vary dramatically, both within and between studies. The extent to which antidepressant medications may interact with cognitive function has not been clearly established, as discussed in major reviews.[38,39] Those antidepressants with anticholinergic properties reliably affected cognitive function, but effects of other antidepressants were less clear. In fact, different studies have reported beneficial or detrimental effects, both, or neither.

While the cognitive effects of individual drugs have not been reliably distinguished, it seems that, generally, most traditional tricyclic antidepressants can disrupt aspects of cognition, particularly processing speed. However, less pronounced effects are reported for selective serotonin reuptake inhibitors (SSRIs)[40–44] or monoamine oxidase inhibitors (MAOIs).[45] Differential effects of different antidepressants on cognition are an important consideration in comparing studies of cognitive performance in depression, and may account for some of the discrepancies between them.

Hospitalization

Another treatment factor that may impinge on neuropsychological performance in depression is hospitalization. Depression is routinely managed on either an inpatient or an outpatient basis. Neuropsychological studies generally assess different proportions of these groups, and it is possible that hospitalization status is a factor in inter-study discrepancies. In a recent study,[18] subgroups of in- and outpatients were compared on tests of memory and executive function. Inpatients performed significantly worse than outpatients, even though clinical severity, assessed on various rating scales, did not differ between the two groups. In a study using the same tests with a purely outpatient sample, Purcell et al[37] reported less global impairment than Elliott et al,[18] though this may be confounded by age differences. Interestingly, though, Purcell et al reported that patients with a history of inpatient episodes performed worse on some measures than those without. Thus, there is some evidence that hospitalization may be an important factor in neuropsychological profile, to an extent not accounted for by differences in severity. However, it is not clear whether neuropsychological impairment is an important indicator for hospitalization (possibly as important as clinical severity), or whether factors related to hospitalization may exacerbate cognitive deficits.

State vs. trait factors in depression

The evidence discussed above suggests that various clinical factors are important in determining neuropsychological profile in depression, though the inter-relationships are complex. These issues also pertain to a fundamental question of whether neuropsychological deficits in depression are state factors (manifest only during a current depressive episode) or trait factors (apparent in individuals vulnerable to depression, even when they are not currently depressed). This question has typically been addressed empirically by assessing patients longitudinally, in both the clinically depressed and recovered states. The majority of studies indicate that there is a marked improvement in cognitive performance on symptomatic recovery.[18,30,46] However, residual impairments relative to controls were also demonstrated in all these studies. Convergent findings have been reported in patients with seasonal affective disorder[47] and with pronounced diurnal variation in mood.[21] Kuny and Stassen[48] charted the progress of cognitive impairment of 30 recovering patients and concluded that cognitive and clinical recovery were largely independent. Their contention was that cognitive impairment may represent an independent syndrome in depression. All of these findings suggest that aspects of cognitive impairment may represent both state and trait factors in depression. It remains to be seen whether any consistent pattern may emerge in what appears to be marked individual variation.

This discussion of how cognitive deficits depend on various clinical parameters has been based on the rather general neuropsychological profile typically observed. However, it is important to consider whether any specificity can be observed in the generalized pattern of impairment; a question that becomes particularly relevant when considering the neural basis of cognitive deficits.

General versus specific deficits in depression

This is an issue with both practical and theoretical significance, but one that remains largely unresolved. The discussion has been framed in a number of different ways, and four of the currently influential debates are highlighted here.

Biases towards mood-congruent information

This debate follows closely from a discussion of the extent to which neuropsychological deficits may relate to clinical symptoms. The contention is that performance may vary with the affective or emotional tone of material being processed. Patients with depressed mood may be differentially sensitive to negatively toned information and process it more effectively. This account has clear implications for the maintenance, and possibly the etiology, of depression; a bias towards negative information may reinforce depressed mood. Bias in information processing has been particularly studied in the context of memory, with numerous studies showing that depressed patients show a tendency to recall negatively, rather than positively, toned material.[49–53] It has even been demonstrated that this bias may be, at least partially, unconscious and thus seen in the context of implicit memory. Watkins et al[54] found that depressed patients showed greater priming of negative than positive words, the reverse of the pattern shown by control subjects. It should be noted however, that not all studies have reported these implicit biases in depression.[55]

While the studies of memory biases predominate, there is also evidence of mood-congruent biases in attentional studies.[52,56] For example, depression-related words cause interference in a Stroop task, while neutral and happy words do not.[57,58] A recent study of an emotional no-go task also found a bias towards negative information in depression,[8] and, interestingly, a contrasting bias towards positive information in patients with mania. The approach of studying emotional biases has the advantage of explicitly linking mood and cognition, which can be related to cognitive-behavioral theories of depression, on which treatment strategies have been based.[59] A related approach, again emphasizing the clinical relevance of neuropsychological impairment, is to attempt to relate cognitive deficits to particular symptoms.

Neuropsychological impairments and specific symptoms

Certain of the clinical symptoms of depression may have a direct causal effect on performance. It is common for subjects to report difficulties in concentration and sustaining attention to cognitive tasks. Indeed, impairments of concentration represent one of the standard operational criteria for a diagnosis of depression (DSM IV).[1] Attentional deficits have been reported in depression,[60] although they have not been widely studied. Another area where the boundary between clinical symptom and neuropsychological deficit is blurred is the issue of motivation. An absence of motivation is one of the clinical symptoms of depression and can play a causal role in a whole range of neuropsychological impairments. In fact, some have argued that all the cognitive deficits of depression could be attributable to motivational factors.[61]

The concept of motivation is somewhat general, and recent studies have discussed more specific forms of motivational deficit in relation to neuropsychological performance. In a study of elderly patients with depression, Beats et al[30] described a 'catastrophic response to perceived failure' on the Tower of London (TOL) task, such that, once patients made an initial error, subsequent performance deteriorated rapidly. In a more explicit test of this hypothesis in younger patients, Elliott et al[18,62] described an abnormal response to failure on two contrasting tests. This abnormality was found to be less that patients performed worse after a failure, but rather that patients failed to use negative feedback as a motivational boost to improve subsequent performance. Control subjects, and also neurological and neurosurgical patients with similar overall deficits, were far less likely to make an error after a preceding error. It is possible that this difference could be due to the expectations of failure and feelings of worthlessness that form part of the clinical profile of depression. Channon[63] also reported an inefficient use of feedback to improve performance on a card-sorting test in patients with dysphoria. This deficit has the advantage of being directly related to aspects of symptomatology and also to influential cognitive and psychological accounts of the disorder.[64-66] However, some attempts to replicate this finding have failed,[37,67] perhaps due to demographic differences in the populations studied.

Mood-congruent biases and specific motivational deficits are important ways of relating clinical symptoms to neuropsychological deficits. However, these factors can only explain certain aspects of the cognitive profile in depression. Depressed patients are impaired on tasks where the material to be processed is emotionally neutral and no error feedback is provided. Therefore, it is also important to consider other ways to characterize the neuropsychological profile of depression.

Effortful versus automatic processing

This is the subject of a long-established debate, focused on the hypothesis that depressed patients are more impaired on effortful than on automatic tasks.[68] This hypothesis would predict deficits cutting across traditionally demarcated cognitive domains (memory, executive function, attention etc.), but dependent instead on how demanding the specific tasks assessed are. To address this hypothesis empirically, it is necessary to demonstrate whether patients show selective impairments on tasks that can be defined as more effortful. For example, one prediction of the hypothesis is that explicit memory (relatively effortful) will be more impaired in depressed patients than implicit memory (relatively automatic). Inevitably, the evidence is inconclusive, with some studies supporting the prediction,[69-72] but others failing to do so.[73,74] The jury is therefore still out on the cognitive effort hypothesis, although it continues to receive support.[75] However, it is not always clear to what extent cognitive effort is a useful concept for explaining neuropsychological impairments in depression, with a danger of the argument becoming circular.

Selective impairments in specific cognitive domains

The cognitive effort hypothesis proposes deficits dependent on the difficulty of tasks rather than domain-specific impairments. However, in recent years, the question of whether the deficits in depression may be specific to a particular domain has also been considered. Two aspects of function that have been experimentally dissociated in patients with neurological and neurosurgical damage are memory and executive function. These dissociations are discussed elsewhere in this book. Evidence for a selective deficit in one or other domain could have neurobiological as well as neuropsychological implications for theories of depression.

The many neuropsychological studies of depressed patients have clearly established that they are impaired on aspects of memory and learning (visual and verbal, short-term and long-term),[14,17,18] as well as various types of executive function.[30,76,77] The exact pattern of deficits may vary between studies, depending on both the particular tests used and the clinical characteristics of the sample population. However, impairment is typically seen across a broad range of cognitive domains.[17,18,21,30,31] The key question is not whether deficits exist in some domains and not others, but whether the deficits are more pronounced in a particular domain. One recent meta-analysis of all studies published since 1975[78] concluded that the neuropsychological deficits in depression are not more pronounced in any particular aspect of function, but are 'consistent with global-diffuse impairment in brain functions'. However, another recent comprehensive review[79] challenged this position, concluding that while deficits are undoubtably present across cognitive domains, executive deficits are particularly prominent. Since executive tasks are, almost by definition, effortful, this view is to some extent consistent with the effortful-processing account discussed above. A number of recent studies support this view. Degl'Innocenti et al[80] report differential deficits in tests of executive function, and Channon and Green[81] have suggested that these impairments may represent a failure to use appropriate strategies. Interestingly, executive deficits have been demonstrated in unmedicated patients,[82] indicating that they are unlikely to be a consequence of medication. At present, therefore, it appears that although depressed patients are impaired on a wide range of tasks, executive deficits may stand out as particularly marked. The concept of 'executive function' has been used almost interchangeably with that of 'frontal lobe function', and therefore specific deficits in these domains would suggest prefrontal pathology in depression. Recent developments in structural and functional neuroimaging have allowed this prediction to be assessed directly.

Neural correlates of neuropsychological deficits

Structural abnormalities

There has been much discussion over the years concerning whether depression may be associated with structural changes in the brain. Convergent evidence suggests that there may be structural abnormalities in elderly patients that relate to degree of cognitive impairment[79] (review: Robbins et al[83]), although the evidence is less conclusive in younger patients. It has recently been argued, however, that structural abnormalities may be associated with depression duration rather than age; obviously, the two are likely to covary in many cases but they are conceptually distinct. Sheline et al[84] found that duration of illness, but not age, predicted loss of hippocampal volume. Several recent studies have attempted to relate structural abnormalities with cognitive deficits. Hickie et al[85] found a correlation between subcortical white matter hyperintensities and psychomotor slowing. Deep white matter hyperintensities have also been associated with various indices of learning and memory,[86,87] as well as aspects of language and executive function.[87] Meanwhile, Shah et al[88] demonstrated an association between verbal memory and density of gray matter in the left hippocampus, a structure typically associated with mnemonic function. These various findings suggest a relationship between neuropsychological deficits and structural abnormalities in at least some subgroups of depressed patients. However, this relationship needs to be characterized more fully before definitive conclusions can be drawn.

Functional abnormalities

During the past few years, functional neuroimaging using positron emission tomography (PET), single photon emission computed tomography (SPECT) and functional magnetic resonance imaging (fMRI) has been used to identify functional abnormalities associated with depression.

Resting state studies

In these studies, patients are scanned at rest and their functional anatomy compared to that of controls. Studies taking this approach identified a number of regions that are abnormal in patients with depression. Probably the most widely replicated finding is of hypofrontality, involving abnormal blood flow in prefrontal cortex. Medial regions of the frontal cortex have been particularly implicated.[89–94] Another functional abnormality that has been reported in several studies is decreased striatal blood flow.[89,95,96] These striatal findings, combined with the prefrontal abnormalities, provide support for the popular theory that depression may involve dysfunction in the frontosubcortical circuitry.[79,83,97,98] This account would be consistent with the neuropsychological evidence for particularly pronounced impairments on tests of executive function. The cognitive effort hypothesis would also predict prefrontal abnormality since increasing task difficulty has been associated with prefrontal activity.[99]

While findings of prefrontal and striatal abnormalities in resting state studies of depression are consistent with the neuropsychological profile, it is possible to look at this relationship more directly. One approach is to use correlational studies, explicitly assessing the extent to which neuropsychological deficits co-occur with functional abnormalities. Bench et al[100] used factor analysis to relate regional cerebral blood flow (rCBF) to clinical features. One of the factors revealed by the analysis had a high loading for cognitive performance and was positively correlated with rCBF in the medial prefrontal cortex. More specifically, Dolan et al[101] followed up this study with a principal components analysis on neuropsychological data. Principal components emerged with high loadings for memory and attention, and both of these were significantly correlated with rCBF in the medial prefrontal cortex and frontal pole. Goodwin[79] also described a correlation between cognitive impairment and hypofrontality.

Activation studies

While the resting state studies described above provide important clues as to the relationship between neuropsychology and brain function, they are not the most direct way to address the issue. In resting state studies, subjects are typically scanned while relaxing with their eyes closed, a rather poorly controlled state. The alternative approach of cognitive activation studies is to scan subjects during the explicit performance of a specific cognitive task, which gives much greater control over their mental processes. The regions activated in response to a cognitive challenge may not be the same as those activated in the resting state. Thus this approach provides a direct assessment of the neural correlates of cognitive impairments. However, it has the important caveat that it can be empirically difficult to establish a causal relationship between reduced neural function and impaired performance. If a subject shows reduced blood flow in response to a task they perform poorly, it is not clear whether they perform poorly because of the neural dysfunction or whether the reduced neural response is a consequence of the below par performance. Regardless of the causality issue, the evidence for a relationship between cognitive impairment and functional abnormality has not always been consistent. Berman et al[102] scanned depressed patients during performance of the classic executive task, the Wisconsin Card Sorting Test, and found no evidence of abnormal prefrontal blood flow. By contrast, two more recent studies have shown reduced frontal blood flow, particularly in the anterior cingulate, during performance of other established executive tasks, the Stroop test[103] and a version of the TOL.[104] Figure 13.2 shows medial prefrontal activation associated with performance of the TOL planning task. A different focus of medial prefrontal dysfunction was found in a recent study,[105] which demonstrated the highly specific response to feedback effect described above, to be dependent on focal functional abnormality in the medial orbitofrontal cortex (OFC). This region has also been highlighted in recent studies of response to treatment,[106] demonstrating an important

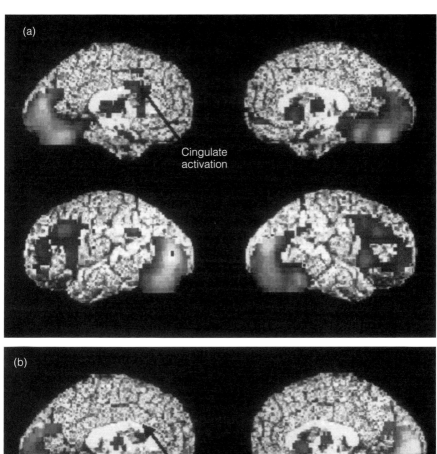

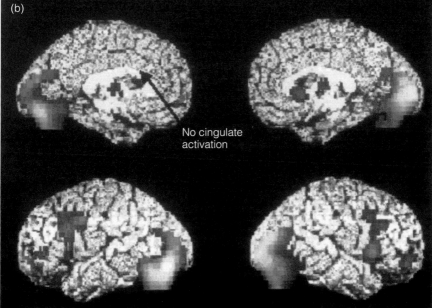

Figure 13.2

Activations associated with the performance of an executive task (the Tower of London) in (a) controls and (b) depressed patients. The activation is shown superimposed on a standard MRI template. Note the absence of anterior cingulate activation in patients.

role for neuroimaging in assessing the issue of abnormal neurotransmission. The OFC is a region where serotonin receptor density may be reduced in depression.[107]

Medial prefrontal dysfunction in depression: a possible unification?

The most reliable finding of the functional neuroimaging literature is thus of prefrontal abnormalities, particularly in medial regions; anterior cingulate (AC) extending to medial OFC. This is clearly a plausible account of the neuropsychological evidence for prominent executive dysfunction in depression. However, prefrontal dysfunction may also contribute to memory deficits, particularly on more 'effortful' mnemonic tasks. The prefrontal cortex has been implicated in aspects of working memory[108] and memory-related control processes.[109] However, depressed patients also show deficits in the simple recognition tasks, more traditionally associated with the function of the temporal lobes. While temporal regions are clearly important substrates of recognition memory, functional neuroimaging has also demonstrated a role for the AC in short-term visual recognition.[110,111] Thus, functional abnormalities of AC may explain mnemonic as well as executive impairments in depression. The medial prefrontal cortex is also implicated in attentional function, which accords with the difficulties in sustaining attention reported by depressed patients. Further, it is a region that has been associated with emotional responses, in both normal subjects and depressed patients.[112] A fundamental pathology in regions of the medial prefrontal cortex may underpin both the clinical features and cognitive deficits seen in depression. It is possible that this pathology may involve both functional and structural abnormalities. A recent study by Drevets et al[94] reported both types of abnormality in the subgenual cingulate, a ventromedial region lying between the AC and OFCs. The medial prefrontal cortex is a region with extensive interconnections and dense ennervation by neurotransmitters, particularly serotonin, believed to be implicated in depression. It is therefore entirely plausible that dysfunction in this region may be fundamental to depression, a disorder characterized by a complex interaction of affective and cognitive disturbance. Figure 13.3 provides a schematic representation of this hypothesis. It remains to be seen, however, whether medial prefrontal abnormality is a predisposing factor to depression, or whether it only becomes manifest with the onset of the disorder. This is one of a number of issues and questions that remain to be addressed in the search for a coherent framework to understand this challenging disorder.

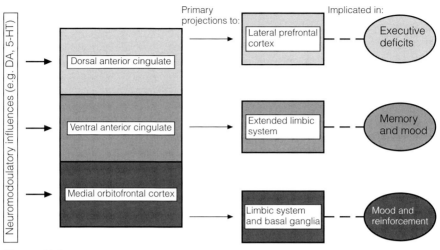

Figure 13.3

Schematic diagram of the role of medial prefrontal cortex in depression.

Acknowledgments

My thanks go to Dr Barbara J Sahakian and Professors Ray Dolan and Bill Deakin for helpful discussion and comments.

References

1. American Psychiatric Association. *Diagnostic and Statistical Manual of Mental Disorders*, 4th edn (Washington DC: APA, 1994).

2. Friedman AS. Minimal effects of severe depression on cognitive functioning. *J Abnorm Social Psychol* (1964) **69:** 237–43.

3. Miller WR. Psychological deficit in depression. *Psychol Bull* (1975) **82:** 238–60.

4. Taylor MA, Abrams ER. Cognitive dysfunction in mania. *Comp Psychiatry* (1986) **27:** 186–91.

5. Johnson MH, Magaro PA. Effects of mood and severity on memory processes in depression and mania. *Psychol Bull* (1987) **101:** 28–40.

6. Bulbena A, Berrios GE. Cognitive function in the affective disorders: a prospective study. *Psychopathology* (1993) **26:** 6–12.

7. Bruder GE, Schnur DB, Fergeson P et al. Dichotic-listening measures of brain laterality in mania. *J Abnorm Psychol* (1994) **103:** 758–66.

8. Murphy FC, Sahakian BJ, Rubinsztein JS et al. Emotional bias and inhibitory control processes in mania and depression. *Psychol Med* (in press).

9. Fuster JM. *The Prefrontal Cortex* (New York: Raven Press, 1989).

10. Malloy P, Bihrle A, Duffy J, Cimino C. The orbitomedial

frontal syndrome. *Arch Clin Neuropsychol* (1993) **8:** 185–201.

11. Nelson EB, Sax KW, Strakowski SM. Attentional performance in patients with psychotic and nonpsychotic depression and schizophrenia. *Am J Psychiatry* (1998) **155:** 137–9.

12. Simpson S, Baldwin RC, Jackson A, Burns A. The differentiation of DSM III-R psychotic depression in later life from nonpsychotic depression: comparison of brain changes measured by multispectral analysis of magnetic resonance brain images, neuropsychological findings and clinical features. *Biol Psychiatry* (1999) **45:** 193–204.

13. Basso MR, Bornstein RA. Neuropsychological deficits in psychotic versus nonpsychotic unipolar depression. *Neuropsychology* (1999) **13:** 69–75.

14. Austin MP, Ross M, Murray C et al. Cognitive function in major depression. *J Affect Disord* (1992) **25:** 21–30.

15. Smith MJ, Brebion G, Banquet JP, Allilaire JF. Experimental evidence for two dimensions of cognitive disorders in depressives. *J Psychiatr Res* (1994) **28:** 401–11.

16. Boone KB et al. Cognitive functioning in older depressed outpatients: relationship of presence and severity of depression to test scores. *Neuropsychology* (1995) **9:** 390–8.

17. Brown RG, Scott LC, Bench CJ, Dolan RJ. Cognitive function in depression: its relationship to the presence and severity of intellectual decline. *Psychol Med* (1994) **24:** 829–47.

18. Elliott R, Sahakian BJ, McKay AP et al. Neuropsychological impairments in unipolar depression: the role of perceived failure on subsequent performance. *Psychol Med* (1996) **26:** 975–89.

19. Hamilton M. A rating scale for depression. *J Neurol Neurosurg Psychiatry* (1960) **23:** 56–62.

20. Montgomery SA, Asberg M. A new depression scale designed to be sensitive to change. *Br J Psychiatry* (1979) **134:** 382–9.

21. Moffoot APR, O'Carroll RE, Bennie J et al. Diurnal variation in mood and neuropsychological function in major depression with melancholia. *J Affect Disord* (1994) **32:** 257–69.

22. Porterfield T, Cook M, Deary IJ, Ebmeier KP. Neuropsychological function and diurnal variation in depression. *J Clin Exp Neuropsychol* (1997) **19:** 906–13.

23. Gottfries CG. Is there a difference between elderly and younger patients with regard to the symptomatology and aetiology of depression? *Int Clin Psychopharmacol* (1998) **13(suppl 5):** S13–18.

24. Robbins TW, Elliott R, Sahakian BJ. Neuropsychology—dementia and affective disorders. *Br Med Bull* (1996) **52:** 627–43.

25. Van Reekum R, Simard M, Clarke D et al. Late-life depression as a possible predictor of dementia: cross-sectional and short-term follow-up results. *Am J Geriatr Psychiatry* (1999) **7:** 151–9.

26. Kiloh LG. Pseudo-dementia. *Acta Psychiatr Scand* (1961) **37:** 336–60.

27. Rosenstein LD. Differential diagnosis of the major progressive dementias and depression in middle and late adulthood: a summary of the literature of the early 1990s *Neuropsychol Rev* (1998) **8:** 109–67.

28. Bassuk SS, Berkman LF, Wypij D. Depressive symptomatology and incident cognitive decline in

an elderly community sample. *Arch Gen Psychiatry* (1998) **55:** 1073–81.

29. Yaffe K, Blackwell T, Gore R et al. Depressive symptoms and cognitive decline in nondemented elderly women: a prospective study. *Arch Gen Psychiatry* (1999) **56:** 425–30.

30. Beats BC, Sahakian BJ, Levy R. Cognitive performance in tests sensitive to frontal lobe dysfunction in the elderly depressed. *Psychol Med* (1996) **26:** 591–603.

31. Palmer BW, Boone KB, Lesser IM et al. Neuropsychological deficits among older depressed patients with predominantly psychological or vegetative symptoms. *J Affect Disord* (1996) **41:** 17–24.

32. Martin DJ, Oren Z, Boone K. Major depressives' and dysthmics' performance on the Wisconsin card sorting test. *J Clin Psychol* (1991) **47:** 684–90.

33. DeLuca J, Johnson SK, Beldowicz D, Natelson BH. Neuropsychological impairments in chronic fatigue syndrome, multiple sclerosis and depression. *J Neurol Neurosurg Psychiatry* (1995) **58:** 38–43.

34. Albus M, Hubman W, Wahlheim C et al. Contrasts in neuropsychological test profile between patients with first episode schizophrenia and first episode affective disorder. *Acta Psychiatr Scand* (1996) **94:** 87–93.

35. Tarbuck AF, Paykel ES. Effects of major depression on the cognitive function of younger and older subjects. *Psychol Med* (1995) **25:** 285–96.

36. Robbins TW, James M, Owen AM et al. Cambridge Neuropsychological Battery (CANTAB): a factor analytic study of a large sample of normal elderly volunteers. *Dementia* (1994) **5:** 266–81.

37. Purcell R, Maruff P, Kyrios M, Pantelis C. Neuropsychological function in young patients with unipolar depression. *Psychol Med* (1997) **27:** 1277–86.

38. Thompson PJ, Trimble MR. Non-MAOI antidepressants and cognitive functions: a review. *Psychol Med* (1982) **12:** 539–48.

39. Amado-Boccara I, Gougoulis N, Poirier Littre MF et al. Effects of antidepressants on cognitive functions: a review. *Neurosci Biobehav Rev* (1995) **19:** 479–93.

40. Moon CAL, Vince M. Treatment of major depression in general practice: a double-blind comparison of paroxetine and lofepramine. *Br J Clin Practice* (1996) **50:** 240–4.

41. Kerr JS, Hindmarch I. Citalopram and other antidepressants: comparative effects on cognitive function and psychomotor performance. *J Serotonin Res* (1996) **3:** 123–9.

42. Kerr JS, Hindmarch I. The effects of reboxetine and amitryptaline, with and without alcohol on cognitive function and psychomotor performance. *Br J Clin Pharmacol* (1996) **42:** 239–41.

43. Fairweather DB et al. Citalopram compared to dothiepin and placebo: effects on cognitive function and psychomotor performance. *Human Psychopharmacol* (1997) **12:** 119–26.

44. Orengo CA, Kunik ME, Molinari V, Workman RH. The use and tolerability of fluoxetine in geripsychiatric inpatients. *J Clin Psychiatry* (1996) **57:** 12–16.

45. Roth M, Mountjoy CQ, Amrein R. Moclobemide in elderly patients with cognitive decline and depression: an international, double-blind placebo-controlled

trial. *Br J Psychiatry* (1997) **168:** 149–57.

46. Abas M, Sahakian BJ, Levy R. Neuropsychological deficits and CT scan changes in elderly depressives. *Psychol Med* (1990) **20:** 507–20.

47. O'Brien JT, Sahakian BJ, Checkley SA. Cognitive impairment in patients with seasonal affective disorder. *Br J Psychiatry* (1993) **163:** 338–43.

48. Kuny S, Stassen HH. Cognitive performance in patients recovering from depression. *Psychopathology* (1995) **28:** 190–207.

49. Lloyd GG, Lishman WA. Effect of depression on the speed of recall of pleasant and unpleasant experiences. *Psychol Med* (1975) **5:** 173–80.

50. Clark DM, Teasdale JD. Diurnal variation in clinical depression and accessibility of memories of positive and negative experiences. *J Abnorm Psychol* (1982) **91:** 87–95.

51. Bradley BP, Mogg K, Millar N. Implicit memory bias in clinical and non clinical depression. *Behav Res Ther* (1996) **34:** 865–79.

52. Williams JMG, Watts FM, Macleod C, Mathews A. *Cognitive Psychology and Emotional Disorders*, 2nd edn (Chichester: John Wiley & Sons, (1997).

53. Blaney PH. Affect and memory: a review. *Psychol Bull* (1986) **99:** 229–46.

54. Watkins PC, Vache K, Verney SP et al. Unconscious mood congruent memory bias in depression. *J Abnorm Psychol* (1996) **105:** 34–41.

55. Isley JE, Moffoot APR, O'Carroll RE. An analysis of memory dysfunction in major depression. *J Affect Disord* (1995) **35:** 1–9.

56. Mogg K, Bradley BP, Williams R. Attentional bias in anxiety and depression: the role of awareness. *Br J Clin Psychol* (1995) **34:** 17–36.

57. Gotlib IH, Cane DB. Construct accessibility and clinical depression: a longitudinal investigation. *J Abnorm Psychol* (1987) **96:** 199–204.

58. Segal ZV, Gemar M, Truchon C et al. A priming methodology for studying self-representation in major depressive disorder. *J Abnorm Psychol* (1995) **104:** 205–13.

59. Teasdale JD. Negative thinking in depression: cause effect or reciprocal relationship? *Adv Behav Res Ther* (1983) **5:** 3–25.

60. Mialet JP, Pope HG, Yurgulen-Todd D. Impaired attention in depressive states: a non-specific deficit? *Psychol Med* (1996) **26:** 1009–20.

61. Schmand B, Kuipers T, Van der Gaag M et al. Cognitive disorders and negative symptoms as correlates of motivational deficits in psychotic patients. *Psychol Med* (1994) **24:** 869–84.

62. Elliott R, Sahakian BJ, Herron JJ et al. Abnormal response to negative feedback in unipolar depression: evidence for a disease-specific impairment. *J Neurol Neurosurg Psychiatry* (1997) **63:** 74–82.

63. Channon S. Executive dysfunction in depression: the Wisconsin Card Sort test. *J Affect Disord* (1996) **9:** 107–14.

64. Beck AT. *Depression: Clinical, Experimental and Theoretical Aspects* (New York: Harper and Row, 1967).

65. Teasdale JD, Barnard PJ. *Affect, Cognition and Change* (Hove: Lawrence Erlbaum Associates, 1993).

66. Lewinsohn PM, Youngren MA, Grosscup SJ. Reinforcement and depression. In Depue RA (ed.) *The Psychobiology of Depressive Disorders* (New York: Academic Press, 1979): 291–316.

67. Shah PJ, O'Carroll RE, Rogers A et al. Abnormal response to negative feedback in depression. *Psychol Med* (1999) **29:** 63–72.

68. Hasher L, Zacks RT. Automatic and effortful processes in memory. *J Exp Psychol* (1979) **108:** 356–88.

69. Danion J-M, Willard-Schroeder D, Zimmermann MA et al. Explicit memory and repetition priming in depression. *Arch Gen Psychiatry* (1991) **48:** 707–11.

70. Denny EB, Hunt R. Affective valence and memory in depression: dissociation of recall and fragment completion. *J Abnorm Psychol* (1992) **101:** 575–80.

71. Bazin N, Perruchet P, De Bonis M, Feline A. The dissociation of explicit and implicit memory in depressed patients. *Psychol Med* (1994) **24:** 239–45.

72. Georgieff N, Dominey PF, Michel F et al. Semantic priming in major depressive state. *Psychiatry Res* (1998) **78:** 29–44.

73. Elliot CL, Greene RL. Clinical depression and implicit memory. *J Abnorm Psychol* (1992) **101:** 572–4.

74. Watkins PC, Mathews A, Williamson DA, Fuller RD. Mood-congruent memory in depression: emotional priming or elaboration. *J Abnorm Psychol* (1992) **101:** 581–6.

75. Hartlage S, Alloy LB, Vazquez C, Dykman B. Automatic and effortful processing in depression. *Psychol Bull* (1993) **113:** 247–78.

76. Dalla Barba G, Parlato V, Iavarone A, Boller F. Anosog-nosia, intrustions and 'frontal' functions in Alzheimer's disease and depression. *Neuropsychologia* (1995) **33:** 247–59.

77. Moreaud O, Naegele B, Chabannes JP et al. Frontal lobe dysfunction and depressive state: relation to endogenous character of depression. *Encephale* (1996) **22:** 47–51.

78. Veiel HOF. A preliminary profile of neuropsychological deficits associated with major depression. *J Clin Exp Neuropsychol* (1997) **19:** 587–603.

79. Goodwin GM. Neuropsychological and neuroimaging evidence for the involvement of frontal lobes in depression. *J Psychopharmacol* (1997) **11:** 115–22.

80. Degl'Innocenti A, Agren H, Backman L. Executive deficits in major depression. *Acta Psychiatr Scand* (1998) **97:** 182–8.

81. Channon S, Green PS. Executive function in depression: the role of performance strategies in aiding depressed and non-depressed participants. *J Neurol Neurosurg Psychiatry* (1999) **66:** 162–71.

82. Merriam EP, Thase ME, Haas GL et al. Prefrontal cortical dysfunction in depression determined by Wisconsin Card Sorting Test performance. *Am J Psychiatry* (1999) **156:** 780–2.

83. Robbins TW, Joyce EM, Sahakian BJ. Neuropsychology and neuroimaging of affective disorders. In Paykel ES (ed.) *Handbook of Affective Disorders* (London: Churchill Livingstone, 1992).

84. Sheline YI, Sanghavi M, Mintun MA, Gado MH. Depression duration but not age predicts hippocampal volume loss in medically healthy women with

recurrent major depession. *J Neurosci* (1999) **19:** 5034–43.

85. Hickie I, Scott E, Mitchell P et al. Subcortical hyperintensities on magnetic resonance imaging: clinical correlates and prognostic significance in patients with severe depression. *Biol Psychiatry* (1995) **3:** 151–60.

86. Jenkins M, Mally P, Salloway S et al. Memory processes in depressed geriatric patients with and without subcortical hyperintensities on MRI. *J Neuroimaging* (1998) **8:** 20–6.

87. Kramer-Ginsberg E, Greenwald BS, Krishnan KR et al. Neuropsychological functioning and MRI signal hyperintensities in geriatric depression. *Am J Psychiatry* (1999) **156:** 438–44.

88. Shah PJ, Ebmeier KP, Glabus MF, Goodwin GM. Cortical grey matter reductions associated with treatment-resistant chronic unipolar depression. Controlled magnetic resonance imaging study. *Br J Psychiatry* (1998) **172:** 527–32.

89. Bench CJ, Friston KJ, Brown RG et al. The anatomy of melancholia — focal abnormalities of cerebral blood flow in major depression. *Psychol Med* (1992) **22:** 607–15.

90. Drevets WC, Videen TO, Price JL et al. A functional anatomical study of unipolar depression. *J Neurosci* (1992) **12(9):** 3628–41.

91. George MS, Ketter TA, Post RM. SPECT and PET in mood disorders. *J Clin Psychiatry* (1993) **54(suppl):** 6–13.

92. Goodwin GM, Austin MP, Dougall N et al. State changes in brain activity shown by the uptake of 99m Tc-exametazime with single photon emission tomography in major depression before and after treatment. *J Affect Disord* (1993) **29:** 243–53.

93. Ebert D, Ebmeier KP. The role of the cingulate gyrus in depression: from functional anatomy to neurochemistry. *Biol Psychiatry* (1996) **39:** 1044–50.

94. Drevets WC, Price JL, Simpson JR et al. Subgenual prefrontal cortex abnormalities in mood disorders. *Nature* (1997) **382:** 824–7.

95. Buchsbaum M, Wu J, DeLisi LE et al. Frontal cortex and basal ganglia metabolic rates assessed by positron emission tomography with [18F]2-deoxyglucose in affective illness. *J Affect Disord* (1986) **10:** 137–52.

96. Cohen R, Semple WE, Gross M et al. Evidence for common alterations in cerebral glucose metabolism in major affective disorders and schizophrenia. *Neuropsychopharmacology* **2:** 241–54.

97. Mega MS, Cummings JL. Fronto-subcortical circuits and neuropsychiatric disorders. *J Neuropsychiatry Clin Neurosci* (1994) **6:** 358–70.

98. Cummings JL. Anatomic and behavioral aspects of fronto-subcortical circuits. *Ann NY Acad Sci* (1995) **769:** 1–13.

99. Barch DM, Braver TS, Nystrom LE et al. Dissociating working memory from task difficulty in human prefrontal cortex. *Neuropsychologica* **35:** 1373–80.

100. Bench CJ, Friston KJ, Brown RG et al. Regional cerebral blood flow in depression measured by positron emission tomography: the relationship with clinical dimensions. *Psychol Med* (1993) **23:** 579–90.

101. Dolan RJ, Bench CJ, Brown RG et al. Neuropsychological dysfunction in depression: the relationship to regional cerebral

blood flow. *Psychol Med* (1994) **24:** 849–57.

102. Berman KF, Doran AR, Pickar D, Weinberger DR. Is the mechanism of prefrontal hypofunction in depression the same as in schizophrenia? Regional cerebral blood flow during cognitive activation. *Br J Psychiatry* (1993) **162:** 183–92.

103. George MS, Ketter TA, Parekh PI et al. Blunted left cingulate activation in mood disorder subjects during a response interference task (the Stroop). *J Neuropsychiatry Clin Neurosci* (1997) **9:** 55–63.

104. Elliott R, Baker SC, Rogers RD et al. Prefrontal dysfunction in depressed patients performing a planning task: a study using positron emission tomography. *Psychol Med* (1997) **27:** 931–42.

105. Elliott R, Sahakian BJ, Michael A et al. Abnormal response to feedback on planning and guessing tasks in patients with unipolar depression. *Psychol Med* (1998) **28:** 559–71.

106. Mayberg HS, Brannan SK, Mahurin RK et al. Cingulate function in depression: a potential predictor of treatment response. *Neuroreport* (1997) **8:** 1057–61.

107. Biver F, Wikler D, Lotstra F et al. Serotonin 5-HT2 receptor imaging in major depression: focal changes in orbito insular cortex. *Br J Psychiatry* (1997) **171:** 444–8.

108. Dolan RJ, Paulesu E, Fletcher PC. Human memory systems. In Frackowick RSJ et al (eds) *Human Brain Function* (Academic Press, 1997): 367–404.

109. Fletcher PC, Frith CD, Grasby PM et al. Brain systems for encoding and retrieval of auditory verbal memory: an in vivo study in humans. *Brain* (1995) **118:** 401–16.

110. Paulesu E. Functional anatomy of working memory: the visuospatial 'sketchpad'. *J Cerebral Blood Flow Metab* (1993) **13:** S551.

111. Elliott R, Dolan RJ. Differential neural responses during performance of matching and non-matching to sample tasks at two day intervals. *J Neurosci* (1999) **15:** 5066–73.

112. Beauregard M, Leroux JM, Bergman S et al. The functional neuroanatomy of major depression: an fMRI study using an emotional activation paradigm. *Neuroreport* (1998) **9:** 3253–8.

14
Cognitive theories of autism

James Russell

It is obvious even to the casual observer that the past 15 or so years have witnessed an explosion of interest in the cognitive psychology of autism, engendered by the appearance of a single hypothesis. All cognitive theories of autism that have emerged since the mid-1980s have been defined in relation to it. This hypothesis states that the core cognitive deficit in autism is lack of (or delayed or deviant development of) an innately specified 'module' for conceptualizing mental states—the so-called 'theory of mind mechanism' (ToMM). I will begin by assessing this position and then set it beside two further theories, one that emphasizes impairment in integrating elements into wholes (weak central coherence theory) and one that emphasizes impaired executive functioning (executive dysfunction (ED) theory.)

The ToMM-deficit theory

First, why use the term 'theory' of mind? Consider introspection. When we take ourselves to be (say) thinking that X or hoping that Y, we are applying concepts—the concept of thought and the concept of hope. And if we are to understand and use the English words 'think' and 'hope', we require the concepts THINK and HOPE. Moreover, mental concepts, just like any other kind of concept, require expertise in their application; and so they can be misapplied. Given this, children must acquire—perhaps they need innate cognitive apparatus to guarantee that they acquire— these concepts. Children are not, after all, *taught* them, any more than they are taught how to speak or to walk. Moreover, it is sometimes useful to think of concept acquisition in terms of theory acquisition, for the following reason. Some concepts are not explanatory. Thus, 'chair' simply means a portable seat for one. These concepts are stipulative. But certain other concepts implicitly tap into what philosophers call 'folk theories' of why phenomena occur. Thus, 'Why did Moira go to the kitchen?' Because she *wanted* a Martini and *believed* that there was a bottle of gin in the fridge. This explains why Moira did what she did in terms of two theoretical postulates and a practical inference.

The theory implicitly being used here (that thoughts and desires, when appropriately combined, cause action) might be wrong; and vulnerability to disconfirmation is the mark of a true theory. Some philosophers do indeed believe that our folk psychological explanations are misconceived, rather in the way in which our earlier attempts to explain schizophrenia in terms of possession by demons were misconceived. But as far as psychology is concerned, this does not matter, because mental evolution could have established in humans an essentially false but heuristically invaluable explanatory system—a ladder which an evolved science will later encourage us to throw away. Evolution will thus have brought it about that the theory is innately present in children. The ToMM-deficit theory states that this theory is *not* innately present in children with autism (or at least not in its normal form), and that once we view these children as lacking it, we will be well placed to explain why certain signs and symptoms co-occur in the disorder. The term 'module' is used to capture the claim that the cognitive machinery necessary for the theory is *sui generis* and that it can be lacking while other important cognitive skills are intact.

The ToMM-deficit theory famously claims to be able to account for the fact that the following two deficits coexist in autism: lack or paucity of pretend play (play in which the child, alone or with others, deliberately takes an object to be other than it is) and difficulty with the so-called *false belief task*. In the false belief task, devised by Wimmer and Perner,[1] children hear a story about a character who places a valued object (e.g. some chocolate) at one place (A) and then departs. In his absence, the object happens to be transferred from place A to another place (B). The character returns, wanting his chocolate, and the child is asked either where the character thinks it is or where the character will look for it (it matters little which form of the question is used). Normally developing children pass this task (i.e. say that the character will look at place A) at about age 4, whereas the average 3-year-old is likely to say that the character will look in the place to where the object has been moved (B)—and will think it is there.

Wimmer and Perner[1] (Wimmer and Perner have diverged somewhat in their views of this transition; the position being reported here is to be found in Perner[2]) explain these data in the following way. What is essential to a theory of mind (ToM) is possessing the insight that the mind is a representing device and that its representations, like all representations, can be false as well as true. What is also essential to a ToM is appreciating that a false representation is no less likely to drive behavior than a true one (for example, we look for things where we think they are—not where they really are). In short, an understanding of false beliefs and of their power to cause behavior is the *sine qua non* of possessing a ToM. This appreciation—the data suggest—does not come to fruition until 4 years. Baron-Cohen et al[3] report that individuals with autism are severely challenged by the false belief task, requiring a verbal mental age of about 8 years (on average) to pass it. Even if they do pass it, of course, this does not necessarily mean that they have 'acquired' a ToM rather late in the day. Rather, they may have learned how to 'hack out' a solution to it—in Frith and Happé's[4] phrase.

How might one account for the coexistence in autism of paucity of pretend play and difficulty with false belief? Leslie[5] argued that both of them exemplify the ability to copy a literal, or first-order, perceptual representation of the way the world is into a second-order representation—a representation, in Leslie's own metaphor, in quotation marks. This is a representation that is neither true nor false: that can be operated on with truth-value bracketted off. He originally called this capacity 'metarepresentation'. (He later changed the term to M-representation, in order to avoid confusion with Perner's rather different use of the term.) This is clearly at stake in the false belief task, insofar as understanding what it means to hold a belief requires the individual to understand the status of a representation that is neither true nor false in itself—only in the running for truth. Meanwhile, the metarepresentational nature of pretend play is most easily appreciated in the case of joint pretense (sharing a pretend game with another); indeed, Leslie himself described it in this context. In his example, the toddler might see his mother putting a banana to her head and talking into it as if it were a telephone. The child's appreciation of what is going on here would seem to depend upon his or her ability to grasp that mother is not entertaining a literal representation of the banana, but that she is bracketting truth-value and taking the banana to be just what she wants it to be. But note that Leslie's claim was not that metarepresentation is only required for pretend *communications* of this kind: it is also necessary for *solo* pretense. I will return to this point.

A moment's thought tells us, however, that there is nothing specifically mental about the capacity for metarepresention, if this is supposed to mean no more than 'representing the world non-literally or non-veridically', because drawings, sentences, films, scale models and, of course, photographs all do it too. So is the claim that autism is a difficulty with metarepresentation of all kinds, or is that it is only the *mental* form of metarepresentation that is impaired in autism? (In Perner's view, what is acquired by normally developing children around 4 years is an insight not into *mental* representation, but into the representation-referent relation in all domains.) An experiment forced a resolution of this ambiguity. Leslie and Thaiss[6] and Leekam and Perner[7] demonstrated that children with autism are *not* challenged by the so-called false photograph task, whose narrative structure is similar to that of the false belief task but in which the child is asked about an out-of-date (and therefore 'false') photograph of a situation. In other words, children with autism seem to be challenged by tasks that require them to understand the representing function of minds, not of *any* medium. Leslie argued that the capacity to grasp *mental* metarepresentation lies at the heart of ToMM.

When it first appeared, the ToMM-deficit view seemed to be remarkably successful at explaining the constellation of symptoms in autism—a constellation that, on the surface, lacks a common denominator. Indeed, the claim was that the theory explains Wing and Gould's[8] 'triad' of symptoms, which are:

- impairment in social behavior (the 'aloof', the 'passive' and the 'odd');
- impairment in verbal and non-verbal communication;
- paucity of imagination.

Children impaired in (as it came to be called) 'mentalizing' would be expected to engage in deviant kinds of social behavior and to fail to communicate with others adequately. But the particular strength of Leslie's hypothesis was that it explained why impairments in imagination, exemplified by a lack of solo pretense, are found together with the first two kinds of impairment.

For a number of years, the ToMM-deficit theory of autism seemed to be the only one available. Perhaps one reason for its hegemony was that the research program for those choosing to work in this area almost wrote itself: identify ToM tasks failed by normally developing under-4s, and give them to children with autism and to a control group of non-autistic mentally handicapped children.

We now turn to the shortcomings of this theory.

Problems with Leslie's metarepresentation hypothesis

Leslie claimed that the onset of pretend play marks the maturation of the ToMM. In other words, the reason why children begin to pretend is that they are becoming able to metarepresent, with pretend play being a symptom or spin-off of this. Such a view would look more plausible, however, were it not for the fact that it is *solo* pretense that arrives at 18 months. Joint pretense (exemplified by the banana scenario) comes later.[9] Moreover, recent research has suggested that children do not have the *concept* of pretending until they are 4[10] or even 5[11] years of age. This puts severe pressure on Leslie's position, suggesting that the act of pretending in toddlerhood may not in fact be a sign of mental-concept understanding; and if it is not, then Leslie's claim about the core deficit in autism is weakened. One of the main attractions of this theory, recall, was that it seemed to explain why poor performance on tests of mental state understanding coexist with lack of *solo* pretend play in the disorder. Leslie has further work to do to persuade us that solo pretense, as well as joint pretense, requires metarepresentation (see below).

Also note that Leslie's hypothesis is that pretense is absent or impoverished in autism because these children lack a concept rooted in the metarepresentational capacity. If so, they should not only fail to generate pretense but should also fail to take what might be called the pretend-stance when encouraged to do so. But it turns out that they are as able as are non-autistic, mentally handicapped children to use pretend props (e.g. a pen standing for a toothbrush) when the context makes this appropriate[12].

Finally, it may be that Leslie's analysis of solo pretense in terms of metarepresentation is flawed.[13] In a nutshell, the pretending toddler might represent himself to himself in the following way: I PRETEND—(of)—the banana—(that) 'It is a telephone'. But might such an act not be entirely 'first order', requiring no reflexive awareness of what one is engaged in? In fact, what is wrong with the venerable Piagetian idea that pretend play is a matter of children's sensorimotor categories ('schemes') becoming sufficiently independent of the current state of physical reality to allow them to take a liberal view of what will count as an X—anything roughly (say) telephone-shaped will do? If so, the advent of pretend play comes to look more like a flourishing of executive control or autonomy than the arrival of a new insight into the nature of mental representation.

What is the third member of the 'triad'?

Recall that lack of imagination is the third member of Wing's triad. How-ever, what Wing was trying to capture in her taxonomy was not a simple absence but a definite presence: the presence of a narrow, repetitive range of activities. (Wing[14] writes in reference to the original classification that Wing and Gould 'found that this kind of abnormality of social inter-action was closely associated with impairment of communication and imagination, the latter resulting in a narrow, repetitive pattern of activi-ties.'). That is to say, what belongs in the third place of the triad is some explicit reference to the fact that individuals with autism are fundamen-tally unspontaneous, being severely rule-bound and novelty-shunning. Indeed, it has to be said that Wing is somewhat unusual in stressing imagination per se and in her view that lack of imagination *causes* repeti-tive behavior. (Rutter's[15] third behavioral criterion is "insistence on same-ness" as shown by stereotyped play patterns, abnormal preoccupations or resistance to change, while Ishii and Takahashi's[16] third criterion is 'insistence on the preservation of sameness or resistance to change'.)

In short, not only does the ToMM-deficit hypothesis fail adequately to account for the paucity of pretend play in autism, but, in its original form at least, it simply ignored one of the major behavioral manifestations of autism—behavioral rigidity. This is not to deny, however, that an enthusi-ast for this theory could make a plausible attempt to explain such rigidity in terms of impaired mentalizing capacities. This is, in fact, what is attempted by the philosopher Peter Carruthers,[17] who argues that impaired ToM will deny children with autism proper access to their *own* mental states, and thus result in failure to assess what will and will not be fun to do or be worth doing. Meanwhile, Perner[18] argues that difficulties with inhibition in early childhood (and by extension in autism) might be caused by lack of insight into the nature of mental representation.

What is a 'module'?

All three theories we shall be considering assume that autism is associated with a lack of insight into, or at least lack of fluency with, mental concepts. So if that is all the ToMM-deficit theory is saying, then it is little more than a description. What makes the theory distinctive, however, is its reference to a mental *module*. Indeed, Leslie is best understood as saying that the disorder of autism is evidence for ToMM itself: nature's demonstration that humans can lack ToMM *while lacking no other significant psychological function.* As we have just seen, however, the failure to account for behavioral rigidity undermines this claim.

What's more, one dissociation does not make a module. The fact (if it *is* a fact; see below) that children with autism are challenged by the false belief task and not challenged by the false photograph is not even evidence for a double dissociation, given that no report has appeared of a clinical population that has impaired understanding of out-of-date pictorial representations but is perfectly good at answering questions about out-of-date mental representations.

Baron-Cohen[19] tried to bolster the modularity claim by reference to the philosopher JA Fodor's[20] influential criteria for modularity. However his decision to jettison three of the nine criteria on rather ad hoc grounds does not inspire confidence. Moreover, one of these three would appear to lie at the very heart of Fodor's program. This is the criterion of 'informational encapsulation', meaning that a module's operation is uninfluenced by top-down or adjacent processing (for example, we know that the two lines in the Müller–Lyer illusion are really equal but we still see them as unequal). What this boils down to is the fact that the computations within a module are *sui generis*, which is to say that they cannot be influenced by what is going on elsewhere in the system; otherwise they would be sharing representations with other systems—something that will disqualify them from being modules. 'The informational encapsulation of the input systems,' Fodor writes, 'is, or so I shall argue, the very essence of their modularity.'[20] However Baron-Cohen rejects this criterion because 'this seems to me to prevent the quite useful possibility that modules interact with one another in a way I will suggest some of those in the Mindreading System do'.[19] Thus unencumbered, he suggests there is a nest of precursor modules maturing before the full-blown ToM module matures. These are the intention detector (ID) and the eye direction detector (EDD), which together channel information into the shared attention mechanism (SAM), after which the ToMM is activated. (The recent work of Leekam[21] and her colleagues casts doubt on the claim being made here that failing to follow gaze adequately in autism is in fact due to failing to share attention. It may be due to failing to benefit from attentional cueing.)

Those who find this way of theorizing problematical may prefer to focus on another of Fodor's nine criteria—'associated with a fixed neural architecture'. If it could be shown that (1) the computing of mental concepts has a determinate neuroanatomical locus, and (2) that this does not function in the normal way in autism, then the ToMM-deficit theory would gain in plausibility. The neuroimaging of brain activity when subjects are thinking about mental states has, however, yielded somewhat contradictory results. Baron-Cohen et al[22,23] implicated the right frontal orbitomedial cortex. Fletcher et al,[24] meanwhile, found that the region covered by Brodmann's areas 8/9 (otherwise the 'paracingulate cortex') was active when drawing inferences about other people's mental states, an area that overlaps with the medial frontal lobe (with left predominance), which Goel et al[25] found to be active in similar circumstances. (For recent imagining data on social perception, see chapters by Firth et al and by Perrett in Baron-Cohen et al.[26]) In a follow-up to the Fletcher et al study, Happé et al[27] demonstrated that individuals with Asperger's syndrome did not show the same pattern of brain activity as that shown in the normal volunteers. The only safe conclusion at this time is 'watch this space', coupled with the caution that it would be unwise in the extreme for psychologists to allow their explanatory categories to be determined for them by neuroanatomy alone. Behavioral and cognitive criteria for modularity cannot be ignored. Moreover, it is important to bear in mind that whether there is a 'social brain' (to which the answer must surely be 'Of course!'), whether this may or may not be activated in the normal ways in autism, whether there is a mental module for computing mental concepts, and whether neuroimaging work has demonstrated that this is impaired in autism, are quite separate questions.

What is 'mental'?

Leslie was very precise about what it means (or was supposed to mean) to possess a ToM. For while the term 'metarepresentation' can be taken in a number of ways (for example, some workers—Frith[28] and, to some extent Leslie[5]—take it to be a neurocognitive mechanism, while others (notably Perner[2]) regard it as a form of explicit knowledge) it does at least focus the research program on the capacity for constructing a particular kind of mental representation. Minds have a number of functions, and erecting representations that are only in the running for truth is but one of them. In contrast to this commendable clarity, what characterizes more recent research on ToM in autism is a very relaxed attitude—perhaps a fatally relaxed one—towards what is to count as the content of a ToM.

Thus, Baron-Cohen et al[29] used the so-called 'language of the eyes' test to identify mentalizing impairments in autism. In this test, a subject views a face, or just its eyes, which has been cut out of a magazine (sometimes the expression is posed) and is asked to decide whether the face is expressing (say) a 'serious message' or a 'playful message'. A panel of four people will have already decided that the facial expression is showing (say) the playful message. Adequate performance on this test means giving a judgment that concurs with the panel's.

We are dealing here with an entirely different domain of mental state understanding than that discussed by Leslie. While facial expressions *may* be categorized as displaying purely cognitive states (e.g. incomprehension, having the 'ah-ha!' experience), more often than not they are expressions of demeanor—as are ways of walking, sitting, speaking and so forth. A person's demeanor is both unintended and intimately linked with his or her affective state. Given this, what such work is doing is embellishing a picture previously drawn by the research of RP Hobson during the early 1980s (reviewed in Hobson[30]), showing that children with autism are poor at categorizing facial expressions of emotion and poor at making cross-modal judgments about emotional expression (e.g. vocal/facial/bodily). Also see the work of Yirmiya et al.[31]

Hobson argues forcefully that the ability to parse (let alone 'resonate to') the emotional expressions of others is not something reducible to purely cognitive and representational abilities: the emotional is not grounded in theory, however we interpret that term. Hobson fields certain Wittgensteinian ideas in favor of this view, and certainly it is Wittgenstein to whom one turns for the reasons why emotional understanding cannot be reduced to the ability to compute the right 'theory'. Wittgenstein[32] invites us to consider the case of a mother whose *first thought* on seeing her child cry as if in pain is 'Is he really in pain?' His point is that it is language-based systems that are theoretical, in the sense of opening up the possibility of doubt and questioning. But these theory-exercising systems must be grounded in something immediate (i.e. not conceptually mediated) and unquestioning.

My concern here is not with questions of causal primacy between affective and mentalizing impairments in autism, so much as with the fact that affective impairments exist—the existence of the 'aloof' subtype of social abnormality points to this—and how their existence is dealt with by what might be called the second wave of ToMM-deficit theorizing. For Baron-Cohen,[33] the ability to read the 'language of the eyes' is explicable in terms of the fact that the superior temporal sulcus and the amygdala are elements of the neural system responsible for the operation of the EDD module, itself part of the 'mind-reading system'. In other words, the neural mechanisms responsible for social understanding are colonized as ToMM's neural substrate in the service of explaining autism. But (in contrast to the Leslie position) it is difficult to see how this way of proceeding has any real explanatory value. It is difficult to see, indeed, how it could be disproved. Everybody accepts that neural mechanisms mediate social understanding, and describing what we know about these and then saying that they make up the 'mind-reading system' and that this is impaired in autism fails to bolster the ToMM-deficit view of autism, given that so much about the disorder remains unexplained (see the next two theories).

Considerations such as these have led to the ToMM-deficit position losing popularity in recent years. Many of those who work on autistic cognition are now more concerned with aspects of the disorder that this theory ignores, in the hope that these aspects may help us to understand the mentalizing deficits themselves. This research program is, in fact, less quixotic than it sounds.

The weak central coherence theory

In his influential book *The Modularity of Mind*,[20] Fodor considered the *fate* of information picked up by the input systems (also known as 'modules'). It was supposed to travel upwards in informationally encapsulated isolation to the so-called *central systems*, about whose working, Fodor despairingly concluded, we know almost nothing. Whether or not the despair was justified, it is incontestible that any account of cognitive architecture whose only constituents are modules is doomed to fail, given that thinkers integrate information across domains, act on and frame beliefs about information from multiple sources, and move both metaphorically and literally from domain to domain (analogical reasoning was for Fodor the quintessential central capacity). What then would be the consequences of possessing adequately functioning input modules (even including, perhaps, the ability to parse others' social behavior as, say, 'intentional' versus 'unintentional') while lacking whatever kind of neural architecture it is that enables global and domain-general cognition? Frith[34] argued that the consequence would be something like autism. This is the weak central coherence (WCC) theory.

Note that what is distinctive to this theory is that it not only predicts the kind of tasks that will challenge individuals with autism, but also predicts that in some areas individuals with autism will *outperform* control subjects. This is because some kinds of task require us to set aside our natural inclination to (say) pick up the gist of a text rather than process it sentence by sentence, to attend to the meaning of an event rather than the elements that make it up—to see a wood rather than some trees. Individuals who have weakly functioning central systems might be expected to have highly efficient input systems and so will inevitably be good at finding the elemental needle in the global haystack. In fact, autobiographical accounts of their disorder written by high-functioning adults with autism typically carry reports of a fragmented phenomenal life.[35]

There is an array of evidence for this theory (succinctly reviewed in Happé[36]). I will briefly mention some of it.

Using context to interpret speech

An excessively bottom-up cognitive style might reasonably be thought to cause the individual to struggle with figurative language. Thus, someone who processes speech sentence by sentence and ignores the surrounding verbal and social context will interpret 'He is as strong as an ox' or 'Well played!' (after being clean-bowled first ball) literally. Individuals with autism do indeed find figurative speech hard to understand.[37] (In fact, one of the defining features of autism is an excessively pedantic and 'robotic' style of speech.) In fact, this neglect of context goes down to the level of word pronunciation. For example, Happé[38] showed that a group of high-functioning individuals with autism failed to use previous sentential context to disambiguate homographic words like 'tear'. Thus, when reading 'In her dress there was a big tear' they would say the final word so as to rhyme with 'teer', as this is the pronunciation commonly given when the word is presented alone.[39]

Perceiving parts within wholes

Certain IQ subtests require people to detect elements within wholes, either as an end in itself (the Embedded Figures Test) or as a stage in constructing a target whole from elements (the Blocks Design Test). In the first case, individuals may have to detect a triangle within a drawing of a pram; in the second case, they may have to configure a group of four bricks to represent a black triangle with a yellow surround—something that cannot be achieved unless one initially perceives the whole as made up of four elements of a certain kind. Individuals with autism outperform control subjects on the Embedded Figures Test.[40,41] Shah and Frith[42] also showed that the frequently reported supranormal performance of people with autism on the Blocks Design Test is due to their excellence at performing the initial segmentation of the target shape.

Visual illusions

Many visual illusions are encouraged by the immediate visual context. Consider Titchener circles in which two circles that otherwise look (and are) equal in size look as though they are of different size when one is surrounded by larger circles and one is surrounded by smaller circles. Happé[43] showed that individuals with autism are less subject to such context-induced illusions than are controls. This outcome is likely to have been due to their tendency to dis-embed elements, given that the control groups' performance was improved by highlighting the target lines, while the performance of the autistic group was not.

Savant skills

Savant skills are common, though by no means universal, in autism, and at least two of these can be viewed as the outcome of excessively local processing styles. Perfect pitch is over-represented in the disorder, something that might be regarded as being due to a heightened sensitivity to a note's particular character, as distinct from its place on the scale. Also, Pring et al[44] concluded from their research into the nature of savant-like drawing abilities in autism that it seems to be due to their ability to break up wholes into parts.

Relation to theory of mind

The WCC theory predicts, of course, that an association will be found between good performance on tasks like the Embedded Figures Test and Blocks Design and poor performance on ToM tasks. The evidence is somewhat equivocal. Happé[45] reports that the minority of individuals with autism who pass ToM tests are just as likely to show weak central coherence as are those who fail them. However, Jarrold et al[46] report an inverse relationship between speed of completing the Embedded Figures Test and performance on ToM tasks. As we shall be discussing later with regard to the ED theory, however, this kind of work also inspires questions about whether tests like false belief are indeed dipstick indicators of the depth at which mental concepts are understood.

It has to be said, however, that the a priori case for linking weak central coherence and weak ToM is less than overwhelming. While it is true that mind-reading in real time requires the ability to assess current context, it obviously requires much else besides. Alternatively, one might construct a causal–developmental account, saying that a child's early experience of self and others being fragmented will impede the acquisition or maturation of such a theory; but claims of this kind are notoriously difficult to test.

More promising than this is a recent attempt to give a cognitive neuropsychological underpinning to the coexistence of weak central coherence and poor mentalizing. This account integrates evidence from two sources. On the one hand, it has been long believed that the right hemisphere is responsible for global, context-sensitive processing; while on the other hand, Happé et al[47] have recently reported that patients with acquired lesions of the right hemisphere (compared with left-hemisphere patients) are likely to have severe social–pragmatic problems and are likely to be impaired on adult-appropriate ToM tasks.

Failure of global integration or oversensitivity to differences between stimuli?

I turn finally in this section to a recent sceptical response to WCC theory—a response that can also be regarded as a cognitive theory of autism in its own right. It starts with the thought that while phenomena of the kind just reviewed do indeed cluster under a 'failure-of-global-processing' umbrella, the WCC theory is *itself* too global. Like the ToMM-deficit theory, it is a high-level account of the deficit couched in terminology used by a philosopher to describe cognitive architecture. What is required instead—this view says—is a theory that starts from an information-processing account of how stimulus categorizing is achieved in the normal case (both human and animal), considers how this might break down, and then predicts the strengths and weaknesses that individuals with autism will be seen to have on simple learning and attentional tasks—predictions that might diverge from those derived from those of WCC theory. Note that this approach also makes a clear contrast between failing to integrate stimuli or their elements (as in WCC theory) and adequate integrative ability coupled with *supra*normal ability at discriminating between stimuli and their elements.

Broadly speaking, this is the research strategy adopted by Plaisted. With reference to discrimination abilities, she notes that we have a successful associative account of a discrimination phenomenon called 'perceptual learning', first reported by Gibson.[48] In contemporary perceptual learning experiments, subjects are initially faced with a discrimination between two exemplars, A1 and A2, that have been generated from a single prototype, A. When this discrimination has been learned, they are then given two new exemplars drawn from the same prototype, A3 and A4, and their ability to make this discrimination is assessed against their ability to learn to discriminate between stimuli of a similar kind but which have been drawn from a different prototype—B3 versus B4. (A second group will have experienced this process in reverse, with stimuli drawn from prototype B being seen initially.) The perceptual learning effect is exemplified by subjects benefiting from pre-exposure to stimuli drawn from the same prototype.

McLaren et al[49] explain this effect in the following way. On the assumption that stimuli consist of elements, presenting two similar stimuli to subjects, as in the present case, results in their being exposed to sets of elements that are (1) unique to A1, (2) unique to A2, and (3) common to both. The associative model that underlies this need not detain us, except for us to note its assumption that the common elements have reduced salience because their associative value is at asymptote (it is, as it were, 'exhausted'), thus affording the *unique* elements *increased* salience. Then, when A3 and A4 are seen, the same kind of process can take place, given that, because they are drawn from the same prototype, they will have very similar sets of common elements. These common elements will have reduced salience, something that will inevitably boost the salience of each set of unique elements. It is evident that this is not only a theory of perceptual learning but a general account of perceptual categorization. Note, by the way, that insofar as it would assume that the initial discrimination is made by globally categorizing A1 versus A2, WCC theory does not predict the perceptual learning effect itself.

Plaisted et al[50] report that high-functioning adults with autism were better than controls at learning the discrimination in the pre-exposure phase but that they did not, unlike controls, show perceptual learning. In other words, they were better than normal at perceiving unique properties and worse than normal at extracting the prototype from which the initial pair of stimuli was derived and generalizing this to new cases. Common features are poorly processed, while unique stimulus features are processed supranormally.

In another study, using children this time, Plaisted et al[51] made a more direct comparison between predictions derived from their theory and from WCC theory. This was a study of visual search. It it well known that search for targets in a field of distractors that are specified by a conjunction of features is slow compared to search for targets that have a single, unique feature. For example, a green X placed in a field with distractors made up of green Ts and red Xs is defined by the conjunction of the feature 'green' (shared with one set of distractors) with the feature X (shared with another). By contrast, a green S would be uniquely defined. In the latter case, the target is reported to 'pop out'. Treisman and Gelade[52] famously argued that in the conjunctive case, focal attention is required if one is to achieve *integration of features*.

Weak central coherence theory would seem to predict that individuals with autism will be even more challenged than are normal subjects by conjunctive search tasks, if indeed the integration of elements is required. By contrast, if individuals with autism are super-good at detecting differences between stimuli, then they should be better than normal at conjunctive search. This latter prediction was borne out. Plaisted et al found that children with autism were not, unlike the control children, significantly slowed in the conjunctive (as against the feature) search task: they were faster than the controls (Figure 14.1). Next: what is the role of number of features that have to be integrated as compared to the perceptual similarity between target and distractors? A subsequent study by O'Riordan and Plaisted[53] varied the two factors independently, and found that in both children with autism and controls it was perceptual similarity (not number of features) that had the greater, retarding influence on reaction time. They were, as before, super-good at discriminating between similar stimuli.

Finally, how might this approach explain ToM impairments? As ever with theories that posit low-level impairments, there are causal–

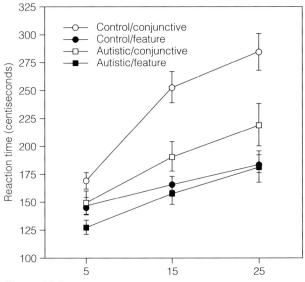

Figure 14.1

Typical data from Plaisted's visual search studies showing reaction times in centiseconds to detecting the presence or absence (two data sets combined) of targets under conjunctive and feature conditions in individuals with autism and normal controls. The horizontal axis shows the number of distractor stimuli.

developmental stories that one can tell about how the early appearance of these impairments might impede the development of mentalizing capacities. Plaisted[54] suggests that if prototype extraction is impaired, then so too will be face perception (faces being the prototypical proto-type)—and thus *social* perception. This may be the case. Or one might, once more, take a cognitive–neuropsychological tack and consider the possible contribution of impaired right-hemisphere processing. If the left hemisphere is relatively more responsible for stimulus processing in individuals with autism, then, given that the neurons in the left hemisphere are more attuned to high spatial frequencies,[55,56] it can be conjectured that this difference is responsible for the supranormal ability to detect fine differences in individuals with autism which Plaisted and her colleagues have unearthed.

The ED theory

This theory adopts what used to be the poor relation of the impairment triad—behavioral rigidity. Needless to say, disorders of spontaneity point directly to the presence of executive disorders.

There are several ED theories, most of which are represented in a recently published book.[57] (Somebody whose work could not be included in this book is Claire Hughes, who has collected important data on the broad phenotype of autism.[58,59]) What I will do in this final section is focus on the version of ED theory which I have been developing, partly because this ED theory makes the strongest claims about the influence of executive impairments on ToM development in autism.

The evidence for ED in autism

It is difficult to define the executive functions in a non-tendentious way. For the time being, therefore, we will work with the broad and intuitive definition of 'the appropriate initiation and inhibition of physical and mental action', noting that this obviously means that many forms of processing must contribute—such as working memory and self-monitoring. Here is a selection of evidence for ED in autism (for an exhaustive review see Pennington and Ozonoff,[60] and chapters in Russell[57]).

- high-level strategic planning;[61,62]
- low-level motor planning;
- categorical set-shifting;[61,62]
- shifting of visual attention on-line;[61,62,64]
- generating novel and random actions;[65–67]
- simultaneously maintaining a rule in working memory and inhibiting a prepotent response;[68,69]
- monitoring negative feedback;[70]
- working memory[71] (but see Russell et al;[72])
- monitoring the visible outcome of actions[73–75] (see later in the text for evidence of lack of impairment in action monitoring—for reasons that I do not have space to discuss, the negative evidence is the more persuasive);
- discriminating one's own from another's actions at recall.[76]

It is also worth noting that Hughes reports that parents[58] and siblings[59] of children with autism are likely to perform poorly on tests of set-shifting, while performing normally or supranormally on certain non-executive measures. Moreover, other workers have suggested links between executive and social skills. McEvoy et al[77] demonstrated an inverse relationship, in a group of non-retarded children with autism, between joint attention skills and the tendency to make perseverative responses on the Spatial Reversal Task (a measure of set-shifting): the less joint attention, the more perseveration. The authors plausibly argue that the ability to shift cognitive set is a necessary condition for successfully sharing attention with another person. On the same theme, Berger et al[78] showed, in a prospective study of high-functioning adolescents with autism, that cognitive set-shifting skills predicted later progress in social understanding (as measured by social comprehension tests); measures of general intelligence, however, did not.

The executive demands made by ToM tasks

Many, though not all, formal tests of executive functioning require subjects to do the following two things at the same time: inhibit a prepotent response and hold in working memory some action-relevant information. Many, though not all, ToM tasks make similar demands. This is clearly the case with respect to the false belief task, insofar as the child has to refrain from telling the experimenter what he or she knows to be true (chocolate at B) while framing an answer to the question in terms of the protagonist's state of belief. Given this, it may turn out that the reason why children with autism are so dramatically impaired on ToM tasks is that they are faced with the joint problem of mentalizing plus executive demands. Moreover, it may be the case that certain kinds of social impairment are not due to a failure to mind-read so much as failure to inhibit the wrong kind of behavior and engage the right kind (witness the Berger et al study referred to above).

I turn now to the evidence for ToM tasks challenging children with autism in virtue of the executive demands that they make. First, we know that children with autism are poor at strategic deception,[79] while everyday observation shows them to be lacking in guile. This could be because their fragile understanding of mental states makes it difficult for them to implant false beliefs into another's mind, or it could be that they are challenged by the executive requirement to disengage from known reality while holding non-veridical information in mind.

My colleagues and I[69] have tried, using the so-called Windows Task, to tease apart the executive and mentalizing requirements in strategic deception, both in normally developing pre-school children and in children with autism. In the Windows Task, the child plays a game against an opponent to win sweets. In the first phase, he or she points to one of two, closed, opaque boxes (one of which contains a sweet) as a way of telling the opponent where to look. The child learns, post hoc and trial-by-trial, that it is in his interests to point to the empty box, because if the opponent visits that one the child wins the sweet from the other box—otherwise it goes to the opponent. In the next phase, the boxes are changed to ones containing windows. These face towards the child and away from the opponent, so that now the child can see which box is empty. Our original concern was with whether subjects can draw the inference that they should point to the empty box *although they have never been reinforced for doing so*. Broadly speaking, the under-4s point to the baited box and the over-4s point to the empty box. Moreover, children with autism are much more likely to point to the baited box than are ability-matched mentally handicapped children. What is more, it is not uncommon for the young pre-school children and the children with autism to continue to point to the baited box (thus losing the sweet each time) for at least 20 trials.

This pattern of autistic responding on the Windows Task certainly looks more like a case of perseveration with a prepotent response than a failure to implant a false belief into the mind of an opponent. Indeed, we later found that this pattern of perseverative responding continues both in normal children[80] and in children with autism[68] when there is no opponent to deceive: the child merely has to point to the empty box with the experimenter sitting next to him.

In a second set of studies, we asked whether children with autism have specific problems understanding the *representing* function of minds, in contrast to experiencing an executive difficulty with juggling competing mental representations. In the first place, it is necessary to note that it is equally accurate to call the false belief task a 'competing belief task', because at the time of being asked the question the child can be said to have in mind two competing representations: his or her own true belief and another's false belief. The first of these might be called 'strong and wrong' and the second 'weak and right', with the executive demand being to suppress the first and frame an answer on the basis of the second. Such an analysis allows us to pose the following question. Beliefs are of course *representational* mental states; to hold a belief is to represent the world as being a certain way. Desires, however, need not be representational. So when I say 'I want a cheeseburger', this implies nothing about how I take the world to be. This is why the sentence 'I believe a cheeseburger' makes no sense: to believe X implies that the world is being represented as being a certain way (you believe a cheeseburger *what*?). Given this, one can ask whether children with autism are challenged by conflicting desire experiments to the same extent as they are challenged by conflicting belief experiments. If they are, then one might suspect that their problem centers on the conflict between 'strong and wrong' versus 'weak and right', not with understanding what it means for mental states to represent. In a task that replicated the narrative and executive structure of the false belief task but with a desire content we were able to show that children with autism were indeed equally challenged by conflicting desire. (In the conflicting desire task, the child plays a game against a puppet in which the first player to complete a jigsaw of a frog wins. The players take it in turns to turn over colored cards, with each color representing a piece of the jigsaw. At time-one they both want the same color and at time-two they want different colors because the child has gained the color he wants. The child is asked the color of the card that the *puppet* wants. As in the false belief task, the other person's mental state stays the same while the child's changes; except that in this case, the relevant mental state is desire rather than belief.)[81]

Finally in this section, the fact that children with autism are not challenged by the false photograph task would *appear* to impede any attempt to explain their failure on false belief tasks in executive terms. This is because the false photograph task might be said to set up a similar kind of 'strong and wrong' versus 'weak and right' conflict to that engendered by the false belief task. But does it? While cautioning that the notion of 'prepotency' has a rather intuitive basis, it can nonetheless be said that one's current true belief (on being asked about another's out-of-date belief) about where a desired object is located is likely to be a more potent lure than one's seeing that a toy cat is now sitting on a toy bed rather than on a toy chair when being asked about an out-of-date photograph.[6] Accordingly, we devised a modified version of the false photograph task intended to boost the prepotency of the wrong information. In this, there was *no* focal object before the camera when the picture was taken (only a screen), and the object (Action Man or Cindy) arrived on the scene while this photograph was developing. In this case, children with autism did indeed perform at a lower level than controls.[81]

In the rest of the chapter I will discuss developmental ideas about how executive dysfunction might impact upon theory of mind.

Relation to ToM (1): The discriminant validity problem

Children with autism do not form the only clinical group with executive problems, and so any ED-to-mentalizing-deficit causal theory must face the challenge of identifying those forms of ED that are special to autism, together with the challenge of saying why these in particular should impact upon mentalizing capacities. This is an aspect of (what workers in this area call) the 'discriminant validity problem',[82,83] discriminating autistic ED from those of other groups.

I will give just two examples of areas in which this discrimination is achieved. First, in a series of studies, Ozonoff and her colleagues succeeded in discriminating children with autism from children with attention deficit hyperactive disorder (ADHD) and Tourette's syndrome (ED has been reported in both) on the basis of the fact that the primary executive disorder within the autistic group, but not within the other groups, was in flexibly switching from one rule to another. They[84,85] tested three groups with the Go–No Go task. There are three phases of this task: (1) respond to one stimulus (e.g. circle) (2) stop responding to this stimulus and respond to another (e.g. square) (3) deal with frequent shifting from one target stimulus to the another. Children with autism performed adequately on (1), performed somewhat worse than controls on (2) and were strongly challenged by (3). In contrast, the ADHD children performed poorly on all phases, while children with Tourette's syndrome were adequate at all phases.

In a second example, we consider a form of executive task that does *not* challenge children with autism but does challenge a population of children with mild frontal deficits—children with early-treated phenyl-ketonuria (PKU). Piagetian search tasks such as A-not-B (with visible or invisible displacement) are executive tasks in the sense that a previously established response has to be over-ridden and a new piece of action-relevant information held in working memory. This task is passed (in its visible displacement form) at about 12 months of age by normally developing children. Diamond et al[86] report that PKU infants perform less well than controls on the visible-transfer version of the A-not-B task, whereas it is well known that young children with autism (matched against mentally handicapped controls) perform adequately on tasks of this kind.[83] Would not any theory proposing a causal linkage between early executive impairments and later mentalizing impairments find this an uncomfortable piece of evidence? On this view, PKU children should be found to have ToM probiems; and nobody has reported these.

Two points can be made in reply. First, the degree of developmental delay in Piagetian search shown by PKU children is actually very modest. Diamond compares the groups in terms of the number of seconds' delay above which the error (return to A) is made. At 12 months (when the error begins to fall away in the normal case) this is only a difference between around 10 s in controls and just below 8 s in PKU (with high phenylalanine levels). It is not as if these children continue to make the error after 12 months. Moreover, at 15 months there are no group differences on the invisible displacement version of the task (although group differences seemed to emerge later). Second, any theory claiming that early executive impairments impact upon ToM development must say which of the many aspects of executive functioning are the crucial ones. Accordingly, it is open to a supporter of such a causal theory to say that Piagetian search tasks do not tap the kinds of executive abilities that strongly impact upon the development of mental concepts. We now encounter one such theory—and its empirical shortcomings.

Relation to ToM (2): A causal–developmental theory assessed

In this section I will briefly review the evidence for a hypothesis of my own about how early executive impairments might impact upon the development of mental concepts.[87,88] Its inspiration was Piagetian. Piaget argued that if a child is to gain a conception of the external world (the other face of which is an experience of the *embodied self*) he or she must be an agent. Lying at the heart of the Piagetian view of agency is the ability to *alter one's perceptual inputs at will*. Next, the child's altering perceptual inputs at will ensures that he or she encounters data that cannot be altered; these data are thus experienced as objective, 'external' to the self, and mind-independent. Given this, impairment in the ability to initiate, inhibit and monitor actions (all of which enable the self-determination of perceptual inputs) can plausibly be said to distort the development of the child's experience of self-hood—as that which determines experience of an objective universe. While having such experiences does not require (it is assumed) the exercise of concepts—it is 'pre-theoretical' in this sense—the later theory-like experience of self (and thus of others) depends on its developing successfully.

How does this theory fare against the evidence? First, it deals with the previously mentioned finding that children with autism are not impaired on Piagetian search tasks by pointing out that Piagetian search skills have generally developed before autism is diagnosed.[89] In the second place, it claims that the aspect of executive functioning whose impairment is most likely to affect ToM development is *action-monitoring*. At its most basic, this means the production of efference copies (also known as 'corollary discharge') of basic actions, but it also encompasses the monitoring of thoughts, at which level it becomes more appropriate to refer to it as 'self-monitoring' (as discussed by workers in schizophrenia[29,90]). The claim is that if children fail to develop (between about 12 and 18 months or so) the ability to monitor actions, intentions and mental episodes (or perhaps if they lose monitoring capacities which they once had), they will fail to develop the kind of experience of self on which the development of an explicit theory of mind depends.

My colleagues and I have recently been testing this conjecture by asking whether children with autism are indeed impaired in the monitoring of basic actions and higher-level intentions. We found no evidence of such impairment. (I had earlier predicted[88] that such impairments would be found, based on the evidence that had been collected to date.[73–75]) With regard to basic actions, children with autism are perfectly good at detecting which moving stimulus on a screen among similarly-moving distractor stimuli they are controlling (Russell and Hill, unpublished data). With regard to higher-level intentions they are also able to describe their original intention when this does not match the outcome. (We used the Transparent Intentions Task here. In this, the child completes an unfinished drawing on a transparency of the kind used for overhead projection. For example, he or she draws an ear on a picture of a boy's head. But, unknown to the child, this transparency has been laid on top of another, so when the top transparency is removed it can be seen that the child has in fact drawn the handle of cup (one drawing had been superimposed on another). Questions are then posed about what the child thought he was drawing (ear or cup) and what he meant to draw.) With regard to the latter finding, the fact that children with autism can characterize their intentions when these conflict with outcomes ('What did you think you were doing?' or 'What did you mean to do?') is a finding that challenges both the ToMM-deficit theory and this version (at least) of the ED theory. I now turn to our latest attempt at an ED theory of autism.

Relation to ToM (3): ED in autism as failures of 'frame control'

It is necessary to distinguish between two kinds of executive task: those in which the subject has to follow an arbitrary rule and those in which he or she has instead to update a mental model of the physical world. It appears that it is only on the former kind of task that individuals with autism are impaired. This may have something important to tell us about how executive and mentalizing impairments are related within the disorder.

Frequently used 'frontal' tasks like Tower of London and Wisconsin Card Sorting Test require subjects to follow a rule that is 'arbitrary' in the following sense. Moving tiles from one configuration to another under certain constraints and sorting cards by (say) color rather than by shape is following a rule without a rationale. That is to say, there is no reason why the tiles should be moved in just this way and no reason why cards should be sorted under one category or another. The situation is quite different in those executive tasks where the necessary action is taken for a reason untraceable to the demands imposed by the experimenter. In search tasks, for example, it cannot be said to be an 'arbitrary rule' that subjects must look in the last place that they saw the object. I will refer to the former type of executive task as 'rulebound' and the latter type as 'non-rulebound'.

With this distinction in mind, I will describe an executive task of each type, each of which is generally failed by normally developing children below the age of about 3 years. (Note that this is well above the age at which autism typically develops, so the fact that children with autism are not impaired on one of the two tasks cannot be explained in terms of age of acquisition (unlike their adequate performance on *Piagetian* search tasks).) See Figure 14.2 for a drawing of the apparatus used in the rule-bound task. This is the 'box task' devised by Hughes and Russell.[68] In the crucial condition, the child must inhibit the prepotent response of reaching through the aperture in the box to obtain a reward (e.g. a marble) and first throw the switch on the side of the box. Reaching without switching first will break a light beam and thereby trigger the mechanism that makes the marble disappear inside the plinth. The switch act has no rationale; or at least it has one only to somebody who understands about light beams and triggering mechanisms.

By contrast, in the second kind of executive task (non-rulebound), the action-relevant information to be held in mind involves not an arbitrary rule but new physical information. In the 'tubes' task (Figure 14.3) devised by Hood,[91] the child sees a ball dropped into the opening of the opaque tube, and has to retrieve the ball. The error that younger children make is to search for the ball in the catch-tray directly beneath the opening—despite the fact that this is not even connected to the tube. One is justified in calling this a 'prepotent error', insofar as it might be said to be

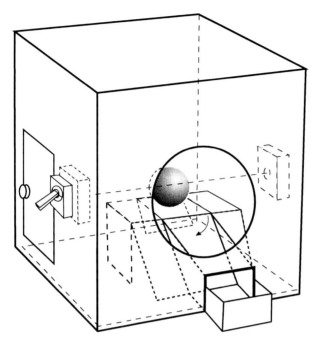

Figure 14.2
A drawing of the box task.

due to the overlearned principle that things fall vertically. Viewed execu-
tively, the child must inhibit acting on this principle and act on the basis
of a representation of the ball's movement. (It is very unlikely that this is a
conceptual failure, given that children can search after invisible displacement at 18 months of age.[92]) We found that while children with autism are
dramatically impaired on the box task,[68] they perform perfectly well on
the tubes task.[93] Furthermore, note that our evidence for intact ability in
action- and intention-monitoring is consistent with the possibility that it is
only rulebound executive tasks that challenge these children.

If further research confirms an autism-specific deficit with ruleboud
executive tasks, what would this imply? It would imply that autism
involves not a generalized executive difficulty, but rather a specific difficulty with moving from one rule to another—an extreme conservativism
about rule-following. But we need to dig deeper to avoid the accusation
(a familiar one in this chapter) of producing a merely descriptive account.

Peterson[94] has recently viewed the profile of cognitive impairments in
autism from the perspective of philosophy and computer science, and
what he suggests certainly illuminates the present data. He notes that
although acting and thinking require us to follow rules, almost all the rules
we follow—those of mathematics and logic are the exceptions—are

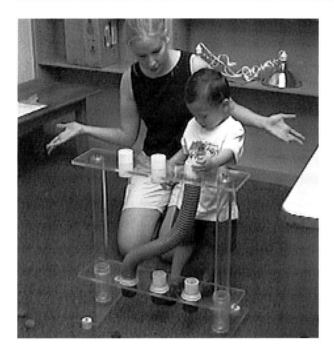

Figure 14.3

A child performs the Tubes task.

defeasible, meaning that they admit of exceptions and that they can be revised in the light of new information. (For example, even the rule that water boils at 100°C is defeasible: it does not do so at the top of Mount Everest.) Accordingly, taking what one might call a 'defeasibility stance' towards rules is an innate human endowment—and thus one that might be innately lacking. Peterson draws an analogy between this rigid rule-following and the so-called 'frame problem' in artificial intelligence. The frame problem is a term used by workers in robotics, a thought experiment to capture the fact that a robot governed by sets of programmed 'if-then' rules will inevitably fail to behave like a human being. For example, a robot might be programmed to collect A-things on its trolley and avoid B-things. Imagine some of the ways in which humans can overcome the frustration of this aim. For example, if a B-thing is tied to the trolley on which the A-thing is being transported, we might cut or untie the string. The robot will need to have this practical knowledge (in the form of 'if-then' rules) programmed in if it is to behave like us. If the string only *rests on* the trolley rather than being attached to it, we will ignore it. How do we ensure that the robot will? It illustrates the impossibility of programming in a set of rules applicable in all possible contingencies: doing so would inevitably lead to a combinatorial explosion. Given this, humans appear to possess a capacity—whatever that is—for abandoning one relatively entrenched rule for some novel ad hoc procedure. The claim can be made, therefore, that this capacity is lacking in autism, and it is this that gives rise to failures on 'frontal' tasks—not to mention the behavioral rigidity that individuals with the disorder show outside the laboratory. There are several ways in which this theory can be tested. For example, it suggests that individuals with autism will be more affected by functional 'fixedness manipulations'[95] than will controls. To illustrate, subjects find it difficult to appreciate that an object can be used as a weight if they had previously been using it as a transformer: they are functionally fixated on it under this aspect. Successful action requires them to move from the electrical domain to the weighing domain. The theory also implies that children with autism will fail to perform on tasks that require an appreciation of the defeasibility of rules like 'sparrows can fly'.

What does this view have to say about the relation between executive and mentalizing impairments in the disorder? I consider (Peterson's views are different) that the link may be made in the following way. Everyday thought involves moving between cognitive frames; it is a matter of ranging across domains in which different rules apply. Unless we are analytical philosophers, scientists or technicians trying to solve clearly circumscribed problems, our minds travel from scenario to scenario in a relatively unconstrained manner. But an individual whose mind did not have this capacity, whose mind was excessively focused and rule-governed, would lack the normal first-person experience of thinking— would have a relatively weak grasp of what we take thinking to be.

Finally, recall my earlier reference to Fodor's notion of the 'central systems' in which domain-general cognition is carried forward. This immediately suggests another prediction that the present theory makes: that individuals with autism will be impaired on tests of analogical reasoning. Scott and Baron-Cohen[95] presents evidence which is supposed to show that such reasoning is intact in autism. However, in their study all the subjects had to do was to draw a parallel between (say) cut Playdough and a cut apple: they remained within the domain of cutting. An appropriately challenging task, however, would require them to see the analogy between cutting and another kind of clean separation, such as divorce. Fodor also characterized central-system thought as 'global'. It is certainly difficult at this point to resist the temptation to refer to right-hemisphere impairments and also to resist the speculation that the neural impairment that underlies autism might be regarded as a general weighting of left-hemisphere against right-hemisphere processing. Such a deficit would be one in overall brain organization rather than one that can be tied to a specific locus. If this is so, the fact that nobody has succeeded in identifying a circumscribed locus of impairment in the autistic brain (see Robbins[97] for a review) looks unsurprising.

There certainly appears to be, then, some scope for rapprochement between WCC and ED theories. And one can say with still more certainty that we are not going to run out of questions.

Acknowledgements

I am very grateful to the following people for their comments on a draft of this chapter: Robert Hanna, Francesca Happé, and Elisabeth Hill.

References

1. Wimmer J, Perner J. Beliefs about beliefs: representational and constraining function of wrong beliefs in young children's understanding of deception. *Cognition* (1983) **13:** 103–28.

2. Perner J. *Understanding the Representational Mind.* (Cambridge MA: MIT Press, 1991).

3. Baron-Cohen S, Leslie A, Frith U. Does the autistic child have a theory of mind? *Cognition* (1985) **21:** 37–46.

4. Frith U, Happé FGE. Autism: beyond 'theory of mind'. *Cognition* (1994) **50:** 115–32.

5. Leslie AM. Pretence and representation: the origins of 'theory of mind'. *Psychol Rev* (1987) **94:** 412–26.

6. Leslie AM, Thaiss L. Domain specificity in conceptual development: neuropsychological evidence from autism. *Cognition* (1992) **43:** 225–51.

7. Leekam SR, Perner J. Does the autistic child have a metarepresentational deficit? *Cognition* (1991) **40:** 203–18.

8. Wing L, Gould J. Severe impairments of social interaction and associated abnormalities in children: epidemiology and classification. *J Aut Child Schiz* (1979) **9:** 11–29.

9. Howes C, Matheson CC. Sequences in the development of competent play with peers: social and pretend play. *Dev Psychobiol* (1992) **28:** 961–74.

10. Josef RM. Intention and knowledge in preschoolers' conception of pretence. *Child Dev* (1998) **69:** 966–80.

11. Lillard A. Young children's conceptualisation of pretence: action or mental representational state? *Child Dev* (1993) **64:** 372–86.

12. Jarrold C, Smith PK, Boucher J et al. Comprehension of pretence in children with autism. *J Aut Dev Disord* (1994) **24:** 433–55.

13. Jarrold C, Carruthers P, Smith PK et al. Pretend play: is it metarepresentational? *Mind Lang* (1994) **9:** 445–68.

14. Wing L. The definition and prevalence of autism: a review. *Eur Child Adol Psychiatry* (1993) **2:** 61–74.

15. Rutter M. Diagnosis and definition. In Rutter M, Schopler E (eds) *Autism: A Reappraisal of Concepts and Treatment* (New York: Plenum Press, 1978): 1–25.

16. Ishii T, Takahashi O. The epidemiology of autistic children in Toyota, Japan: Prevalence. *Jap J Child Adol Psychiatry* (1993) **24:** 311–21.

17. Carruthers P. Autism as mindblindness: an elaboration and partial defence. In Carruthers P, Smith PK (eds) *Theories of Theories of Mind* (Cambridge: Cambridge University Press, 1996): 257–76.

18. Perner J. The meta-intentional nature of executive functions and theory of mind. In Carruthers P, Boucher J (eds) *Thought and Language: Interdisciplinary Perspec-*

tives (Cambridge: Cambridge University Press, 1998): 270–83.

19. Baron-Cohen S. How to build a baby that can read minds: cognitive mechanisms in mindreading. *Cahiers de Psy Cog* (1994) **13:** 513–52.

20. Fodor JA. *The Modularity of Mind.* (Cambridge MA: MIT Press, 1983).

21. Leekam SR, Hunniset E, Moore C. Targets and cues: gaze-following in children with autism. *J Child Psychol Psychiatry* (1998) **39:** 951–62.

22. Baron-Cohen S, Ring H, Moriarty J et al. Recognition of mental state terms: a clinical study of autism and a functional neuroimaging study of normal adults. *Br J Psychiatry* (1994) **165**; 640–9.

23. Baron-Cohen S, Ring H, Wheelright S et al. Social intelligence in the normal and autistic brain: an fMRI study. *Eur J Neurosci* (1999) **11:** 1891–8.

24. Fletcher PC, Happé F, Frith U et al. Other minds in the brain: a functional imaging study of 'theory of mind' in story comprehension. *Cognition* (1995) **57:** 109–28.

25. Goel V, Grafman J, Sadato N et al, Modelling other minds. *Neuroreport* (1995) **6:** 1741–6.

26. Baron-Cohen S, Tager-Flusberg H, Cohen D (eds) *Understanding Other Minds*, 2nd edn. (Oxford: Basil Blackwell, 2000).

27. Happé F, Ehlers S, Fletcher P et al. 'Theory of mind' in the brain. Evidence from a PET scan study of Aspberger Syndrome. *Neuroreport* (1996) **8:** 197–201.

28. Frith CD. *The Cognitive Neuropsychology of Schizophrenia* (Hove: Lawrence Erlbaum Associates, 1992).

29. Baron-Cohen S, Jolliffe T, Mortimore C et al. Another advanced test of theory of mind: evidence from very high functioning adults with autism or Asperger syndrome. *J Child Psychol Psychiatry* (1997) **38:** 813–22.

30. Hobson RP. *Autism and the Development of Mind* (Hove: Lawrence Erlbaum Associates, 1993).

31. Yirmiya N, Sigman MD, Kasari C et al. Empathy and cognition in high-functioning children with autism. *Child Dev* (1992) **63:** 150–60.

32. Wittgenstein L. Cause and effect: intuitive awareness. *Philosophia* (1976) **6:** 413–31.

33. Baron-Cohen S. *Mindblindness.* (Cambridge MA: MIT Press, 1995).

34. Frith U. *Autism: Explaining the Enigma.* (Oxford: Basil Blackwell, 1989).

35. Grandin T. My experiences as an autistic child and a review of the selected literature. *J Orthomolecular Psychiatry* (1984) **13:** 144–75.

36. Happé FGE. Autism: cognitive deficit or cognitive style? *Trends Cogn Sci* (1999) **3:** 216–22.

37. Happé FGE. Communicative competence and theory of mind: a test of relevance theory. *Cognition* (1993) **48:** 101–19.

38. Happé FGE. Central coherence and theory of mind in autism: reading homographs in context. *Br J Dev Psychol* (1997) **15:** 1–12.

39. Snowling M, Frith U. Comprehension in 'hyperlexic' readers. *J Exp Child Psychol* (1986) **42:** 392–415.

40. Jolliffe T, Baron-Cohen S. Are people with autism and Asperger syndrome faster than normal on the Embedded Figures Test? *J Child Psychol Psychiatry* (1997) **38:** 527–34.

41. Shah A, Frith U. An islet of ability in autistic children: a research note. *J Child Psychol Psychiatry* (1983) **24:** 216–20.

42. Shah A, Frith U. Why do autistic

individuals show superior performance on the Blocks Design test? *J Child Psychol Psychiatry* (1993) **34:** 1351–64.

43. Happé FGE. Studying weak central coherence at low levels: children with autism do not succumb to visual illusions. *J Child Psychol Psychiatry* (1996) **37:** 873–7.

44. Pring L, Hermelin B, Heavey L. Savants, segments, art, and autism. *J Child Psychol Psychiatry* (1995) **36:** 1065–76.

45. Happé FGE. Central coherence and theory of mind in autism: reading homographs in context. *Br J Dev Psychol* (1997) **15:** 1–12.

46. Jarrold C, Butler DW, Cottington EM et al. Linking theory of mind and central coherence bias in autism and in the general population. *Dev Psychol* (2000) **36:** 126–37.

47. Happé FGE, Brownell H, Winner E. Acquired 'theory of mind' impairments following stroke. *Cognition* (in press).

48. Gibson JJ, Gibson EJ. Perceptual learning—differentiation or enrichment? *Psychol Rev* (1955) **62:** 32–41.

49. McLaren IPL, Kaye H, Mackintosh NJ. An associative theory of representation of stimuli: applications to perceptual learning and latent inhibition. In Morris RGM (ed.) *Parallel Distributed Processing: Implications for Psychology and Neurobiology* (Oxford: Clarendon Press, 1989: 889–909).

50. Plaisted K, O'Riordan M, Baron-Cohen S. Enhanced discrimination of novel, highly similar stimuli by adults with autism during a perceptual learning task. *J Child Psychol Psychiatry* (1998) **39:** 765–75.

51. Plaisted K, O'Riordan M, Baron-Cohen S. Enhanced visual search for a conjunctive target in autism:

a research note. *J Child Psychol Psychiatry* (1998) **39:** 777–83.

52. Treisman A, Gelade G. A feature integration theory of attention. *Cogn Psychol* (1980) **12:** 97–136.

53. O'Riordan, Plaisted K. Enhanced discrimination in autism. Manuscript submitted for publication.

54. Plaisted K. Aspects of autism that theory of mind cannot explain. In Baron-Cohen S, Tager-Flusberg H, Cohen D (eds) *Understanding other Minds*, 2nd edn (Oxford: Basil Blackwell, 2000).

55. Christman S, Ketterle FL. Hemispheric asymmetry in the processing of absolute versus relative spatial frequency. *Brain Cogn* (1991) **16:** 62–73.

56. Sergent J. The cerebral balance of power: confrontation or cooperation? *J Exp Psychol: Hum Percept Perform* (1982) **11:** 846–61.

57. Russell J (ed.) *Autism as an Executive Disorder* (Oxford: Basil Blackwell, 1997).

58. Hughes C, Leboyer M, Bouvard M. Executive function in parents of children with autism. *Psychol Med* (1997) **14:** 275–300.

59. Hughes C, Plumet M-H, Leboyer M. Towards a cognitive phenotype for autism: increased prevalence of executive dysfunction and superior spatial span amongst siblings of children with autism. *J Child Psychol Psychiatry* (1999) **40:** 705–18.

60. Pennington BF, Ozonoff S. Executive functions and developmental psychopathology. *J Child Psychol Psychiatry* (1996) **37:** 51–88.

61. Ozonoff S, Pennington BF, Rogers S. Executive deficits in high-functioning autistic children: relationship to theory of mind. *J Child Psychol Psychiatry* (1991) **32:** 1081–105.

62. Hughes C, Russell J, Robbins TW. Evidence for executive dysfunc-

tion in autism. *Neuropsychologia* (1994) **32:** 477–92.

63. Hughes C. Planning problems in autism at the level of motor control. *J Child Psychol Psychiatry* (1993) **26**; 99–107.

64. Wainwright-Sharp JA, Bryson SE. Visual orienting deficits in high-functioning people with autism. *J Aut Dev Disord* (1993) **23:** 1–13.

65. Boucher J. Alternation, sequencing behaviour, and response to novelty in autistic children. *J Child Psychol Psychiatry* (1977) **18:** 67–72.

66. Frith J. Cognitive mechanisms in autism: experiments with colour and tone sequence production. *J Aut Child Schiz* (1972) **2:** 160–72.

67. Turner M. Towards an executive dysfunction account of repetitive behaviour in autism. In Russell J (ed.) *Autism as an Executive Disorder* (Oxford: Oxford University Press, 1997) 57–100.

68. Hughes C, Russell J. Autistic children's difficulty with disengagement from an object: its implications for theories of autism. *Dev Psychol* (1993) **29:** 498–510.

69. Russell J, Mauthner N, Sharpe S et al. The Windows Task as a measure of strategic deception in preschoolers and autistic subjects. *Br J Dev Psychol* (1991) **9:** 331–49.

70. Prior M, Hoffman W. Brief report: neuropsychological testing of autistic children through an exploration of frontal lobe tests. *J Aut Dev Disord* (1990) **20:** 581–90.

71. Bennetto L, Pennington BF, Rogers SJ. Intact and impaired memory functions in autism. *Child Devel* (1996) **67:** 1816–35.

72. Russell J, Jarrold C, Henry L. Working memory in children with autism and with moderate learning difficulties. *J Child Psychol Psychiatry* (1996) **37:** 673–86.

73. Frith U, Hermelin B. The role of visual and motor cues for normal,

74. Hermelin B, O'Connor N. Location and distance estimates by blind and sighted children. *Q J Exp Psychol* (1975) **27:** 295–301.

75. Russell J, Jarrold C. Error-correction problems in children with autism: evidence for a monitoring impairment? *J Aut Dev Disord* (1998) **28:** 177–88.

76. Russell J, Jarrold C. Memory for actions in children with autism: self versus other. *Cogn Neuropsychiatry* (1999) **4:** 303–31.

77. McEvoy RE, Roger SJ, Pennington BF. Executive function and social communication deficits in young autistic children. *J Child Psychol Psychiatry* (1993) **34:** 563–78.

78. Berger HJC, van Sapaendonck KPM, Horstick B et al. Cognitive shifting as a predictor of progress in social understanding in high-functioning adolescents with autism: a prospective study. *J Aut Dev Disord* (1993) **23:** 341–59.

79. Sodian B, Frith J. Deception and sabotage in autistic, retarded and normal children. *J Child Psychol Psychiatry* (1992) **33:** 591–605.

80. Russell J, Jarrold C, Potel D. What makes strategic deception difficult—the deception or the strategy? *Br J Dev Psychol* (1994) **12:** 301–14.

81. Russell J, Sattmarsh D, Hill E. What do executive factors contribute to the failure on false belief tasks by children with autism? *J Child Psychol Psychiatry* (1999) **40:** 859–68.

82. Ozonoff S. Components of executive dysfunction in autism and other disorders. In Russell J (ed.) *Autism as an Executive Disorder* (Oxford: Oxford University Press, 1997: 143–78).

83. Pennington BF, Rogers SJ, Ben-

netto L. Validity tests of the executive dysfunction hypothesis of autism. In Russell J (ed.) *Autism as an Executive Disorder* (Oxford: Oxford University Press, 1997: 143–76).

84. Ozonoff S, Strayer DL, McMahon WM et al. Executive function abilities in children with autism and Tourette syndrome: an information-processing approach. *J Child Psychol Psychiatry* (1994) **35:** 1015–32.

85. Ozonoff S, Strayer DL, McMahon WM et al. Inhibitory deficits in Tourette syndrome: a function of co-morbidity and symptom severity. *J Child Psychol Psychiatry* (1998) **39:** 1109–18.

86. Diamond A, Prevor MB, Callender G et al. Prefrontal cortex cognitive deficits in children treated early and continuously for PKU. *Monogr Soc Res Child Dev* (1997) **62:** (Serial Number 252).

87. Russell J. *Agency: Its Role in Mental Development* (Hove: The Psychology Press, 1996).

88. Russell J. How executive disorders can bring about an inadequate theory of mind. In Russell J (ed.) *Autism as an Executive Disorder* (Oxford: Oxford University Press, 1997): 256–304.

89. Bailey A, Phillips W, Rutter M. Autism: towards an integration of clinical, genetic, neuropsychological, and neurobiological perspec-
tives. *J Child Psychol Psychiatry* (1996) **37:** 89–126.

90. Feinberg J. Efference copy and corollary discharge: implications for thinking and its disorder. *Schiz Bull* (1978) **4:** 636–40.

91. Hood BM. Gravity rules for 2–4 year olds? *Cogn Dev* (1995) **10**; 577–98.

92. Piaget J. *The Child's Construction of Reality* (London: Routledge and Kegan Paul, 1955).

93. Russell J, Jarrold C, Hood BM. Two intact executive capacities in children with autism: implications for the core executive dysfunctions in the disorder. *J Aut Dev Disord* (1999) **29(2):** 103–12

94. Peterson D. Dialogical processing and autistic bias. Manuscript available from Department of Computer Science, Birmingham University.

95. Dunkler K. On problem solving. *Psychol Monogr* (1945) Number 270.

96. Scott FJ, Baron-Cohen S. Logical, analogical, and psychological reasoning in autism: a test of Cosmedes theory. *Dev Psychopathol* (1996) **8:** 235–45.

97. Robbins TW. The neurobiology of autism. In Russell J (ed.) *Autism as an Executive Disorder* (Oxford: Oxford University Press, 1997): 21–56.

15
Cognitive dysfunction in tuberous sclerosis and other neuronal migration disorders

John E Harrison and Patrick F Bolton

Introduction

The consequences for cognitive ability of neuronal migration disorders (NMDs) remain a relatively unexplored area of neuropsychological research. One possible reason for this is the strong a priori probability that considerable variations in cognitive competence can be expected in patients who are united by a diagnostic category but who may have markedly different neural lesion sites. In addition to wide variation in the location of brain lesions, considerable variation with respect to lesion size and number has also been acknowledged in individuals with NMDs. The impact of the characteristic lesions seen in NMDs is further complicated by the possibility that lesions may also be epileptogenic foci. Given this variability and complexity, dissociating and quantifying the contribution of epilepsy and brain lesions to cognitive dysfunction has remained a substantial challenge.

The lesions seen in patients with NMDs occur in utero during neuronal migration. The brain is broadly acknowledged to have considerable plasticity during its early development, and so it is conceivable that some reorganization of cognitive ability may occur in patients who acquire lesions early in life. Thus a combination of functional neuroanatomy and neuropsychological assessment with NMD patients may provide a fruitful model for further exploring the 'Kennard effect', the phenomenon by which cognitive function is subserved by untypical neural substrates. In our discussion of the various forms of NMD we will further allude to this possibility.

Lissencephaly

This is a malformation of the brain caused by the failure of nerve cells to migrate and form a normal cortical mantle. This often means that sulci and gyri fail to develop resulting in a smooth rather than convulated cortex; hence the name lissencephaly, taken from the Greek *lissos* (smooth) and *enkephalos* (brain). Children born with lissencephaly will have severe retardation and may experience frequent seizures. Lissencephaly is a feature of a number of syndromes, the most common being isolated lissencephaly sequence, Miller–Dieker syndrome and Walker–Warburg syndrome.

Polymicrogyria

As the name suggests, polymicrogyria is characterized by the presence of increased numbers of small gyri, again due to abnormal neuronal migration. Rather than exhibit the normal six-laminar architecture of normal cortex, the wormlike gyri seen in this disorder usually exhibit either a two- or four-laminar structure. Polymicrogyria can involve the whole brain, but more often involves parts of the brain symmetrically or asymmetrically. This variation in abnormal pathology is reflected cognitively and behaviorally in degrees of mental retardation and seizures.

Schizencephaly

Again, the name of this disorder gives clues to nature. Schizencephaly is characterized by a cleft that extends from the subarachnoid space to the subependyma of the lateral ventricles, caused by the failure of neurons to migrate from the germinal matrix. Clefts can be narrow and closed (type 1) or open and wide (type 2) and are usually located near the pre- or post-central gyri. Schizencephaly almost always leads to severe intellectual impairment.

Heterotopias

These form a group of disorders that feature brain abnormalities due to unsuccessful neuronal migration. Broadly categorized into 'focal' and 'diffuse', heterotopias are associated with mental retardation and epilepsy.

Dysplasia 'not otherwise classified'

This constitutes the general catch-all category for dysplasias that cannot be categorized using the taxonomy that includes heterotopia, lissencephaly, schizencephaly, etc.

A general characteristic of all the foregoing NMDs is that they usually give rise to severe mental retardation that is often accompanied by epilepsy and spasticity. Thus the typical NMD patient has low levels of cognitive function and is generally untestable using anything but the most basic cognitive assessments. Consequently, there are few reported studies of cognitive function in these patient groups. However, the neuronal migration disorder of tuberous sclerosis (TS) is often present in patients who are unaware that they have the disorder until the onset of symptoms quite late in life or when they have children who are more obviously affected by the disease. The most severely affected patients exhibit mental retardation so profound as to rival that seen in the previously discussed NMDs. However, many are free of the behavioral difficulties seen in many patients with the disease and can be of demonstrably normal intellect. In spite of this, very little research has been carried out to investigate cognitive abilities in individuals with TS. In the rest of this chapter we shall review the brief literature detailing cognition in TS.

Tuberous sclerosis

The French neurologist Bourneville (1880) first coined the term 'sclérose tubéreuse', to describe the potato-like growths (hence 'tubers') evident in the brains of patients with the condition. He realized that the epilepsy associated with TS often had a focal origin in one of the tubers and also described the characteristic facial rash ('adenoma sebaceum', now more properly referred to as facial angiofibroma). Interestingly, it would appear that Bourneville thought this coincidental, supposing the rash to be caused by the ingestion of large amounts of bromide, the medication used for treating epilepsy at that time. The prevalence of TS has been estimated to be about 1 in 10 000, whereas the birth incidence is thought to be 1 in 5800.[1]

The causes of brain lesions in TS

The great diversity of manifestations and the marked variation in expression of the disease has always been a challenge to explain in pathophysiological terms. However, with recent advances in the delineation of the genetic basis of TS, a model of pathogenesis that accounts for these puzzling features has begun to emerge. The model is a two-hit model that was first propounded to explain carcinogenesis.[2] According to this model, a mutation in one of the two copies of either of the TSC genes is associated with no or minimal problems, simply because the other normal copy of the gene provides sufficient back-up (i.e. the mutation is recessive). However, during embryogenesis, random somatic mutations (mutations that develop during mitotic cell division) by chance knock out the one remaining functional copy of the TSC gene. As a result, the progeny of this mutated cell grow and divide abnormally and give rise to hamartomas. The brain lesions are therefore believed to develop in the following way. During normal brain development, precursor neuronal cells are located in the ventricular and subventricular zones.[3] They divide and give rise to neurons that then migrate along radial glial lines to the cortical plate, which eventually develops into the laminar cortex.[3] The progeny of any one precursor cell may migrate to widely dispersed cortical regions, particularly if the precursor cell or one of its daughters migrates tangentially in the ventricular zone before migrating radially to the cortical plate.[4] Hence, a second hit in one of the precursor cells can give rise to cell progeny that result in tubers in several different locations. Some support for this model of abnormal neurogenesis is provided by the presence of radial migration wedges on MRI scans.[5] These are wedge-shaped areas of abnormality that have their apex at the ventricles and then fan out to the tuber located on the surface of the cortex. Further support for the two-hit model of pathogenesis comes from molecular genetic studies of tissue from various types of TS lesion. These investigations have shown that the chromosomes in cells from the lesion exhibit loss of heterozygosity.[6] That is to say, there are microdeletions in one copy of the chromosome in the regions 16p13 or 9q34. These microdeletions are thought to be the signs of the somatic mutation. The other copy of the gene may then be found to have a point mutation.

The brain lesions characteristic of TS

Brain lesions of one form or another occur in over 95% of cases. They develop in early fetal life and then usually seem to stay static.[7] The commonest abnormality comprises the so-called subependymal nodules (SENs). These are typically found along the walls of the ventricles, frequently in the striathalamic groove between the caudate nucleus and the thalamus. Histologically, they are composed almost entirely of astrocytes. The clearest images of SENs are obtained using computerized tomography (CT) due to their tendency to calcify, even in very young patients (after about 12 months). In general, SENs are benign; however, in approximately 5–10% of cases they develop into subependymal giant-cell astrocytomas (SEGAs). These may grow and block the foramen of Munro, leading to interference in the circulation of cerebrospinal fluid and hence raised intracranial pressure.

The other common brain lesion is the cortical tuber. Histologically, tubers are composed of the same combination of abnormal glial and neural cells as SENs and exhibit similar signs of demyelination. Physically, the potato-like growths are paler and slightly firmer than normal. The vast majority of tubers are found at the gray–white matter interface, where they disrupt normal cortical structure. Otherwise, the size, number and cortical location of tubers vary greatly from patient to patient.

Identifying TS brain lesions

Cortical tubers are best visualized using magnetic resonance imaging (MRI) scans and usually show up on T2-weighted and proton density images, where they appear hyperintense to the surrounding tissue. Several neuroimaging studies have reported on the distribution of cortical tubers. The large-scale MRI studies of clinic populations have differed somewhat in the distribution pattern.[5,8] In both series, tubers were most common in the frontal and parietal lobes, then the temporal lobes, and lastly the occipital lobes and cerebellum. In the clinic series of Braffman, 40% of patients had between 1 and 10 tubers; 33% 11–20; 14% 21–30, and 5% more than 31.[8] There is only one report of brain scan findings in an epidemiological series of cases, and this was based on CT scan findings, so the results are difficult to compare directly,[9] but, predictably, fewer tubers were found. Thus, in 47 TS patients, 23 (49%) had fewer than two tubers and only one patient had more than 11 tubers. The frontal lobes were involved in 44%, parietal in 34%, temporal in 15% and occipital in 6%. Extremely rarely, tubers may develop in the spinal cord.[7] The reason for this pattern of tuber distribution by lobe is uncertain, but a possible explanation might be that the pattern simply reflects a correlation with the size of these structures.

Studies of cognitive dysfunction in TS

Mental retardation, epilepsy and facial angiofibroma were originally identified as the classic triad of TS signs. However, it has become clear that mental retardation is not a necessary consequence of the disorder. The general literature on mental retardation in TS indicates a level of mental retardation of about 60%. However, this figure is likely to be an overestimate of the true rate, as the more mildly affected cases are unlikely to have been completely ascertained. A figure of 40% is likely to be the most accurate, as it is based on studies of patients largely ascertained through the investigation of relatives of proband cases of TS. This estimate is likely to be more accurate, as the population they ascertained is more likely to include the mild cases that were probably missed by other studies. One study also suggested that the prevalence of mental retardation was significantly greater in males than in females, a finding that the investigators suggested might be explained by the greater vulnerability of male brains to developmental problems.[9] This sex difference has not been reported in other studies.

The clinical diagnosis of mental retardation in these studies was usually based not upon standardized assessments of IQ, but instead on IQ estimates based on the individual's range of function, educational level, and self-help and social skills. Few detailed studies of cognitive function have been conducted, presumably because the profundity of lesions has been presumed to cause substantial global deficits. As a consequence the few existing studies of cognition have been restricted to IQ assessments. For example, Miller[10] found low IQ levels in two TS patients. A later study of 23 child patients[11] showed that seven had normal intelligence, 10 had mental retardation and six both mental retardation and autism. However, even among the seven participants with normal intelligence, four had specific developmental disorders, exhibiting dyspraxia, dyscalculia, speech delays and visuomotor disturbance. This variety in outcome and observed cognitive deficit might well be expected in a heterogeneous disorder such as TS. Classical neuropsychology suggests that lesions in different brain locations are likely to give rise to specific cognitive deficits, dependent upon the location of the lesion. This classical view can be successfully applied to the findings of Jambaque et al,[11] who cite the presence of a sole, left parietal lobe lesion as the likely cause of a case of constructive apraxia in a subject with a measured IQ of 107. The findings and observations of the Jambaque study confirm that in the absence of data collected via formal psychological testing, we cannot be certain that apparently normal patients are indeed free of cognitive deficits.

It was on the basis of a clinical judgment about the presence of mental retardation that Webb et al[12] concluded in their 1991 study that a group of TS patients, secondarily ascertained via a proband case, were of normal intellect. We recently had the opportunity to determine the veracity of this claim by revisiting this family to conduct detailed psychological assessments. The challenge at the outset of this study was the selection of suitable psychological tests for use with a group of patients likely to exhibit considerable variation with regard to lesion number and location. MRI data collected as part of the 1991 study protocol suggested that lesions to prefrontal lobe regions were common in this group (Table 15.1).

We therefore selected a battery of tests, including a number known to be sensitive to lesions to the prefrontal regions, comprising the following tasks.

Controlled Word Association (CWA)

Verbal fluency (VF) tests for the letter 'B' (phonological VF) and the category 'animals' (semantic VF) were administered using instructions similar to those suggested by Lezak.[13] Scores were interpreted with reference to norms collected by one of us.[14] Poor performance on the phonological version of this task has been associated with damage to the anterior portion of what Mesulam[15] had described as a language network. Lesions to the left inferior frontal gyrus tend to give rise to poor performance.[16,17] By contrast, poor performance on semantic versions of the task has been associated with damage to the temporal lobes.[18]

Table 15.1 Distribution of MRI-detected tuberous lesions.[12]

Subject	Age	BDI[1]	Frontal		Parietal		Occipital		Temporal		SEN[2]
			Right	Left	Right	Left	Right	Left	Right	Left	
1[a]	11	NA	2	1	2	–	–	–	–	–	5
2[a]	13	NA	1	1	1	1	1	2	1	1	5
3	17	2	1	–	2	3	–	2	–	–	4
4	30	4	4	–	–	–	–	–	–	–	0
5[a]	43	5	1	–	1	2	–	–	–	–	2
6	43	5	–	–	2	–	1	–	–	1	4
7	56	22	1	1	–	1	–	–	–	–	1
Total		38	10	3	8	7	2	4	1	2	21

[a]History of epilepsy.
BDI, Beck Depression Inventory.
SEN, subependymal nodules.

Hayling Sentence Completion Test (HSC)[19]

This test measures (a) latency of completion of everyday sentences with a word missing at the end. Subjects are then tested for the ability to inhibit an automatic response and generate nonsense words to complete similar sentences (measured as an error score).

Eye Emotion Test (EET)

Given the prevalence of autism in sufferers from TS, we included this test, which has been shown to be sensitive to dysfunction in individuals with autistic signs. This test requires the subject to study pictures of the peri-ocular area of a face from which they must infer a mental state.

Spatial span (SSP)

This is a test analogous to the Corsi block-tapping test,[20] in that it requires subjects to monitor and recall a sequence of blocks that change color.

Spatial Working Memory (SWM)

This task tests a subject's ability to retain information regarding memory for locations previously visited. Errors are scored according to the number of occasions on which the subject returned to a box in which a blue token had already been found. An efficient means of completing the test is to follow a predetermined search sequence, starting with a particular box and then returning to that same box once a token has been found. This yields a 'strategy' measure, obtained by counting the number of occasions upon which the subject does not begin with the previously chosen starting box. Thus a high score implies low use of strategy and a low score an effective use of strategy.

Stockings of Cambridge task (SOC)

This is a modified version of the Tower of London spatial planning task[21] which allows for the measurement of both speed and accuracy of thinking.

Pattern recognition (PRM)

In this task, subjects are presented with two series of 12 abstract patterns and are instructed to remember them. After a 5-s delay, each pattern, paired with a novel pattern, is presented in reverse order and subjects are instructed to touch the pattern they have previously seen.

Spatial recognition (SRM)

In this task, five squares are presented sequentially in different locations around the screen. Subsequently, in the recognition phase, each square is presented with a novel location and subjects are asked to touch the location they have previously seen a square appear in. This procedure is repeated a further three times.

IDED shifting task (IED)

This task requires subjects to learn a series of nine two-alternative, forced-choice discriminations using feedback provided automatically by computer. Two critical stages occur within the test, one at the 6th rule change, when subjects must shift to new exemplars of the most recent dimension, and a second at the 8th rule change, where subjects must shift to a second dimension. This protocol provides two popularly used outcome measures, 'stages completed' and total errors'.

Mini-Mental State Examination (MMSE)[22]

This is a quick and broad assessment of cognitive dysfunction whose utility lies in suggesting areas of dysfunction that might then be further explored. It also functions as a test of both language reception and production, and so can be used as a quick test of the subject's ability to both receive and produce linguistic information.

Raven's Advanced Progressive Matrices (RAPM)[23]

This is a non-verbal test of intellect. Recent research has suggested that it seems sensitive to impairments of fluid intelligence and frontal lobe damage.[24] Interpretation of performance was made with reference to the norms published in the Warrington Recognition Memory Test.[25]

The National Adult Reading Test (NART)[26]

This has been shown to be a relatively robust indicator of premorbid intelligence, relying upon a correlation between vocabulary size and general intelligence.

Beck Depression Inventory (BDI)[27]

Depression has been shown to have a deleterious effect on cognitive performance, a possible confound we sought to control for by using this instrument.

Patient performance was first compared with that of the control group. As expected, no significant differences were seen in the performance of the two groups, consistent with the thesis that any cognitive deficiencies in the patient group would be highly variable, with patient profiles differing markedly from one another. The failure to find differences between the two groups extended to comparisons based on age and IQ, with the patient group recording a mean IQ (99.3, SD = 13) very close to the population mean of 100. In order to test the theory that isolated deficits would be found in individual patients, the authors then conducted single-case assessments, comparing individual performance on the administered tests with normative data sets (full details of this methodology are given in Chapter 1). Performance at or below the 5th percentile level was taken as evidence of dysfunction, a procedure that yielded clear evidence of dysfunction in all but two of the patients tested. As predicted from the pattern of lesion location, performance on tests traditionally shown to be sensitive to prefrontal lesions was the most commonly observed pattern of deficit. The two most sensitive tests to dysfunction were the Stockings of Cambridge and ID/ED shift tests from the CANTAB battery. Poor performance on the former test has been shown to be a common difficulty in patients with lesions to prefrontal regions, a pattern broadly found in the Harrison et al study.[14] Less obvious is a satisfactory explanation for poor performance on the ID/ED set-shifting test. The usual neural correlate of poor performance on this task is the presence of lesions in the basal ganglia. For example, patients with Huntington's disease (HD) are well known to have difficulties at the extradimensional set-shifting stage of this task. Recent research has also shown that patients undergoing bilateral pallidotomy for the amelioration of the signs and symptoms of late-stage Parkinson's disease (PD) are entirely robbed of this skill by the procedure.

A later, larger study by the same group yielded similar findings in a group of 19 patients, again selected on the basis of a clinical judgment of normal intellect confirmed by IQ testing. The pattern of results seen in this wider group was essentially similar to those reported by Harrison et al.[14] However, on this occasion the number of patients performing poorly on the ID/ED task was sufficient to reach statistical significance. This second observation confirming the tendency of some patients to perform the ID/ED task poorly tempted the authors into considering the possible neural abnormalities underlying poor performance on this task.

Previous research using the ID/ED shift task has suggested that patients with basal ganglia[28] or prefrontal lobe[29] dysfunction seem prone to deficits on this task, though probably for different reasons.[30] An issue in much neuropsychological assessment is the sensitivity of tests to patients with specific patterns of dysfunction. In this regard, ID/ED shift deficits are found more reliably in patients with HD than in PD patients. Lawrence et al.[31] suggested on the basis of the performance of HD patients that damage to the caudate nuclei was the likely cause of dysfunction. Both bilateral and unilateral lesions to the caudate nucleus are extremely rare, and so no opportunity exists to test how critical this structure is for successful ID/ED shift completion. However, among the small number of caudate lesion studies reported, a number have suggested dysfunction on tests analogous to the ID/ED shift, specifically the Wisconsin Card Sorting Test (WCST). In fact, of the two reports to discuss the use of the WCST with caudate lesioned patients, Mendez[32] found marked impairment in patients with caudate lesions. More recently, Petty[33] has reported a case of bilateral caudate damage whose WCST deficit was so pronounced that he failed to achieve even one category and made 48 errors.

As discussed above, impaired ID/ED shift performance can be due to a number of possible cognitive deficits. Equally, it follows that lesions to a number of different brain loci can cause these cognitive deficits. However, what is notable about the ID/ED shift is that neuropsychiatric disease categories without frontostriatal involvement do not exhibit impaired performance. So, for example, patients with temporal lobe lesions, depression, mild dementia of the Alzheimer type and undergoing surgical removal of the amygdala and hippocampus are comparable in performance to neurologically normal controls. On the face of it, it seems odd that such a large proportion of TS patients of normal intellect should exhibit dysfunction, especially given the lack of imaging evidence of tuber involvement. However, TS brain lesions are not confined to tubers; in fact, SENs are found in a greater proportion of patients than tubers and are likely to be present in a large proportion of patients in our study sample. Although these lesions are generally believed to be benign, given that they are most often found in the striathalamic groove, between the head of caudate and thalamus, it seems possible that the ID/ED shift deficits seen in TS are due to the presence of these calcified lesions found proximal to the caudate nucleus. Clearly, such a possibility must remain speculative until evidence in support of this assertion is obtained.

Future directions

Cognitive deficits and epilepsy?

An outstanding issue is the currently uncertain relationship between epilepsy and cognitive dysfunction. The relationship between mental retardation and epilepsy is very strong, and particularly so with infantile spasms.[34] In fact, it is very rare for a mentally retarded child with TS not to have a history of epilepsy. Moreover, in those with mental retardation, seizures start significantly earlier than in the intellectually normal. These findings have led to speculation that the mental retardation may, in part, be due to epilepsy. As a consequence, some commentators have suggested that early treatment may improve the prognostic outlook[35] and so recommend prompt, effective management. However, it is also evident that the types of seizure and their age of onset are associated with the number of tubers as well as the characteristics of the brain abnormality.[5] It is possible that the observed association reflects the nature of the underlying brain abnormality, rather than a direct effect of the seizure disorder on intellectual development. This issue clearly warrants investigation.

Is there a shift in the IQ distribution in TS, or is it bimodal?

There has been some speculation that the levels of intelligence found in apparently cognitively normal patients with TS might be generally lower than that of the normal population.[36,37] This line of theorizing asserts that IQ is necessarily lower in individuals who fulfill the diagnostic criteria for the disorder. Thus, if one were able to plot the IQ levels of the TS population against that of the normal population the distributions would be similar to those shown in Figure 15.1a. An alternative perspective, about which there has been much speculation in the literature, is that the IQ distribution for patients with TS is bimodally distributed, perhaps similar to the distribution shown in Figure 15.1b. This thesis provides for the existence of two subgroups within the population of TS patients, one with normal levels of IQ and the other with a shift of the distribution to the left.

Evidence suggesting this to be the case has recently been obtained by Joinson et al.[38] In this study more than 100 TS patients were assessed

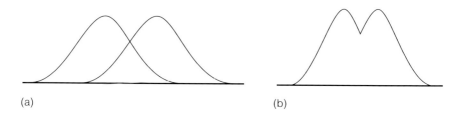

Figure 15.1

(a) Hypothetical TS versus controls distributions and (b) bimodal TS distributions.

and their IQ levels determined. The analysis revealed a bimodal distribution for the TS group, which the authors interpreted as statistical support for the existence of two discrete populations within the TS group, a normal ability group and a group with learning disability. A comparison of the mean IQ of the normal ability group with that of a group of unaffected sublings yielded a statistical significant advantage for the sibling group. This suggests a 'leftward' shift in the mean IQ of even relatively unimpaired TS patients, perhaps similar to the IQ shift reported in cognitively normal patients with neurofibromatosis 1.[39]

Brain–behavior correlates?

Further uncertainties are evident over the detailed pattern of intellectual and cognitive impairments associated with TS. It is, for example, not known whether TS is associated with a general decrement in IQ or whether verbal or performance skills may be more severely affected, according to the location of the tubers. Likewise, it is not known whether individuals with TS of normal intelligence are prone to specific cognitive deficits such as developmental language disorders or specific reading difficulties. The very limited evidence suggests that there may be additional subtleties of these kinds to explore. Furthermore, Baltaxe studied a volunteer sample of 34 TS children. She found that most subjects had expressive language difficulties and problems in auditory language processing and pragmatics. This applied to those with normal as well as near-normal intelligence. However, both of these studies were conducted on clinic and volunteer samples and neither had a control group for comparison, so the findings are difficult to interpret, although they clearly indicate the importance of systematically investigating the issues, using standardized measures.

The relationship between the number of locations of lesions and their consequences for normal function remains uncertain. A major limitation in this regard is the reliability with which lesions can be identified using the various methods of brain imaging. Studies have shown that, of the available techniques, fluid attenuated inversion recovery (FLAIR) sequences appear to be the most sensitive when cortical tubers are being imaged. As already discussed, the substantial inter-subject variation seen in tuber number and location makes simple explanations difficult to come by. However, an extensive study linking structure to function may identify the critical lesions, or patterns of lesions, that compromise cognitive function.

It is appropriate to remind ourselves that psychological tests comprise a relatively blunt tool when seeking to localize brain lesions. However, a number of tests are known to be sensitive to deficits traditionally caused by lesions to the prefrontal areas of the brain. A wealth of studies now attests to the fact that similar deficits occur when neural structures with connections to prefrontal areas are injured.

References

1. Osborne JP, Fryer A, Webb D. Epidemiology of tuberous sclerosis. *Annals New York Academy of Science* (1991) **615:** 125–7.

2. Knudson AG. *Proceedings of the National Academy of Science* (1971) **68:** 820.

3. Rakic P. Corticogenesis in human and nonhuman primates. In Gazzaniga MS (ed.) *The Cognitive Neurosciences* (Cambridge, MA: MIT Press, 1995): 127–45.

4. Levitt P. Experimental approaches that reveal principles of cerebral cortical development. In Gazzaniga M (ed.) *The Cognitive Neurosciences* (Cambridge, MA: MIT Press, 1995): 147–63.

5. Shepherd CW, Houser OW, Gomez MR. MR findings in tuberous sclerosis complex and correlation with seizure development and mental impairment. *Am J Neuroradiol* (1995) **16:** 149–55.

6. Green AJ, Smith M, Yates JRW. Loss of Heterozygosity On Chromosome 16p13.3 In Hamartomas From Tuberous Sclerosis Patients. *Nature Genetics* (1994) **6(2):** 193–6.

7. Gomez MR. *Tuberous Sclerosis.* (New York: Raven Press, 1988).

8. Braffman BH, Bilaniuk LT, Naidich TP et al. MR imaging of tuberous sclerosis: pathogenesis of this phakomatosis, use of gadopentetate dimeglumine and literature review. *Radiology* (1992) **183:** 227–38.

9. Clarke A, Cook P, Osborne JP. Cranial computed tomographic findings in tuberous sclerosis are not affected by sex. *Developmental Medicine and Child Neurology* (1996) **38:** 139–44.

10. Miller VS, Bigler ED. Neuropsychological aspects of tuberous sclerosis. *Clin Neuropsychol* (1982) **4(1):** 26–34.

11. Jambaque I, Cusmai R, Curatolo P et al. Neuropsychological aspects of tuberous sclerosis in relation to epilepsy and MRI findings. *Dev Med Child Neurol* (1991) **33(8):** 698–705.

12. Webb DW, Thomson JLG, Osborne JP. Cranial magnetic resonance imaging in patients with tuberous sclerosis and normal intellect. *Arch Dis Child* (1991) **66:** 1375–7.

13. Lezak M. *Neuropsychological Assessment* (New York: Oxford University Press, 1976).

14. Harrison JE, Buxton P, Husain M, Wise R. Short test of semantic and phonological fluency: normal performance, validity and test–retest reliability. *Br J Clin Psychol* (2000) **39(2):** 181–91.

15. Mesulam M. Large-scale neurocognitive networks and distributed processing for attention, language and memory. *Ann Neurol* (1990) **28:** 597–613.

16. Benton AL. Differential behavioural effects of frontal lobe disease. *Neuropsychologia* (1968) **6:** 53.

17. Miller E. Verbal fluency as a function of a measure of verbal intelligence and in relation to different types of cerebral pathology. *Br J Clin Psychol* (1984) **23:** 53–7.

18. Hodges JR, Patterson K, Oxbury S, Funnell E. Semantic dementia: progressive fluent aphasia with temporal lobe atrophy. *Brain* (1992) **115:** 1783–806.

19. Burgess PW, Shallice T. Response suppression, initiation and strategy use following frontal lobe lesions. *Neuropsychologia* (1996) **34(4):** 263–73.

20. Milner B. Interhemispheric differences in the localisation of psychological processes in man. *Br Med Bull* (1971) **27:** 272–7.

21. Shallice T. Specific impairments of planning. *Phil Trans R Soc (Lond)* (1982) **298:** 199–209.

22. Folstein MF, Folstein SE, McHugh PR. 'Mini Mental State' a practical method for grading the cognitive state of patients for the clinician. *J Psychiatr Res* (1975) **12:** 189–98.

23. Raven JC. *Advanced Progressive Matrices* (London: HK Lewis & Co., 1958).

24. Duncan J, Emslie H, Williams P et al. Intelligence and the frontal lobe—the organisation of goal-directed behaviour. *Cogn Psychol* (1995) **30(3):** 257–303.

25. Warrington EK. *Recognition Memory Test Manual* (London: NFER-Nelson, 1984).

26. Nelson H. *National Adult Reading Test* (Windsor: NFER-Nelson, 1982).

27. Beck AT. *Beck Depression Inventory* (London: The Psychological Corporation, 1988).

28. Downes JJ, Roberts AC, Sahakian BJ et al. Impaired extra-dimensional shift performance in medicated and unmedicated Parkinson's disease: evidence for a specific attentional dysfunction. *Neuropsychologia* (1989) **27(11–12):** 1329–43.

29. Owen AM, Roberts AC, Polkey CE et al. Extra-dimensional versus intra-dimensional set shifting performance following frontal lobe excisions, temporal lobe excisions or amygdalo-hippocampectomy in man. *Neuropsychologia* (1991) **29(10):** 993–1006.

30. Owen AM, Roberts AC, Hodges JR et al. Contrasting mechanisms of impaired attentional set-shifting in patients with frontal-lobe damage or Parkinsons disease. *Brain* (1993) **116(Pt 5):** 1159–75.

31. Lawrence AD, Sahakian BJ, Hodges JR et al. Executive and mnemonic functions in early Huntington's disease. *Brain* (1996) **119:** 1633–45.

32. Mendez MF, Adams NL, Lewandowski KS. Neurobehavioral changes associated with caudate lesions. *Neurology* (1989) **39(3):** 349–54.

33. Petty RG, Bonner D, Mouratoglou V, Silverman M. Acute frontal lobe syndrome and dyscontrol associated with bilateral caudate nucleus infarctions. *Br J Psychiatry* (1996) **168(2):** 237–40.

34. Webb DW, Fryer AE, Osborne JP. On the incidence of fits and mental retardation in tuberous sclerosis. *Journal of Medical Genetics* (1991) **28:** 395–7.

35. Webb DW, Osborne JP. Tuberous Sclerosis. *Archives Of Disease In Childhood* (1995) **72(6):** 471–4.

36. Gillberg IC, Gillberg C, Ahlsen G. Autistic behaviour and attention deficits in tuberous sclerosis: a population-based study. *Dev Med Child Neurol* (1994) **36:** 50–6.

37. Harrison JE, Bolton P. Tuberous sclerosis. *J Child Psychol Psychiatry* (1997) **38(6):** 603–14.

38. Joinson C, O'Callaghan FJ, Osborne JP et al. Learning disability and epilepsy in an epidemiological sample of individuals with tuberous sclerosis. (Submitted.)

39. Ferner RE, Hughes RA, Weinman J. Intellectual impairment in neurofibromatosis 1. *J Neurol Sci* (1996) **138:** 125–33.

16
Motor neuron disease

Sharon Abrahams and Laura H Goldstein

Summary

Motor neuron disease (MND) is characterized by the progressive degeneration of the upper and lower motor neurons. Approximately 90% of cases are sporadic, with an incidence rate of 1–2/100 000. The disease typically affects adults in late middle life, and 75% of patients present with symptoms in the limbs, while 25% present with bulbar signs. The disease typically progresses to affect other regions, and death usually occurs between 1 and 5 years from the onset of symptoms.

Traditionally, MND has been regarded as a disease of the motor system with no impairment of cognitive abilities. Cognitive deficits were thought to be exclusively associated with a frontotemporal dementia which occurs in approximately 3% of individuals with MND. However, evidence has now accumulated of a pattern of selective cognitive impairment in non-demented MND patients. Despite variable results on specific tests, the majority of neuropsychological studies have revealed predominantly executive deficits, with memory impairment less consistently reported and relative sparing of other cognitive functions. The most striking and consistent deficit is found using verbal fluency (VF) procedures. One of the major problems, which only a few studies have addressed, is how to allow for the range of physical disability, which may exaggerate performance deficits.

The application of both structural and functional brain-imaging techniques has been fruitful in understanding the cerebral dysfunction which underlies these cognitive deficits. A growing number of imaging studies has demonstrated a pattern of extra-motor cortical and subcortical dysfunction in MND patients, with corresponding cognitive impairment. The findings have extensively implicated the frontal cortex, and neuropsychological tests such as verbal fluency have been shown to be a sensitive indicator of such extra-motor involvement. Recent neuropathological evidence has also demonstrated neuronal loss in corresponding extra-motor regions.

Research is now shifting towards determining whether such cognitive and extended cerebral changes are restricted to a subgroup of patients and how MND-associated dementia relates to cognitive impairment in MND without dementia. In addition, the association between cognitive deficits and clinical signs of bulbar dysfunction and emotional lability is being considered, as is the profile of impairment in primary lateral sclerosis. Longitudinal studies combining functional neuroimaging and neuropsychological assessment are being planned.

What is motor neuron disease?

Definitions and terminology

Motor neuron disease is a progressive disorder characterized by degeneration of the upper motor neurons (UMNs) and lower motor neurons (LMNs). In the UK, MND is a more generic term used to include the complete spectrum of the disease. Amyotrophic lateral sclerosis (ALS), originally described by Charcot and Joffroy,[1] is the most common syndrome within the rubric of MND and is defined by degeneration of both UMNs and LMNs.[2] Other rare clinical variants include progressive muscular atrophy, where symptoms and signs remain confined to the LMNs, and primary lateral sclerosis, with only UMN involvement. Progressive bulbar palsy, consisting of bulbar and pseudobulbar palsy, is another syndrome within MND, but largely overlaps with the Charcot-type ALS syndrome. The syndromes of progressive bulbar palsy and Charcot-type ALS are referred to collectively as ALS in North America and in most of Europe, but are referred to as MND in this chapter, according to UK practice.

Epidemiology

The majority of cases of MND are sporadic.[3] However, there exists a familial variant of the disease with an autosomal dominant transmission that affects almost 5% of cases.[4] The incidence of sporadic MND is estimated to be approximately 1–2/100 000, with a prevalence of 4–6/100 000.[5,6] The worldwide incidence is fairly constant, expect for small isolated areas where there is a high incidence of atypical variations of the disease (e.g. Western Pacific Island of Guam). Sporadic MND is generally more common in men than in women, at a ratio of 3 : 2. Onset typically occurs in late middle adult life, and onset prior to the age of 30 is rare. The peak age of onset is between 55 and 75 years of age. Patients with a younger age of onset generally have a better prognosis.[2,7,8]

Diagnostic criteria and clinical presentation

Diagnosis of MND is based on clinical and electrophysiological evidence of a progressive disorder with the characteristic combination of both UMN and LMN signs in the same body region.[9] Research diagnostic criteria embody this approach in the El Escorial criteria.[10] The UMNs (pyramidal tract or corticospinal tract motor neurons) originate in the primary motor cortex and form synapses with the LMNs in the motor nuclei of the brainstem (via the corticobulbar tracts) and in the spinal cord (via the corticospinal tracts). The LMNs directly innervate the muscles, connecting them to the central nervous system, and form the spinal reflex arc. When the LMNs die, there is a reduction in the release of trophic factors into the muscle, resulting in wasting of the muscle tissue. In addition, the reflex arc is broken, reflexes are depressed or absent, muscle tone is flaccid and fasciculations may become apparent. The UMNs serve to modulate the function of the reflex arc. Damage to these neurons causes spasticity and increased sensitivity of the tendon reflexes.

Clinical presentation of a patient with typical MND involves a combination of both upper and lower motor neuron signs, which can affect cranial, limb, thoracic and abdominal muscles. The majority (75%) of MND patients present with symptoms in the limbs, while 25% present with bulbar symptoms (e.g. dysarthria and dysphagia).[5] Regardless of the site of onset, the disease typically progresses to affect the other regions. At present there is no cure, and prognosis is poor. Death usually occurs within 1–5 years from the onset of symptoms (median ~3.5 years), as a result of respiratory failure. However, 20% of patients survive beyond 5 years, and 10% survive beyond 10 years.

Etiology and treatment

Etiology remains unknown, despite a range of hypotheses, which have included excitotoxic neuronal damage via increased levels of glutamate, autoimmune pathogenesis and neurotrophic deficiencies (for reviews see Shaw,[6] Eisen and Krieger[7] and Appel et al[11]). Gene mutations have been identified in the familial variant of the disease, and mutations in the superoxide dismutase (SOD1) gene on chromosome 21 have been suggested to account for approximately 10–20% of all familial cases and 2–3% of all cases.[12,13] In addition, there has been some evidence to link the apolipoprotein E (APOE) gene with the bulbar onset form of MND.[14] Neurofilament gene mutations have also been found in about 1% of sporadic cases.[15]

Clinical trials have recently been conducted on a number of potential therapeutic agents. Riluzole, which inhibits release of glutamate from presynaptic endings, has shown modest effects in prolonging survival.[16] Several neurotrophic factors have also been evaluated, and in one study the insulin-like growth factor 1 produced a positive effect in slowing disease progress,[17] but this has not been replicated.[18]

Neuropsychological investigations in MND

Motor neuron disease has been regarded as a disorder of the motor system, with no associated cognitive impairments. Until relatively recently, cognitive deficits were associated exclusively with approximately 3% of MND patients in whom a frontotemporal dementia occurs[19,20] (this subgroup of patients is described in more detail towards the end of the chapter). However, evidence has now accumulated from neuropsychological investigations that has revealed a pattern of selective cognitive impairments in non-demented patients with typical MND.

Executive functions

The most striking and consistently reported deficit in MND patients has been demonstrated using the VF test.[21-29] Tests of fluency require the person to rapidly generate responses with minimal use of external cues, and hence place heavy demands on executive functions. Typically, impairments have been demonstrated using a spoken letter-based word-generation procedure such as the Controlled Oral Word Association Test, where the participant is required to say as many words as possible, beginning with a given letter, in a limited time period.[21,24-26,28,29] However, such studies have generally not controlled for the degree of dysarthria, which may reduce the rate of speech output and hence exaggerate performance decrements. Deficits have also been demonstrated using a written version of the test, the Thurstone's Word Fluency Test,[30] although this procedure may also be problematic, due to the severity of upper limb involvement in some MND patients and associated writing disabilities. An impairment in MND patients on this test was originally described by Kew et al,[27] who discounted the potential disadvantage caused by writing disabilities by demonstrating that the number of words generated did not correlate with a measure of motor speed.

In an extensive investigation of 52 non-demented patients with MND, a written VF procedure was developed which directly accommodated for writing disabilities.[22] Participants first performed the two standard conditions of Thurstone's procedure (words beginning with letter S in 5 min and four-letter words beginning with C in 4 min). Individual variations in speed of writing were then controlled for by incorporating a copy condition. This enabled the calculation of the 'Verbal Fluency Index' (VFI), which provided an estimate of the average time taken to think of each word ((time allowed for test – time to copy words)/number of words generated). Using this method, a clear VF impairment, independent of physical disability, was demonstrated in non-demented MND patients.[22]

Other fluency procedures have been included less frequently in investigations of MND patients. Abe et al[21] demonstrated an impairment on a category fluency test, in which the participant was required to generate as many examples of animals, fruits and vehicles as possible in 1-min periods. In contrast, Hartikainen et al[31] failed to show a deficit using a simple category fluency procedure in which the participant had to produce as many four-footed animals as possible in 1 min. Once again, these semantic-based word-generation procedures both involved spoken responses and hence were vulnerable to the effects of speech impairments. Ludolph et al[28] demonstrated evidence of a deficit using a non-VF test, in which participants were required to draw as many different figures as possible by connecting five symmetrically arranged dots. MND patients did not show a deficit on the total number of figures drawn, but displayed a significant increase in the number of rule breaks (perseverative errors and incorrectly completed drawings).

The Wisconsin Card Sorting Test (WCST) has also been frequently used to investigate cognitive impairment in MND. This test is widely used in a clinical setting to measure the executive functions of rule deduction and shifting mental set. Abrahams et al[22] demonstrated evidence of a deficit on this test in the group of 52 MND patients, with a significant reduction in the number of categories achieved and an increased number of errors. This finding was consistent with previously reported MND studies, which have used the WCST or a similar shorter modified version.[24,29,32] However, several studies have also failed to replicate these results using the same procedures.[27,28,33] Impairments in shifting mental set have also been revealed using the Alternating S test and Trail Making Test,[31] but both of these measures rely on motor speed and hence may be vulnerable to the effects of disability. Other tests of executive function which have shown some sensitivity to the cognitive impairments in MND include tests of verbal reasoning[25,26] and picture-sequencing, which assesses the ability to plan, organize and monitor one's own performance.[33]

Deficits in attention in MND patients have been revealed using the Verbal Series Attention Test, which includes a range of tests dependent on working memory processes (e.g. counting backwards in threes).[29] Several tests of visual attention have also shown some sensitivity to deficits in MND patients.[24–26,29,34] Chari et al[34] administered a computerized battery of non-verbal tests (Cambridge Neuropsychological Test Automated Battery, CANTAB) to a group of 50 MND patients. The battery accommodated for physical disability by estimating patients' sensorimotor capacity. With this method, evidence of a deficit in focal attention (visual search) independent of physical disability was revealed. In contrast, patients showed unimpaired performance on recognition memory and learning tasks. Finally, an impairment has also been elicited on some measures of selective attention (Stroop;[24] Negative Priming[22]). However, this has not been consistently demonstrated.[27,28]

Memory functions

The findings from investigations of memory functioning in MND have been even more variable, and impairments have not been consistently reproduced. On tests of verbal memory, an impairment in prose recall was reported in one study,[35] but not in others.[31,32] Deficits in word-list and paired associate learning have been more frequently reported,[23,25,29,32] but inconsistently.[27,28] In addition, a word-recognition deficit was demonstrated by two recent investigations,[22,24] but not by earlier studies.[27,29,33]

On visual memory tests, a deficit in object recall was demonstrated using the Kendrick Object Learning Test (KOLT) or similar picture-recall procedures,[23,27,32] but was not replicated elsewhere.[22] An impairment has also been found in the immediate recall of shapes and designs, using the Benton Visual Retention Test,[24] but no deficits were revealed in delayed visuospatial recall, using the Rey Osterrieth Figure.[28,32] Finally, a visual recognition memory deficit was elicited in MND patients using the Kimura recurring figures test,[24] which supported the earlier findings of an impairment in the visual recognition of abstract stimuli,[25] but no deficits have been reported using a number of other measures.[27,33,34]

Language functions

Simple language functions have generally been found to be preserved in MND, with no impairments on tests of naming.[27,29,33] More complex language abilities have been sometimes shown to be impaired, with poor scores on verbal subtests of the WAIS-R,[22,24] although deficits have not been found in other studies.[27,32] Finally, Talbot et al[33] demonstrated a deficit on the token test, a measure of language comprehension. However, the pattern of impairment in MND patients indicated poor self-regulation of performance and executive dysfunction, with an increase in perseverative errors, rather than a primary linguistic disorder.

Strong et al[36] highlighted the need for a comprehensive assessment of language in MND. In addition, they emphasized the difficulty in assessing language functions in MND patients with bulbar involvement and associated dysarthria. This is clearly evident on procedures such as the subtests of the WAIS-R, which require elaborate spoken responses, thereby disadvantaging patients with bulbar dysfunction.[22]

Visuoperceptual functions

Visuoperceptual functions have been found to be relatively intact, with unimpaired performance on tests of fragmented letters,[27] judgment of line orientation[29] and the Dot Counting, Position Discrimination, Number Location and Cube Analysis subtests from the Visual Object and Space Perception battery.[33] In addition, unimpaired performance has been shown on tests of mental rotation.[27] Hartikainen et al[31] reported evidence of a deficit on simple and more complex visuoperceptual functions using the Digit Symbol and Block Design tests of the WAIS-R, although both of these tests rely on motor speed for effective performance and do not allow for upper limb disabilities.

Summary of neuropsychological investigations

Overall, the growing number of neuropsychological studies have produced variable results on specific tests, despite a similar cognitive profile of selective impairments in tests of executive and memory functions, with apparent relative sparing of other cognitive functions. The most consistently reported deficit is found using tests of verbal fluency, indicating underlying dysfunction in executive processes. The investigations also revealed less convincing evidence of a memory impairment across a range of visual and verbal memory procedures, including tests of immediate and delayed recall, and recognition. Language and visuoperceptual functions appear to remain relatively intact. Unfortunately, with the exception of a few recent investigations, these studies have not attempted to control for disabilities in speech and motor functions, which are prevalent in this patient group and which may have served to exaggerate these impairments.

Neuropsychological investigations and brain imaging in MND

The application of recently developed brain-imaging techniques to the study of MND has been fruitful. There is an increasing number of both structural and functional imaging studies, which have provided strong evidence of extra-motor cerebral involvement in non-demented MND patients. Moreover, recent investigations have directly related such findings to a corresponding pattern of cognitive dysfunction.

Structural imaging studies

Early structural imaging studies typically showed atrophy restricted to the motor cortex and corticospinal tracts in non-demented MND patients, using computerized tomography (CT)[26,37] and magnetic resonance imaging (MRI).[38–40] David and Gillham[32] did succeed in detecting cerebral atrophy in 8 of 14 MND patients using CT; however, these data were not quantified, and hence no correlations could be attempted with neuropsychological measures.

The development of more sensitive MRI techniques has provided evidence of extra-motor cortical and subcortical atrophy. Kiernan and Hudson[41] employed volumetric MRI measurements and revealed shrinkage in the volume of the underlying white matter in the anterior frontal cortex in 11 non-demented patients with MND, but no significant frontal cortical atrophy. In a longitudinal study of MND, progressive atrophy of the frontal and temporal regions was demonstrated using serial CT and MRI.[42] Atrophy was initially detected in the frontal and anterior temporal lobes, and then progressed to the pre- and then post-central gyrus, anterior cingulate (AC) and corpus callosum. Three of the patients studied were also demented, but the frontotemporal degeneration was not restricted to these patients. Unfortunately, in neither of these structural imaging investigations were the findings related to neuropsychological data.

A recent study by Frank et al[24] obtained volumetric measures of MRI scans in 74 patients with sporadic MND. When the patients were divided into two groups based on the presence or absence of neuropsychological impairments (with impairment reflecting deficits on tests of VF, visual attention, and visual memory), the impaired group showed more pronounced changes of ventricular enlargement and parenchymal atrophy in cranial magnetic resonance images. Unfortunately, the magnetic resonance volumetric techniques in this study did not allow for the delineation of separate brain regions.

Functional imaging studies

A variety of functional imaging techniques has been employed to investigate cerebral dysfunction in MND. Ludolph et al[28] conducted a positron emission tomography (PET) study of 18 MND patients and demonstrated reduced cortical glucose utilization in the frontal and entire cortex. Neuropsychological assessment undertaken on some of these patients revealed deficits on selective tests of executive function, namely verbal and non-verbal fluency. Talbot et al[33] employed single photon emission computed tomography (SPECT) to demonstrate pronounced reductions in regional cerebral blood flow (rCBF) in frontal and anterior temporal cortex in non-demented patients with MND. These patients also showed evidence of subtle frontal lobe dysfunction, with deficits on picture sequencing and a tendency towards poorer performance on VF and the WCST.

Both SPECT and MRI techniques were used in a recent investigation by Abe et al.[21] Twenty-six MND patients were divided into three groups on the basis of a cluster analysis of a number of neuropsychological measures, including tests of executive function (WCST, VF), attention and memory function. A comparison between the three groups and healthy controls revealed that patients in group 1 were specifically impaired on tests of attention and executive function, patients in group 2 displayed deficits of attention, while patients in group 3 had preserved ability of attention and executive function. In addition, patients in groups 1 and 2 had evidence of corresponding frontal lobe atrophy on MRI scans (detected by visual assessment of the scans) and reduced isotope uptake in frontal regions on SPECT, which was more evident in patients in group 1. These findings suggest that deficits in attention and executive functions may evolve in MND patients in correspondence with pathological changes in the frontal lobes.

A series of studies in MND patients has also made use of PET activation techniques.[23,27,43] Kew et al[43] employed a motor activation paradigm involving the random generation of movements. The task compared rCBF during paced joystick movements in a freely chosen (random) direction to movements only in a forward direction (stereotyped). Abnormalities in rCBF were revealed in the medial prefrontal cortex, AC gyrus and parahippocampal gyrus in a group of 12 MND patients. In a further study,[27] 16 MND patients were divided into two groups (impaired or unimpaired) based on their performance on a written VF test. The two groups, each consisting of five patients, were then compared with healthy controls on the above PET activation paradigm. The results demonstrated that both MND groups showed significant reductions in rCBF in medial prefrontal cortex and parahippocampal gyrus. In addition, MND patients who were impaired on the fluency test showed abnormalities in the AC gyrus and anterior thalamic nuclear complex. The results of these studies suggested that rCBF abnormalities were present along a limbo–thalamo–cortical pathway in some patients. In addition, cerebral dysfunction in these regions was more pronounced in MND patients who performed poorly on the written VF test.[27]

A further PET activation study was then designed to explore more directly the association between deficits on VF tests and frontal lobe cerebral dysfunction in MND.[23] As the activating task, the study employed a VF procedure which compared rCBF during two conditions: letter-based word generation and word repetition. Two groups of MND patients were formed, defined by the presence or absence of impairment on a written VF task (which was adapted to accommodate for writing disabilities). The comparison of rCBF measurements between the two patient groups and healthy age-matched controls during the fluency activation task revealed extensive regions of reduced activation only in the MND patients who were impaired on the written VF test. Significantly impaired activation was found in regions of the dorsolateral prefrontal cortex, lateral and medial premotor cortex, primary motor cortex and insular cortex, bilaterally. In addition, there was again clear evidence of subcortical involvement, with reduced rCBF in the anterior thalamic nuclear complex.[23] Patients with MND who were unimpaired on the written VF test showed relatively normal patterns of rCBF activation. These results were obtained despite matched performance on the fluency task during scanning, and suggest that deficits in VF constitute a sensitive indicator of cerebral dysfunction (predominantly involving the frontal cortex) in MND. It should be noted that a subsequent comparison between the two MND patient groups revealed a number of significant differences on other tests of executive and memory function, including the WCST (number of trials to first criterion), paired associate learning (learning of hard word pairs) and KOLT.

Summary of brain-imaging investigations

The findings of a growing number of structural and functional imaging studies have demonstrated regions of extra-motor cortical and subcortical dysfunction in MND patients with cognitive impairments. These regions have extensively involved the frontal cortex and correspond to the predominance of executive dysfunction found in this patient group. These studies have strongly associated deficits on specific cognitive tests with such cortical and subcortical involvement, and demonstrate that such neuropsychological measures constitute a sensitive indicator of extended cerebral dysfunction.

Neuropathological investigations in MND

Further evidence of the cortical and subcortical dysfunction which may underlie the cognitive deficits in MND patients is beginning to emerge from postmortem neuropathological investigations. Rafalowska and Dziewulska[44] investigated six MND patients and demonstrated white matter changes in the frontal, temporal and parietal lobes. The finding of atrophy in the underlying subcortical white matter is consistent with the structural MRI findings reported by Kiernan and Hudson.[41] In addition, in the study by Abe et al[21] described earlier, in which three groups of MND patients were investigated, subsequent postmortem investigations revealed spongy degeneration and neuronal loss in the frontal lobes in patients with the most severe cognitive impairment (group 1). This patient group was shown to be specifically impaired on tests of attention and executive functions. Hence, these results strongly relate cognitive dysfunction to the underlying cortical and predominantly frontal lobe atrophy in MND.

Neuropathological investigations have also revealed a pattern of subcortical involvement in non-demented MND patients, consistent with the findings of the brain-imaging investigations.[23,27,28,43] Pathological changes have been reported in the limbic structures, with ubiquitin immunoreactive inclusions in the dentate gyrus of the hippocampus and associated entorhinal cortex and in the amygdala in some non-demented MND subjects.[45–48] Such changes in the limbic system may be associated with the memory impairment that is sometimes found in MND patients.[23,27,43] MND has also been associated with thalamic degeneration. Brownell et al[49] reported thalamic gliosis in 53% of 36 cases of non-demented MND patients. In other patient groups, thalamic abnormalities have been related to severe cognitive changes, including memory loss and frontal lobe-type deficits.[50,51]

Cognitive deficits and subgroups of MND

There is now convincing evidence of cognitive deficits and extra-motor cerebral involvement in non-demented patients with MND. Hence research is now shifting towards determining whether such changes are restricted to a specific subgroup of patients and to exploring the relationship between the various clinical presentations of the disease.

MND-related dementia

The relationship between non-demented MND patients and cases of MND-related dementia remains unclear. The dementia may pre-date, follow or develop concurrently with the symptoms of motor neuron degeneration,[52,53] although the cognitive changes commonly constitute the presenting symptoms. These cases are characterized by behavioral and cognitive problems reflecting gross frontal lobe dysfunction with relative preservation of functions of the posterior association cortices.[53,54] Behavioral features include disinhibition, apathy and personality changes.[19,20] Formal neuropsychological testing is often difficult, due to the severity of the disorder. However, some studies have demonstrated gross deficits in verbal fluency, attention and shifting from one line of thinking to another.[33,54] The underlying pathology in these cases of MND-related dementia has been shown to consist of spongiform neuronal degeneration in layers 2 and 3 of the prefrontal cortex,[48,53,55,56] with additional involvement of regions within the limbic system (the hippocampal formation, subiculum and amygdala).[45,47,48,57]

   This profile of predominantly frontal lobe-type cognitive dysfunction with corresponding cortical and subcortical dysfunction parallels that found in non-demented MND patients, although the latter clearly exhibit less severe cognitive deficits and cerebral dysfunction. This finding has led to the suggestion that within MND a spectrum of extra-motor cortical and subcortical involvement exists.[46] Talbot et al[33] employed a battery of neuropsychological tests and SPECT imaging techniques to compare directly patients with classical MND, MND-related dementia and frontal lobe dementia alone. All three groups were shown to have reduced rCBF in frontal and anterior temporal regions, and this was more pronounced in the two dementia groups. The neuropsychological and SPECT findings showed a common pattern of cerebral involvement, indicating that MND-related dementia should be regarded as a clinical variant of disease and that the three disorders represent a clinical range of a pathological continuum. They suggest that patients with classical MND resulting from initial brainstem and spinal cord involvement may only show mild frontal lobe involvement due to poor life-expectancy, which limits the spread of the disease into the frontal lobes. In contrast, in cases of initial extensive frontal lobe-type involvement (frontal lobe-type dementia), the disease may spread to the brainstem, and hence patients may go on to develop symptoms of MND and hence MND-related dementia.

Bulbar dysfunction

Several studies have explored the relationship between cognitive deficits and bulbar involvement in MND. Such investigations stem from the finding that bulbar dysfunction is present in up to 85% of MND-related dementia cases.[19,33,52,56] In addition, an earlier study of non-demented MND patients suggested that cognitive impairment was more likely to be found in patients with bulbar dysfunction.[32] However, this assumption may have been somewhat unfounded, as only three of the total of 14 subjects studied did not show this neurological picture.

Bulbar dysfunction in MND results from UMN (pseudobulbar palsy) and LMN (bulbar palsy) involvement, both of which may produce the characteristic symptoms of dysarthria. In a recent investigation conducted by Massman et al,[29] a very large cohort of 146 participants with sporadic MND was investigated. The battery of tests employed measures of executive function, attention, memory, language and visuoperception. Selective deficits of executive function and attention were found only in a subgroup of 35.6% of patients. In addition, the presence of dysarthria was suggested to be associated with increased risk of being classified as cognitively impaired. This, it was thought, could reflect the possibility that dysarthria was associated with greater cerebral involvement. However, it must be noted that reduced speech output associated with dysarthria would serve to disadvantage patients on a number of neuropsychological measures. More convincingly, Kiernan and Hudson[41] demonstrated a correlation between clinical scores of bulbar function and volumetric measures of underlying white matter in the anterior frontal cortex in 11 non-demented MND patients. This finding indicated that the degree of neuronal degeneration of axons projecting to the frontal cortex was related to the severity of bulbar involvement.

In a recent investigation, we examined whether abnormalities of cognitive function were related to the presence of pseudobulbar palsy (defined by UMN involvement in the bulbar region).[22] The study employed a combination of standard and more experimental tests of executive and memory function to investigate 24 MND patients with pseudobulbar palsy and 28 MND patients without this pseudobulbar involvement. A pattern of cognitive dysfunction which predominantly involved executive processes was revealed in the combined MND patient group. However, several executive deficits were more pronounced in pseudobulbar palsy MND patients. On the written VF procedure described earlier, the pseudobulbar patients tended to be more impaired, and the results revealed a surprisingly strong correlation between the VFI and measures of severity of speech and swallowing disabilities, despite the task being a written one. It is of note that the VFI did not correlate with severity of upper limb weakness, suggesting that the adaptations successfully controlled for patients' motor deficits.

The pseudobulbar patients also demonstrated a deficit on the random movement joystick test, in comparison to MND patients without pseudobulbar involvement. The procedure, based on that used in the PET activation studies,[27,43] is a non-verbal test of intrinsic response generation, in which participants had to generate random sequences of 50 movements with a four-way directional joystick. Subtle impairments in planning were also observed in this subgroup using a computerized version of the Tower of Hanoi test. On this test, the pseudobulbar palsy patients displayed shorter planning times on more complex trials, which required greater flexibility of initiation of response, as the solution was less obvious. On these trials, pseudobulbar palsy patients tended to plan less exhaustively, which may have resulted in the slight decrement in performance that was found. However, cognitive impairment was not exclusive to this subgroup of patients, and the combined MND patient group as a whole demonstrated deficits on VF and the WCST, in addition to a deficit on a word-recognition test and some evidence of an impairment in a test of attention and inhibition (negative priming).

Overall, these few studies demonstrate the presence of some association between cognitive impairment, underlying cerebral dysfunction and the presence of bulbar involvement, particularly pseudobulbar palsy. However, cognitive dysfunction does not appear to be limited to this subgroup.

Emotional lability

Emotional lability is a term used to describe the pathological laughing and crying which may occur in up to 20% of patients with MND.[58] These patients display a reduced threshold for and loss of ability to control episodes of laughing and crying. This phenomenon was originally investigated in MND by Ziegler,[59] who related it to the presence of brainstem lesions, although its etiology still remains unclear. Gallagher[58] found that it increased with disease progression and was more frequently present in patients with bulbar involvement. In a recent investigation,[60] both emotional lability and cognitive impairments were associated with bulbar symptomatology. This study also revealed that MND patients with high scores on an emotional lability measure were more likely to belong to a subgroup of patients who performed more poorly on tests of cognitive ability, including tests of executive function and memory. Little research has been conducted in this area, but this recent investigation suggested, therefore, that some association may exist between emotional lability and cognitive impairment in MND.

Primary lateral sclerosis

Cognitive deficits have also been associated with a distinct clinical variant of MND, primary lateral sclerosis (PLS), where symptoms remain exclusive to UMNs.[61,62] In a group of non-demented PLS patients, Caselli et al[62] reported mild cognitive impairment in eight of the nine patients investigated. Deficits were more commonly, although not exclusively, seen on tests sensitive to executive functions. These included VF, the WCST, the Trail Making Test and the Stroop. In addition, there was also some evidence of impairment on a range of tests of memory. Tests assessing visuospatial functions and basic language processes such as naming appeared to be less sensitive to any impairment. Clearly, this cognitive profile parallels that found with non-demented classical MND patients, which involves degeneration of both UMNs and LMNs, and suggests the possibility of common underlying pathological processes.

Future research directions

This chapter has demonstrated that cognitive deficits and extra-motor cerebral involvement in MND are well established and that the disease must now be regarded as a multisystem disorder. Further research will need to confirm whether the disease does indeed selectively affect the cognitive processes and corresponding cortical and subcortical regions which have been identified, or whether there is evidence of more global involvement. Exploration of a distinct subgroup of MND defined by cognitive and corresponding cerebral changes has yet to be conducted. Longitudinal studies are required in order to determine whether such changes develop in all sufferers as the disease progresses and hence whether they should be regarded as an integral part of the complete spectrum of the disorder. Such prospective studies will elucidate the underlying pathways involved during the progression of the disease. The relationship between cognitive impairment and clinical characteristics of the disease, such as bulbar involvement or emotional lability, remains unclear and the current findings warrant further investigations. In addition, investigations of why some neuropsychological measures are more sensitive than others may indicate which underlying cognitive processes are involved. Finally, these findings have clear implications in terms of the clinical management of such patients, and hence research needs to be directed at determining whether people with MND are aware of such cognitive change and how such impairment impacts on everyday life.

Acknowledgments

We wish to thank Professor Nigel Leigh for his help in the preparation of this text. Much of our group's work has been supported by the Wellcome Trust, the Medical Research Council, and, through the King's MND Care and Research Centre, by the Motor Neurone Disease Association, UK. Additional support has come from the Tregaskis Bequest, University of London.

References

1. Charcot JM, Joffroy A. Deux cas d'atrophie musculaire progressive avec les lesions de la substance grise et faisceaux anterolateraux de la moelle epineire. *Arch Physiol Normal Pathol Paris* (1869) **2:** 354–67, 629–49, 744–60.

2. Mitsumoto H, Chad DA, Pioro E. *Amyotrophic Lateral Sclerosis* (Philadelphia: FA Davis Company, 1998).

3. Norris F, Shepherd R, Denys E. Onset, natural history and outcome in idiopathic adult motor neurone disease. *J Neurol Sci* (1993) **11:** 48–55.

4. De Belleroche J, Leigh PN, Clifford Rose F. Familial motor neuron disease. In Leigh PN, Swash M (eds) *Motor Neuron Disease; Biology and Management* (London: Springer-Verlag, 1995): 35–52.

5. Leigh PN, Ray-Chaudhuri K. Motor neurone disease. *J Neurol Neurosurg Psychiatry* (1994) **57:** 886–96.

6. Shaw PJ. Motor neurone disease: science, medicine and the future. *BMJ* (1999) **318:** 1118–21.

7. Eisen A, Krieger C. *Amyotrophic Lateral Sclerosis: A Synthesis of Research and Clinical Practice* (Cambridge: Cambridge University Press, 1998).

8. Kondo K. Epidemiology of motor neuron disease. In Leigh PN, Swash M (eds) *Motor Neuron Disease; Biology and Management* (London: Springer-Verlag, 1995): 19–34.

9. Swash M, Leigh N. Criteria for diagnosis of familial amyotrophic lateral sclerosis: review. *Neuromuscul Disord* (1992) **2:** 7–9.

10. Brooks BR. World Federation of Neurology Sub Committee on Neuromuscular Diseases. El Escorial criteria for the diagnosis of amyotrophic lateral sclerosis. *J Neurol Sci Suppl* (1994) **124:** 96–107.

11. Appel SH, Engelhart JI, Smith RG, Stephani E. Theories of causation. In Leigh PN, Swash M (eds) *Motor*

Neuron Disease; Biology and Management (London: Springer-Verlag, 1995): 219–40.

12. Radunovic A, Leigh PN. Cu/Zn superoxide dismutase gene mutations in amyotrophic lateral sclerosis: correlation between genotype and clinical features. *J Neurol Neurosurg Psychiatry* (1996) **61:** 565–72.

13. Rosen DR, Siddique T, Patterson D et al. Mutations in Cu/Zn superoxide dismutase are associated with familial amyotrophic lateral sclerosis. *Nature* (1993) **362:** 59–62.

14. Al-Chalabi A, Enayat ZE, Bakker MC et al. Association of apolipoprotein E e4 allele with bulbar onset motor neuron disease. *Lancet* (1996) **347:** 159–60.

15. Al-Chalabi A, Andersen PM, Nilsson P et al. Deletions of the heavy neurofilament subunit tail in amyotrophic lateral sclerosis. *Hum Mol Genet* (1999) **8:** 157–64.

16. Lacomblez L, Bensimon G, Leigh PN et al. ALS/riluzole Study Group II. Dose-ranging study of riluzole in amyotrophic lateral sclerosis. *Lancet* (1996) **347:** 1425–32.

17. Lai EC, Felice KJ, Festoff BW et al. Effect of recombinant human insulin-like growth factor-1 on progression in ALS. *Neurology* (1997) **49:** 1621–30.

18. Borasio GD, Robberecht W, Leigh PN et al. A placebo-controlled trial of insulin-like growth factor-I in amyotrophic lateral sclerosis. European ALS/IGF-I Study Group. *Neurology* (1998) **51:** 583–6.

19. Kew JJM, Leigh PN. Dementia with motor neuron disease. In Rosser M (ed.) *Balliere's Clinical Neurology: Unusual Dementias,* Vol 1. No. 3. (London: Bailliere Tindal, 1992): 611–26.

20. Neary D, Snowden JS. Frontal lobe dementia: nosology, neuropsychology and neuropathol-ogy. *Brain Cogn* (1996) **31:** 176–87.

21. Abe K, Fujimura H, Toyooka K et al. Cognitive function in amyotrophic lateral sclerosis. *J Neurol Sci* (1997) **148:** 95–100.

22. Abrahams S, Goldstein LH, Al-Chalabi A et al. The relationship between cognitive dysfunction and pseudobulbar palsy in amyotrophic lateral sclerosis. *J Neurol Neurosurg Psychiatry* (1997) **62:** 464–72.

23. Abrahams S, Goldstein LH, Kew JJM et al. Frontal lobe dysfunction in amyotrophic lateral sclerosis: a PET study. *Brain* (1996) **119:** 2105–20.

24. Frank B, Haas J, Heinze HJ et al. Relation of neuropsychological and magnetic resonance findings in amyotrophic lateral sclerosis: evidence for subgroups. *Clin Neurol Neurosurg* (1997) **99:** 79–86.

25. Gallassi R, Montagna P, Ciardulli C et al. Cognitive impairments in motor neurone disease. *Acta Neurol Scand* (1985) **71:** 480–4.

26. Gallassi R, Montagna P, Morriale A et al. Neuropsychological, electroencephalogram and brain computed tomography findings in motor neurone disease. *Eur Neurol* (1989) **29:** 115–20.

27. Kew JJM, Goldstein LH, Leigh PN et al. The relationship between abnormalities of cognitive function and cerebral activation in amyotrophic lateral sclerosis: a neuropsychological and positron emission tomography study. *Brain* (1993) **116:** 1399–423.

28. Ludolph AC, Langen KJ, Regard M et al. Frontal lobe function in amyotrophic lateral sclerosis: a neuropsychological and positron emission tomography study. *Acta Neurol Scand* (1992) **85:** 81–9.

29. Massman PJ, Sims J, Cooke N et al. Prevalence and correlates of neuropsychological deficits in

amyotrophic lateral sclerosis. *J Neurol Neurosurg Psychiatry* (1996) **61:** 450–5.

30. Thurstone LL, Thurstone TG. Primary Mental Abilities. (Chicago: Science Research Associates, 1962).

31. Hartikainen P, Helkala EL, Soininen H, Riekkinen P. Cognitive and memory deficits in untreated Parkinson's disease and amyotrophic lateral sclerosis patients: a comparative study. *J Neural Transm* (1993) **6:** 127–37.

32. David A, Gillham R. Neuropsychological study of motor neurone disease. *Psychosomatics* (1986) **27:** 441–5.

33. Talbot PR, Goulding PJ, Lloyd JJ et al. Inter-relation between 'classic' motor neuron disease and frontotemporal dementia: neuropsychological and single photon emission computed tomography study. *J Neurol Neurosurg Psychiatry* (1995) **58:** 541–7.

34. Chari G, Shaw PJ, Sahgal A. Non-verbal visual attention, but not recognition memory or learning processes are impaired in motor neurone disease. *Neuropsychologia* (1996) **34:** 377–85.

35. Iwasaki Y, Kinoshita M, Ikeda K et al. Cognitive impairment in amyotrophic lateral sclerosis and its relation to motor disabilities. *Acta Neurol Scand* (1990) **81:** 141–3.

36. Strong MJ, Grace MG, Orange JB, Leeper HA. Cognition, language, and speech in amyotrophic lateral sclerosis: a review. *J Clin Exp Neuropsychol* (1996) **18:** 291–303.

37. Poloni M, Capitani E, Mazzini L, Ceroni M. Neuropsychological measures in amyotrophic lateral sclerosis and their relationship with CT scan-assessed cerebral atrophy. *Acta Neurol Scand* (1986) **74:** 257–60.

38. Goodin DS, Rowley HA, Olney RK. Magnetic resonance imaging in amyotrophic lateral sclerosis. *Ann Neurol* (1988) **23:** 418–20.

39. Luis ML, Hormigo A, Mauricio C et al. Magnetic resonance imaging in motor neuron disease. *J Neurol* (1992) **239:** 112–13.

40. Ishikawa K, Nagura H, Yokota T, Yamanouchi H. Signal loss in the motor cortex on magnetic resonance images in amyotrophic lateral sclerosis. *Ann Neurol* (1993) **33:** 218–22.

41. Kiernan JA, Hudson AJ. Frontal lobe atrophy in motor neuron diseases. *Brain* (1994) **117:** 747–57.

42. Kato S, Hayashi H, Yagishita A. Involvement of frontotemporal lobe and limbic system in amyotrophic lateral sclerosis: as assessed by serial computed tomography and magnetic resonance imaging. *J Neurol Sci* (1993) **116:** 52–8.

43. Kew JJM, Leigh PN, Playford ED et al. Cortical function in amyotrophic lateral sclerosis: a positron emission tomography study. *Brain* (1993) **116:** 655–80.

44. Rafalowska J, Dziewulska D. White matter injury in amyotrophic lateral sclerosis (ALS). *Folia Neuropathol* (1996) **34:** 87–91.

45. Anderson VER, Cairns N, Leigh PN. Involvement of the amygdala in motor neurone disease. *J Neurol Sci* (1996) **129 (suppl):** 75–8.

46. Leigh PN, Kew JJM, Goldstein LH, Brooks DJ. The cerebral lesions in amyotrophic lateral sclerosis: new insights from pathology and functional brain imaging. In Clifford Rose F (ed.) *ALS—from Charcot to the Present and into the Future* (London: Smith-Gordon, 1994): 191–210.

47. Okamoto K, Hirai S, Yamazaki T et al. New ubiquitin-positive intraneuronal inclusions in the extramotor cortices in patients with

amyotrophic lateral sclerosis. *Neurosci Lett* (1991) **129:** 233–6.

48. Wightman G, Anderson VER, Martin J et al. Hippocampal and neocortical ubiquitin-immunoreactive inclusions in amyotrophic lateral sclerosis with dementia. *Neurosci Lett* (1992) **139:** 269–74.

49. Brownell B, Oppenheimer DR, Hughes JT. The central nervous system in motor neurone disease. *J Neurol Neurosurg Psychiatry* (1992) **33:** 338–57.

50. Speedie LJ, Heilman KM. Amnesic disturbance following infarction of the left dorsomedial nucleus of the thalamus. *Neuropsychologia* (1982) **20:** 597–604.

51. Speedie LJ, Heilman KM. Anterograde memory deficits for visuospatial material after infarction of the right thalamus. *Arch Neurol* (1983) **40:** 183–6.

52. Mitsuyama Y. Presenile dementia with motor neurone disease in Japan: clinico-pathological review of 26 cases. *J Neurol Neurosurg Psychiatry* (1984) **47:** 953–9.

53. Neary D, Snowden JS, Mann DMA et al. Frontal lobe dementia and motor neuron disease. *J Neurol Neurosurg Psychiatry* (1990) **53:** 23–32.

54. Peavy GM, Herzog AG, Rubin NP, Mesulam MM. Neuropsychological aspects of dementia of motor neurone disease: a report of two cases. *Neurology* (1992) **42:** 1004–8.

55. Hudson AJ. Amyotrophic lateral sclerosis and its association with dementia, parkinsonism and other neurological disorders: a review. *Brain* (1981) **104:** 217–47.

56. Wikstrom J, Paetau A, Palo J et al. Classic amyotrophic lateral sclerosis with dementia. *Arch Neurol* (1982) **39,** 681–3.

57. Kato S, Masaya O, Hayashi H et al. Participation of the limbic system and its associated areas in the dementia of amyotrophic lateral sclerosis. *J Neurol Sci* (1994) **126:** 62–9.

58. Gallagher JP. Pathologic laughter and crying in ALS: a search for their origin. *Acta Neurol Scand* (1989) **80:** 114–17.

59. Ziegler LH. Psychotic and emotional phenomena associated with amyotrophic lateral sclerosis. *Arch Neurol Psychiatry* (1930) **24:** 930–6.

60. Newsom-Davis I. Cognitive dysfunction and emotional lability in amyotrophic lateral sclerosis. D. Clin. Psych. thesis, University of London, 1997.

61. Arruda WO, Coelho Neto M. Primary lateral sclerosis: a case report with SPECT study. *Arq Neuropsiquiatr* (1998) **56:** 465–71.

62. Caselli RJ, Smith BE, Osborne D. Primary lateral sclerosis: a neuropsychological study. *Neurology* (1995) **45:** 2005–9.

Index

Notes: page numbers in *italics* refer to tables. Abbreviations used in subheadings are: ACoA = anterior communicating artery; DAT = dementia of the Alzheimer type; ED = executive dysfunction; HD = Huntington's disease; IDED = intradimensional and extradimensional (IDED) shifting task; MND = motor neuron disease; NMDs = neuronal migration disorders; OCD = obsessive–compulsive disorder; PD = Parkinson's disease; ToM = theory of mind; ToMM = theory of mind mechanism; WCC = weak central coherence; WCST = Wisconsin Card Sorting Test.